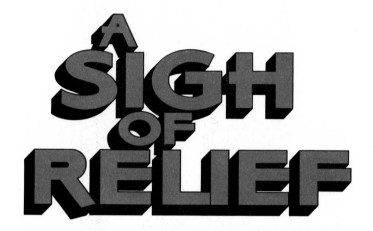

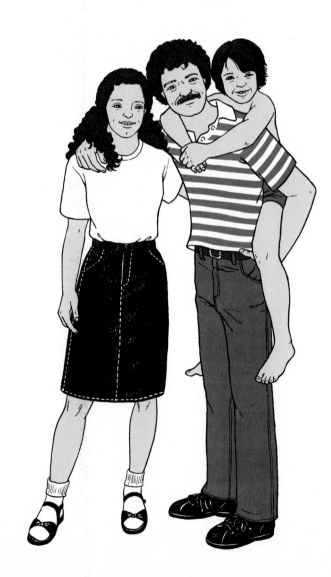

UNANIMOUS ACCLAIM
FOR PREVIOUS EDITIONS OF THIS BESTSELLING CLASSIC

"At last — a first-aid handbook for childhood emergencies that parents can pull out and refer to quickly and easily — when time counts. **A SIGH OF RELIEF** should make all parents sigh with relief."

—MOTHER'S MANUAL

"A must for all homes where active children live and play."   —LOS ANGELES HERALD EXAMINER

"Safeguards and solutions for childhood health and safety."   —TODAY'S CATHOLIC TEACHER

"It's a godsend for anyone with responsibility for children . . . . The tone is supportive but no-nonsense, and above all thorough. The book is lovingly and explicitly illustrated and includes a clever index system for serious emergencies."

—NEWSDAY

"**A SIGH OF RELIEF** is a good thing to have around somewhere near the medicine cabinet."

—THE TODAY SHOW, NBC-TV

" . . . a most valuable book . . . . No family with small children will want to pass this by."

—THE EL PASO TIMES

"The book is extremely valuable for anyone living or working with children . . . . With **A SIGH OF RELIEF** in the house . . . parents will be able to breathe one."   —GANNETT NEWSPAPER CHAIN

"An excellent compendium of safety precautions and emergency instructions."   —LIBRARY JOURNAL

"One of the best things you could have around the house for childhood emergencies is this new quick reference book."   —CHICAGO SUN-TIMES

"[**A SIGH OF RELIEF**] is being hailed by doctors and The National Safety Council as one of the best of its kind."

—SEATTLE POST-INTELLIGENCER

"Guardian Angel of a book . . . unlike any book published to date . . . . Whether you're a parent, grand-parent, or a regular baby-sitter, **A SIGH OF RELIEF** is a must for any household a child visits."

—THE AMSTERDAM NEWS

"Help before you need it is available in **A SIGH OF RELIEF**, with well-illustrated sections."

—MS. MAGAZINE

"**A SIGH OF RELIEF** deserves to be in every family's library, alongside the venerable Dr. Spock . . . an indispensable handbook for parents, grandparents, baby-sitters, teachers — anyone who shares responsibility for small fry."

—DAYTON DAILY NEWS

"**A SIGH OF RELIEF** is perhaps the most practical gift for parents."   —NEWSDAY

"An excellent family reference book."   —PARENTS MAGAZINE

"It tells you what to do until the doctor comes (or you go to the doctor) in great graphic and understandable detail . . . particularly noteworthy."

—BOOKVIEWS

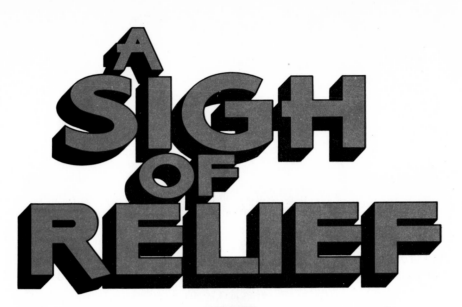

A SIGH OF RELIEF

THE FIRST-AID HANDBOOK FOR CHILDHOOD EMERGENCIES

•

REVISED EDITION

Created, Designed & Produced
by
Martin I. Green

BANTAM BOOKS
NEW YORK • TORONTO • LONDON • SYDNEY • AUCKLAND

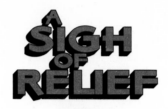

THE
FIRST-AID
HANDBOOK
FOR
CHILDHOOD
EMERGENCIES

·

REVISED EDITION

A Bantam Book/September 1977
Bantam Revised Edition/July 1984
Bantam Revised Edition/September 1989
Bantam Revised Edition/October 1994

Library of Congress Cataloging-in-Publication Data
Green, Martin I.
A sigh of relief: the first-aid handbook for childhood emergencies/
created, designed & produced by Martin I. Green.—
3rd rev. ed.
p.   cm.
ISBN 0-553-35180-X
1. Pediatric emergencies. 2. First aid in illness and injury.
3. Children's accidents—Prevention. I. Title
RJ370.G73 1994
618.92'60252 — dc20   93-8663
                                                        CIP
                                                        r93

Published simultaneously in the United States and Canada.

Bantam books are published by Bantam Books, a division of Bantam Doubleday Dell Publishing
Group, Inc. Its trademark, consisting of the words "Bantam Books" and the portrayal of a rooster, is
registered in the United States Patent Office and in other countries, Marca Registrada. Bantam
Books, 1540 Broadway, New York 10036.

This edition published by arrangement with Martin I. Green and Berkshire Studio.
Printed in The United States of America
0 9 8 7 6 5 4 3 2 1

CREDITS

Created, Designed & Produced by	**MARTIN I. GREEN**
Illustrated & Designed by	**BOBBI BONGARD**
Written by	**ROSS FIRESTONE & MARTIN I. GREEN**
Edited by	**ROSS FIRESTONE**
Editorial Associate & Proofreader	**CIA ELKIN**
Research & Administrative Coordinator	**EILEEN TAFT**
Research Associates	**EILEEN TAFT & CIA ELKIN**
First-Aid Consultant	**JOSEPH A. WALLICK, M.P.H.**
Medical Consultants	**KENNETH JAY SOLOMON, M.D.**
	STEPHEN LUDWIG, M.D.
Mechanical Art	**BOBBI BONGARD**
Color Separations	**CANDACE BARBACCIA & BOBBI BONGARD**
Typesetting	**PAGESPLUS, INC.**

I am forever indebted to the following for their extraordinary support and encouragement:
Leo K. Barnes, Bessie Boris, Martha Donovan, Alan Douglas, Lee Everett, Gail Firestone,
Harvey Rottenberg, Ben Schawinsky, Anne Sipp, Lynne West and Jeff Young.

Finally, I would like to thank my friends at Bantam Books whose enthusiasm and
understanding will always be appreciated: Irwyn Applebaum, Lou Aronica,
Toni Burbank, Tom Dupree and Linda Grey.

MIG

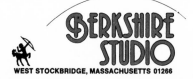

BERKSHIRE STUDIO
WEST STOCKBRIDGE, MASSACHUSETTS 01266

ACKNOWLEDGMENTS

We are most grateful to the following for providing us with information,
for making their facilities available to us,
and for reviewing and commenting on the manuscript during its various phases.

John Ambre, M.D., Ph.D.
Director of Department of Toxicology and Drug Abuse
American Medical Association
Chicago, Illinois

American Academy of Pediatrics
Elk Grove, Illinois

American Association of Poison Control Centers
Washington, D.C.

American Automobile Association
Washington, D.C.

American College of Emergency Physicians
Dallas, Texas

American Diabetes Association
Alexandria, Virginia

American Lung Association of Western
  Massachusetts
Springfield, Massachusetts

American Red Cross
National Headquarters
Washington, D.C.

American Trauma Society
Upper Marlboro, Maryland

Hunt Anderson
Director of Boating Safety Education
United States Coast Guard
Washington, D.C.

Jay M. Arena, M.D.
Professor Emeritus, Department of Pediatrics
Director Emeritus, Poison Control Center
Duke University Medical Center
Durham, North Carolina

Captain George Armstrong, M.P.H., R.Ph.
Chief of Surveillance and Data Processing
Federal Drug Administration
Rockville, Maryland

Joel Bass, M.D.
Associate Pediatrician, Department of Pediatrics
Director of Ambulatory Pediatrics
MetroWest Medical Center
Framingham, Massachusetts

Bikecentennial: The Bicycle Travel Association
Missoula, Montana

Robert Burnside
Director of Health and Safety Services
American Red Cross
National Headquarters
Washington, D.C.

Joy Byers
Director of Public Awareness and Information
National Committee to Prevent Child Abuse
Chicago, Illinois

Richard M. Cantor, M.D., F.A.C.E.P.
Assistant Professor, Department of Emergency
    Medicine
SUNY Health Science Center at Syracuse
Syracuse, New York

Center for Auto Safety
Washington, D.C.

Centers for Disease Control
Atlanta, Georgia

Child Find of America, Inc.
New Paltz, New York

Catherine Christoffel, M.D.
Attending Physician, Division of General and
    Emergency Pediatrics
Children's Memorial Hospital
Chicago, Illinois
Professor of Pediatrics
Northwestern University School of Medicine
Chicago, Illinois

Ray Ciszek
Director
The Safety Society
Reston, Virginia

Committee for Children
Seattle, Washington

Consumer Products Safety Commission
Washington, D.C.

Council on Family Health
New York, New York

C.P. Dail
Manager of Health and Safety Services
American Red Cross European Area Headquarters
Stuttgart, Germany

Richard Dart, M.D.
Director
Rocky Mountain Poison and Drug Center
Denver, Colorado

Alan R. Dimick, M.D., F.A.C.S.
Director of Burn Center
University of Alabama at Birmingham
Birmingham, Alabama

Drowning Prevention and Beach Safety Program
Chicago Park District
Chicago, Illinois

Herta Feely
Executive Director
National Safe Kids Campaign
Washington, D.C.

Susan S. Gallagher, M.P.H.
Director
EDC, Inc.
Newton, Massachusetts

Alan Gelberg, M.S.
Deputy Chief of Surveillance and Data Processing
Federal Drug Administration
Rockville, Maryland

Barbara Ghannam
Director of Research and Development
National Child Safety Council
Jackson, Michigan

Bernard Guyer, M.D.
Professor, School of Hygiene and Public Health
Chairman, Department of Maternal and Child Health
Johns Hopkins University
Baltimore, Maryland

Harvard School of Public Health
Boston, Massachusetts

William Hull
Manager of Children and Youth Studies
Highway Safety Research Center
University of North Carolina
Chapel Hill, North Carolina

Institute for Injury Reduction
Upper Marlboro, Maryland

Insurance Institute for Highway Safety
Arlington, Virginia

Juvenile Products Manufacturers Association
Marlton, New Jersey

Stephen Kaufman, M.D., F.A.C.E.P.
Director of Emergency Services
Columbia-Greene Medical Center
Hudson, New York

Laura Kavanagh
Associate Director
National Center for Education in Maternal and Child
    Health
Arlington, Virginia

C. Henry Kempé Center for the Prevention and
    Treatment of Child Abuse and Neglect
Denver, Colorado

Brad Keshlear
Former President
National Water Safety Congress
Oxford, Mississippi

Katherine Kincaid
Staff Liaison
National Safe Kids Campaign
Washington, D.C.

Toby Litovitz, M.D.
Director
National Capital Poison Center
Washington, D.C.

Anne Marie Lopes
National Safe Kids Campaign
Washington, D.C.

Maryland Poison Information Center
Baltimore, Maryland

Massachusetts Environmental Police
Boating and Recreational Vehicle Safety Bureau
Topsfield, Massachusetts

Massachusetts Society for the Prevention of Cruelty
    to Children
Boston, Massachusetts

Joann McLaughlin
Director of Professional Affairs
Burn Foundation
Philadelphia, Pennsylvania

Sally Metz, M.S.
Former Program Manager
Injury Prevention Resource and Research Center
Dartmouth Medical School
Hanover, New Hampshire

Jeffrey P. Michael, Ed.D.
Office of Occupant Protection
National Highway Traffic Safety Administration
U.S. Department of Transportation
Washington, D.C.

Sylvia Micik, M.D.
Program Medical Director
California Center for Childhood Injury Prevention
San Diego State University
San Diego, California

National Association for the Education of Young
    Children
Washington, D.C.

National Center for Missing and Exploited Children
Arlington, Virginia

National Clearinghouse for Alcohol and Drug
    Information
Rockville, Maryland

National Council on Patient Information and
    Education
Washington, D.C.

National Fire Protection Association
Quincy, Massachusetts

National Head Injury Foundation
Washington, D.C.

National Health Information Center
Washington, D.C.

National Institute of Child Health
Bethesda, Maryland

National Institute on Drug Abuse
Rockville, Maryland

National Jewish Lung Line Information Service
National Jewish Center for Immunology and
    Respiratory Medicine
Denver, Colorado

National Pediculosis Association
Newton, Massachusetts

National Reye's Syndrome Foundation
Bryan, Ohio

Mary Ann O'Connor, M.A.
Former Program Director
Injury Prevention Resource and Research Center
Dartmouth Medical School
Hanover, New Hampshire

Gary Oderda, Pharm.D.
Professor and Chairman, Department of Pharmacy
    Practice
University of Utah
Salt Lake City, Utah
President
American Association of Poison Control Centers
Washington, D.C.

Parents Anonymous National
Los Angeles, California

Pediatric AIDS Foundation
Santa Monica, California

Peter Pons, M.D., F.A.C.E.P.
Medical Director of Denver Paramedic Division
Denver General Hospital
Denver, Colorado

Pittsfield Fire Department
Pittsfield, Massachusetts

Brad Prenney
Director of Childhood Lead Poisoning Prevention
    Program
Massachusetts Department of Public Health
Boston, Massachusetts

Cindy Rodgers, M.S.P.H.
Director of Injury Prevention and Control Program
Massachusetts Department of Public Health
Boston, Massachusetts

Deborah Sherger, R.N.
Rocky Mountain Poison and Drug Center
Denver, Colorado

SIDS Alliance
Columbia, Maryland

Mary Beth Smuts, M.P.H.
United States Environmental Protection Agency
Boston, Massachusetts

Rose Ann Soloway, R.N., M.S.Ed., C.S.P.I.
Education/Communications Coordinator
National Capital Poison Center
Washington, D.C.

Captain Alan M. Steinman, M.D.
United States Coast Guard
Washington, D.C.

John B. Sullivan, Jr., M.D.
Medical Director of the Arizona Poison Center
Director of Clinical Toxicology Program
Director of The University Physicians, Inc.
University of Arizona
Tucson, Arizona

Stephen P. Teret, M.P.H., J.D.
Director of Injury Prevention Center
Johns Hopkins University
Baltimore, Maryland

Theodore G. Tong, Pharm.D.
Associate Dean, College of Pharmacy
Director of Poison and Drug Information Center
University of Arizona
Tucson, Arizona

Toy Manufacturers of America
New York, New York

Linda Tracy
Project Manager
Bicycle Federation of America
Washington, D.C.

Albert K. Tsai, M.D., F.A.C.E.P.
Staff Physician, Emergency Department
Henepen County Medical Center
Minneapolis, Minnesota

United States Cycling Federation
Colorado Springs, Colorado

United States Department of Health and Human
    Services
Washington, D.C.

United States Environmental Protection Agency
Public Information Center
Washington, D.C.

Kathleen Weber
Director of Child Passenger Protection Research
    Program
University of Michigan Medical School
Ann Arbor, Michigan

Mark Widome, M.D.
Professor of Pediatrics
Penn State University College of Medicine
Hershey, Pennsylvania
Past Chairman
American Academy of Pediatrics Accident Prevention
    Committee

Robert Williams, M.D., F.A.C.E.P.
President
American College of Emergency Physicians
Dallas, Texas

Alan Woolf, M.D., M.P.H.
Director
Massachusetts Poison Control System
Boston, Massachusetts

Janice Yuwiler, M.P.H.
Program Director
California Center for Childhood Injury Prevention
San Diego State University
San Diego, California

Israel Zuniga
Health and Safety Associate
American Red Cross
National Headquarters
Washington, D.C.

FOR
MY PARENTS, ANNE AND BEN GREEN,
MARY,
OUR SON, JARED
AND
ALL CHILDREN EVERYWHERE

THIS EDITION IS ESPECIALLY DEDICATED
TO HERBERT H. SIPP,
WHOSE INTEGRITY, TALENT AND FRIENDSHIP
WILL NEVER BE FORGOTTEN.

CONTENTS

PART ONE
PREVENTIONS: REDUCING THE ODDS

PART TWO
BE PREPARED

PART THREE
COMMON CHILDHOOD ILLNESSES & DISORDERS

PART FOUR
EMERGENCIES & MISHAPS: FIRST-AID PROCEDURES

PREFACE

By Stephen Ludwig, M.D.
Division Chief, General Pediatrics, Children's Hospital of Philadelphia
Professor of Pediatrics, University of Pennsylvania School of Medicine

You are now a part of the EMS-C, the Emergency Medical Services System for Children.

The EMS-C is a recently formed system that is developing community-by-community across the United States. Its purpose is to encourage the prompt recognition of a serious illness or injury in a child and the safe, rapid transportation of that child to a center capable of providing the appropriate medical care. The EMS-C involves not only the community hospital emergency department and the regional pediatric medical center, but also emergency medical technicians and paramedics, physicians working in office practice and, most of all, parents, teachers, day-care staff and others who are responsible for the care of children.

Over the past decade there has been a quiet revolution in the way emergency care has been given to children. The revolution has taken place in many hospital emergency departments, in the ambulance services that bring children to the hospitals, as well as in homes, day-care centers and schools. Pediatric Emergency Medicine has emerged as a new medical specialty, and a great deal of new information has been developed about treating the emergencies of pediatric patients. Our goal is to save lives that otherwise might have been lost, and to improve the quality of living for the survivors. There are now more than 500 physicians across the United States who have dedicated their careers to this specialty, and the number is rapidly growing.

In order for the EMS-C to work, someone must take the first steps. Often that is the role of the parents. But before parents and other caregivers can take that first step, they must be prepared with the proper knowledge and skills. **A Sigh of Relief** does just that. It is an outstanding guide. Indeed, it is the most widely used book of its kind. By following its instructions and advice you will be able to recognize when a child is seriously ill or injured. You will know how to provide a prompt and appropriate response. You will know how to access the other components of the EMS-C. You will know when to call for immediate help. Most importantly, you will learn how to prevent many illnesses and injuries from ever occurring.

I want to thank you on behalf of your child and children everywhere. With the knowledge contained in this volume, you have helped them and those of us in Pediatric Emergency Medicine immensely.

INTRODUCTION

By Kenneth Jay Solomon, M.D.
Chief of Neonatology, St. Joseph's Women's Hospital of Tampa, Florida

I am proud to have served as medical consultant for **A Sigh of Relief** since its inception more than 17 years ago. When it was first published back in 1977 it made an immediate impact on the field of childhood emergency care and prevention. No other first-aid guide had ever shown so clearly and thoroughly what to do when faced with a serious emergency, and it was hailed by both medical professionals and the lay public as "the finest book of its kind," "an important handbook" that belongs "on every family's shelf." Since then it has gone through four major editions in the United States and has been published in Japan, France, Italy, Yugoslavia, Germany, Mexico, Israel and numerous other countries, attaining the status of a modern classic.

This new, greatly enlarged and completely revised edition updates the original **A Sigh of Relief** by incorporating the latest research in state-of-the-art management of childhood emergencies. After extensive review by a full range of experts, most of the first-aid and safety procedures have been recast or expanded and many new procedures added. This edition also broadens the scope of the earlier book by adding many valuable new features, such as an extensive section on child abuse, and detailed instructions about how to handle a host of common childhood disorders and illnesses. To make the information it offers easier to use and instantly accessible, the book has also been totally redesigned and printed in two colors. All these improvements make the new **A Sigh of Relief,** in my opinion, even more indispensable than it was before.

And the need for **A Sigh of Relief** has never been greater. Over the past few decades medicine has made remarkable progress in such difficult areas as cancer and leukemia survival and the prevention and treatment of infectious diseases. We have reached something like a 20 percent improvement in the overall mortality rate. Yet so-called "accidents" still account for the greatest proportion of childhood deaths. There is even some indication that the death toll is increasing for certain groups of youngsters, most notably those between 5 and 14. What is responsible for these sad facts, and what can we do to give our children more adequate protection?

As a parent and pediatrician, I feel the main problem is that adults are still so poorly prepared for the steps that must be taken in an emergency. I have been faced countless times with distraught, bewildered parents whose best intentions failed to aid their children because they didn't know what to do. The basic information was not readily available to them in a truly usable form.

Prevention remains our best defense against childhood injuries and illnesses, but we must also know how to respond quickly and appropriately to any emergency situation if it arises. Nothing is more tragic than an emergency made worse by a parent's impulsive and misguided efforts to help the child. Hippocrates articulated the principle when he said, "First, do no harm."

This book has been carefully designed and organized for use by parents, baby-sitters and other caregivers responsible for children's well-being. The unique indexing system on the back cover provides immediate access to guidance on how to handle just about all the major medical emergencies your youngster may encounter. Each first-aid procedure is presented in easy to follow instructions and is supported by clarifying step-by-step illustrations.

I suggest you read through the entire emergency section as soon as possible so you will have some familiarity with the recommended procedures before you ever need to use them. Remember that the basic purpose of first aid is to preserve the child's life and prevent further physical and psychological injury until help arrives. It is never a substitute for professional medical care. Since prevention is always preferable to cure, I also suggest you carefully study the opening section on prevention for the helpful guidance it has to offer. Keep the book in an accessible place known to everyone in your family.

To my knowledge, before **A Sigh of Relief** was published there had never been a handbook for parents that treated both the prevention and management of childhood emergencies in a truly effective manner. I was enormously pleased when this book first came into existence. And I'm even more gratified by the way this new edition has managed to improve on the original achievement.

PART ONE

PREVENTIONS: REDUCING THE ODDS

INTRODUCTION

By Vincent L. Tofany
Past President of the National Safety Council

Prevention is, of course, the single most important element in child safety. When successful, it makes emergency measures unnecessary.

There are few mysteries in accident prevention. The preparations, practices and required actions are usually, if not always, simple, obvious and based upon common sense. But as many writers have pointed out, common sense is an uncommon commodity, and the obvious is often overlooked, so it is always useful to have these basic preventive measures brought to our attention.

And sometimes common sense is not enough. In the more than 75 years that the organized voluntary safety movement has been in existence in the United States, it has developed and tested a great variety of preventive techniques applicable to all ages and activities. The authors of this book have made extensive use of this body of work.

As every safety worker knows, no matter how ardently prevention may be advocated, there will always be failures in prevention that may lead to accidental injuries. It is entirely appropriate, then, that **A Sigh of Relief** goes on to treat emergency management — "first aid" is perhaps the better-known term. The emergency management section of this book has an original and, I believe, useful format designed to supply parents and other responsible adults with the needed information in quickly retrievable, highly graphic form.

Without question, parents who take seriously what they read here will be better able to protect their children from harm. And children reared by safety-minded parents will themselves grow up even more alert and informed about safety than their parents were.

*Excerpted from the first edition of **A Sigh of Relief.***

PARENTS, CHILDREN & "ACCIDENTS"

So-called "accidents" — injuries resulting from carelessness, unawareness or ignorance — are by far the most common type of childhood emergency, the biggest single threat in the first 15 years of a youngster's life. A child is more likely than an adult to have serious injuries because he is not only the victim but often the unconscious cause. It is ironic that the major contributing factors are also some of the most basic, desirable and enjoyable characteristics of childhood.

During infancy a child's environment is necessarily limited, and it is relatively easy for parents to control potential dangers. But as every parent learns, this phase soon ends as a baby begins to turn over, crawl and then walk. This new mobility expands the child's world and exposes her to a greatly increased risk of injury. Yet it is normal for children to explore their new environment, and to want to understand and master it with their newly developing abilities and almost limitless energy. What often places them in situations of high risk is their inexperience.

At the beginning, when your child is young and completely vulnerable, you can protect him from harm by staying physically close. But the development process begun at birth is designed to produce a self-sufficient, independent individual at maturity, and a child's environment must necessarily soon expand beyond the point where you can (or should) be physically present every moment of the day.

Fortunately, about the same time the youngster's world expands, she begins to understand and respond to language. It is usually at this point that the admonition "No!" begins to be used around the home with increasing, sometimes maddening, regularity. The child's ability to respond to simple instructions is what makes it possible for you to protect her from a distance. It also enables you to begin her safety training.

Safety training involves four major steps:

- **Defining** the limits of safe behavior for the large number of threatening situations a child may be expected to encounter. Many injuries are predictable, and with the proper precautions, they can also be averted.
- **Teaching** these limits patiently until she understands and accepts them.
- **Reinforcing** these limits whenever she forgets or ignores them.
- **Making changes** in the child's immediate environment to minimize risks and encourage a more positive attitude.

Consistency is an important factor in this process. It is easier for a child to follow a simple unchanging rule than one that may be altered by parental mood or whim. Restrictions that come and go according to special circumstances present younger children with confusing distinctions and subtleties that may be beyond their scope. The more clear and simple the rule, the more likely the child to abide by it. Safety discussions should be kept at age-appropriate levels. A two-year-old can understand more complicated instructions than a ten-month-old.

Restrictions appropriate at one point in a child's life may become unrealistic and unnecessary only a few months later. A parent must try to strike the fine balance between a youngster's need for reasonable protection from danger and the comparable need for diversity of experience and the freedom to explore.

This is one of the most difficult responsibilities of parenthood, because the balance shifts constantly as a child's judgment and abilities improve. As the years pass, the need for parental guidance slowly decreases until the child becomes autonomous. As this scenario unfolds, you must be able to loosen the limitations imposed upon your child, relaxing them gradually as she demonstrates ever-increasing maturity.

Yet injuries will still sometimes happen because of a child's natural tendency to test all limits. Children are aware of their ongoing physical development and constantly try to master new physical skills. Moreover, parents usually prize their child's achievements, and the youngster is encouraged by this approval to stretch out for new accomplishments.

A child's healthy development also requires a secure and loving environment in which he occupies an important place. To be truly effective, safety training and the discipline that comes with it should always be offered in the spirit of concern, acceptance and love. We must strive to show our children that while we may not approve of certain things **they do,** we do not disapprove of **them.** We can say no to them and love them at the same time. And it will help them understand that, if we explain why something is forbidden instead of just telling them not to do it.

In some households, one or both parents is particularly, even morbidly, fearful for the child's safety and tends to become overly protective. Not infrequently, a parent will have difficulty acknowledging a youngster's improved abilities, to the extent of inhibiting her normal pursuit of experience. The children of neurotically fearful parents are often insecure and profoundly lacking in confidence. Of course we should protect our children from **unreasonably** dangerous situations that have considerable potential for serious injury. Yet it is through systematic exposure to new and demanding experiences that we provide the stimulation and environmental richness essential to a child's ongoing development. We should want to encourage our sons and daughters to operate somewhere near the limits of their capacities without either exposing them to unreasonable danger or smothering them with our own unreasonable fears.

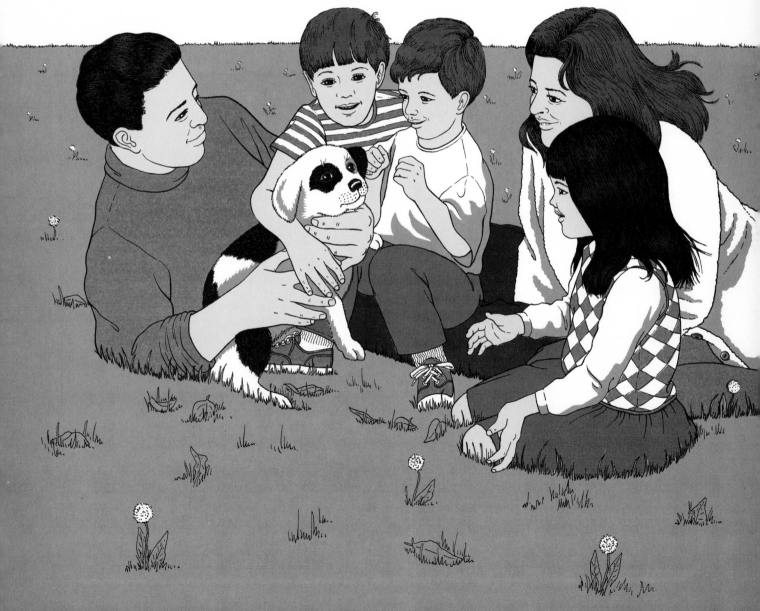

HOME SAFETY

Every parent wants to give his child a safe home, a place to live and grow that is free of foreseeable danger. Your efforts here have a double benefit: they protect your youngster from physical harm and also establish a consciousness about safety she will take out into the world with her wherever she goes.

This chapter discusses the most common kinds of home injuries and the ways they can be prevented. (Drowning, certainly one of the major hazards, is treated on pages 80-93 in the chapter on **WATER SAFETY**.) You'll also find room-by-room suggestions about the specific dangers inherent in each different area of your home.

The risk of injuries increases dramatically once your child is able to crawl and walk. With physical mobility comes an enhanced sense of curiosity and a desire to explore the world. Before she begins to crawl, go through your home at her level — on your hands and knees, or even better, on your stomach — searching out the hazards that might attract her attention. Make your home as safe as possible for your young explorer, so you won't have to keep saying "No!"

A grandparents' home can be an especially dangerous place for young children. If your youngsters spend a lot of time there, help childproof it. If visits are occasional, watch the children carefully and don't leave them unattended. This same precaution applies to any other house they may visit.

Remember that hazards change constantly according to your child's age and development. Safety training and childproofing your home are continuing processes with different requirements for each stage of childhood. Parents must not only recognize present dangers but anticipate those to come.

Remember also that the moods and circumstances of your family have an important influence on your child's safety. Injuries are most likely to occur:
- When children are so hungry or thirsty they are ready to eat or drink anything. Many poisonings take place just before mealtime.
- When children and parents are tired, usually before it's time for a nap, in late afternoon or before bedtime.
- When children are overactive or rushed and don't allow enough time to do things carefully.
- When mothers are pregnant or parents are ill and not able to supervise the children with their usual patience and care.
- When parents quarrel or are under emotional stress and aren't paying adequate attention to their children. A child may react in rebellious or hazardous ways.
- When the family routine is upset by moves, long trips or vacations.
- When baby-sitters or other less-experienced people are supervising the child.

SUFFOCATION

Infants are particularly susceptible to suffocation. An infant's head is large and heavy in proportion to the rest of his body, and his neck muscles aren't developed enough to enable him to pull his head away from an object or space that hampers his breathing.

Parents must stay constantly alert to this danger and learn to take the following precautions:
- Never put your infant to sleep on a waterbed, bean bag cushion or soft pillow. Don't place pillows or large stuffed toys in his crib.

- Keep plastic bags out of your child's reach. Don't use them as waterproof crib sheets or mattress covers. Never let your child play with them or use them to store his toys. Plastic bags should be knotted and thrown out immediately, or stored safely away.
- Don't give a young child soft pillows and other bedclothes that might interfere with his breathing. Tuck the bottom sheet smoothly under the crib mattress. Keep the top sheet away from a baby's face and loose enough to let him move about freely.
- Window blinds or drapery cords should be tied back, well out of reach.
- Never suspend toys across a crib or playpen or tie playthings onto them. Don't tie pacifiers around a baby's neck. Crib mobiles should be kept at a safe distance and removed when she can pull herself up.
- Clothing with hoods or hanging strings can get caught on a crib or playpen and should be taken off before the infant is left alone.
- If using a mesh-sided crib or playpen, don't leave your baby alone with the side down; the mesh forms a pocket that can trap his head and restrict breathing.
- Never leave your infant unattended with a feeding bottle propped up in her mouth.
- Because chewing ability is immature until about age four, round foods present a choking hazard to very young children. Don't give them grapes, hot dogs, hard candies, carrots, seeds, raisins, popcorn, nuts and other foods that are hard to chew.
- Never let your youngster run with food in her mouth or engage in horseplay while eating. Small toys present the same dangers. Make sure she doesn't put small toys or small round objects, like marbles, buttons, coins or pebbles, into her mouth.
- Remove the doors from any unused refrigerators or freezers so that children can't be trapped inside. Picnic coolers should also be stored out of reach.
- A child can be trapped in a toy chest and suffocate. Make sure yours has a safety hinge to prevent sudden drops, and drill a few air holes in the top.
- Scarves can catch on furniture, playground equipment, trees and the like. Young children shouldn't wear them. At the very least, the scarf should be tucked securely inside the child's jacket. Store long scarves, ropes and cords out of reach. Jump ropes are not appropriate toys for children under six. Teach your older children to store them away safely.

FALLS

Falls are common in the home at every age and a major cause of serious injury. Here's what you can do to keep the injuries to a minimum:

- Make sure your floors aren't slippery. Keep them clean and dry, and don't wax them to a high gloss. Wipe up spilled liquids immediately.
- Keep carpets and area rugs anchored firmly in place.
- If you have children under three, install safety gates at the top and bottom of all stairways. (See **INFANT EQUIPMENT**, pages 38-42, for the types of gates to use.)
- Make sure steps and stairways are kept uncluttered and in good repair. They should also be well lit and have handrails on both sides. Unanchored rugs at the top of the landings are especially dangerous. Other hazards include loose or missing handrails, loose carpeting, worn treads, and stairs of unequal height. Keep stairs clear of objects that don't belong there, and don't let your children play or run on them.
- Check that all balconies and high porches are in good condition and enclosed with strong railings. To keep your child from catching her head, the space between the railings shouldn't be any larger than 3 1/2 inches.
- Bathroom falls can be avoided by installing grab bars and rubber mats or abrasive treads inside tubs and showers. Use non-skid bath mats to keep your child from slipping when she steps out. Kids under three should always be supervised in the bathroom.
- Open windows from the top, not the bottom. If you must open a window from the bottom, install a window guard. Most screens can be pushed out with very little pressure; they are designed to keep bugs out, not children in. Don't let your child sit on windowsills or lean against a screen.
- Keep doors leading to the basement or garage locked with a hook and eye latch installed high up out of your child's reach.
- Don't leave toys and other objects lying around on the floor. Toys should be put away promptly after each use so they won't be tripped over.
- All rooms, hallways and stairways should be adequately lit.
- Doorways and halls should be free of obstructions.
- Always fasten safety straps on highchairs, infant seats and changing tables. Never leave your child alone in one, even after you've strapped him in.
- Make sure your child's skirts and pants aren't too long and that shoes aren't too large or left untied. Never let a youngster dress up in a sash, scarf or cape that trails on the floor behind him.
- Keep your youngster away from tabletops and other high surfaces. Don't let a toddler try to climb into his highchair by himself. Bunk beds aren't safe for chil-

dren under six.
- Baby walkers have been the cause of serious falling injuries and shouldn't be used.
- Whenever you put your baby in her crib, be sure you raise the sides to their fullest height and lock them into position.
- Remove sharp-edged furniture, or pad edges and corners. Glass-topped tables are a particular haz-

ard and should not be in a house with children.
- Always push kitchen and dining room chairs under the tables to reduce the chance of children using them to climb to higher places.
- Keep storage areas uncluttered, and never pile things so high they could cave in on the child.
- Discourage roughhousing, bravado and wild play inside the home.

POISONING

Most poisonings take place in the home and involve children under five eating or drinking toxic substances carelessly left within reach. Almost every room in the house contains common substances that can poison a child if ingested:

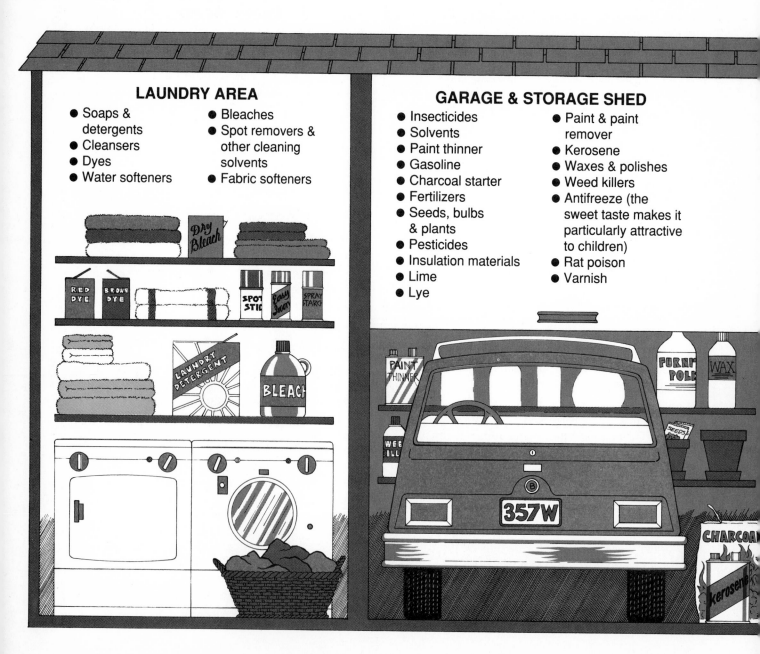

LAUNDRY AREA

- Soaps & detergents
- Cleansers
- Dyes
- Water softeners
- Bleaches
- Spot removers & other cleaning solvents
- Fabric softeners

GARAGE & STORAGE SHED

- Insecticides
- Solvents
- Paint thinner
- Gasoline
- Charcoal starter
- Fertilizers
- Seeds, bulbs & plants
- Pesticides
- Insulation materials
- Lime
- Lye
- Paint & paint remover
- Kerosene
- Waxes & polishes
- Weed killers
- Antifreeze (the sweet taste makes it particularly attractive to children)
- Rat poison
- Varnish

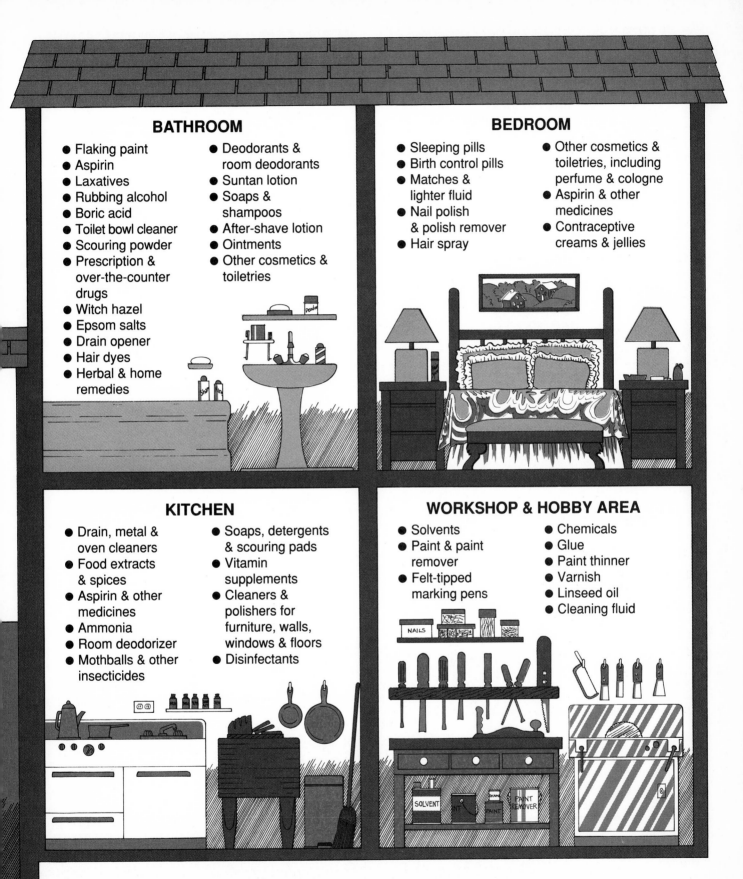

BATHROOM

- Flaking paint
- Aspirin
- Laxatives
- Rubbing alcohol
- Boric acid
- Toilet bowl cleaner
- Scouring powder
- Prescription & over-the-counter drugs
- Witch hazel
- Epsom salts
- Drain opener
- Hair dyes
- Herbal & home remedies
- Deodorants & room deodorants
- Suntan lotion
- Soaps & shampoos
- After-shave lotion
- Ointments
- Other cosmetics & toiletries

BEDROOM

- Sleeping pills
- Birth control pills
- Matches & lighter fluid
- Nail polish & polish remover
- Hair spray
- Other cosmetics & toiletries, including perfume & cologne
- Aspirin & other medicines
- Contraceptive creams & jellies

KITCHEN

- Drain, metal & oven cleaners
- Food extracts & spices
- Aspirin & other medicines
- Ammonia
- Room deodorizer
- Mothballs & other insecticides
- Soaps, detergents & scouring pads
- Vitamin supplements
- Cleaners & polishers for furniture, walls, windows & floors
- Disinfectants

WORKSHOP & HOBBY AREA

- Solvents
- Paint & paint remover
- Felt-tipped marking pens
- Chemicals
- Glue
- Paint thinner
- Varnish
- Linseed oil
- Cleaning fluid

All these substances should be stored where a youngster can't get at them, locked away high up and out of reach. Standard cabinet locks are not really childproof. Hook and eye latches installed out of reach offer much better protection.

To prevent any possible confusion, potentially dangerous substances should be stored separately from food and other things your child might seek out. Children can't always differentiate between containers that resemble each other. A gallon of bleach can easily be mistaken for a gallon of milk. Keep harmful products in their original containers, and don't remove the labels; they often provide information about antidotes. Never store dangerous substances in soda bottles, milk cartons, coffee cans and other familiar containers. Youngsters can swallow a deadly amount of something before they realize it isn't what they expected.

Label each item clearly. Children have a way of prying off so-called child-resistant lids, but they do offer some protection and should always be used. Make sure they've been fastened securely before storing the containers away. And never leave handbags or briefcases lying around; they may contain some of the same dangerous substances found elsewhere in the home.

Most childhood poisonings result from swallowing prescription or over-the-counter medications, so be especially careful about keeping them out of sight and reach. Store them in child-resistant containers, but remember that no container is completely childproof. Children learn by example and imitation, so don't take your medications in front of them, and never call medicine "candy" as a way of getting them to swallow it. Grandparents' medications pose a particular hazard. They are often kept on bedside or kitchen tables or in purses, and frequently dispensed without child-resistant caps in small containers that are attractive to youngsters. Remind older relatives and friends to put their medications away before your children come to visit. When they are visiting you, hide their purses on top of the refrigerator or some other safe place.

Be cautious about using common household products like kitchen or bathroom cleansers and toilet bowl cleaners. Don't leave them out for even a moment when your child isn't safely in her crib or playpen. Baby powder can be dangerous if inhaled, so an open container should never be left within a baby's reach. Perfume and cologne look inviting to a child but are poisonous when swallowed and harmful if inhaled or sprayed in the eyes. Pesticides and insecticides are especially hazardous. Even the fumes can be toxic.

Empty ashtrays promptly, and get rid of the cigarette butts; they are poisonous as well as a choking hazard. Make sure they are fully extinguished before throwing them in the garbage. After entertaining, empty all glasses and store liquor safely away.

Remove poisonous plants or keep them out of reach. Philodendron and dieffenbachia are the two plants that result in most calls to Poison Control Centers. A child can pick up toxic sap just by touching dieffenbachia; if transferred to his mouth it can cause severe burning and choking. Plants with berries and colorful plants like poinsettias are particularly attractive to children. It is helpful to know the names of your plants in case they are eaten.

The severity of childhood poisoning may depend on the speed with which you can obtain expert emergency information and treatment. Get stickers with the telephone number of your local Poison Control Center and put them on every telephone in your home. In case of a poisoning emergency, call the PCC right away, and they will tell you what to do. If you can't get hold of the PCC, dial the Emergency Medical Service at 911 or "O"; see **EMS (EMERGENCY MEDICAL SERVICES),** page 272. In case you are unable to reach either of them for some reason, see **POISONING,** pages 344-352 in the emergency first-aid section.

You should also prepare yourself by having on hand the various recommended antidotes. Syrup of ipecac is available at drugstores without a prescription, but don't use it to induce vomiting unless instructed to do so by the PCC or your doctor. Some poisonous substances can inflict further harm coming back up and have to be treated differently. Also have on hand Epsom salts and activated charcoal, which work as antidotes in certain types of poisonings.

FIRE AND BURNS

Fire poses a serious threat to everyone in your home, adults as well as children. Smoke inhalation is a particular hazard, causing more deaths than burns. Here are some basic measures to minimize the risk of injury:

● Smoke detectors offer your family the single most effective protection. Install one on every level of your home and on the ceiling outside the bedroom area. Test them every six months to be sure they

are working properly, and if they are battery-powered, replace the batteries regularly. Never borrow a battery for some other use.

● Teach your child what to do in case of a fire and review it with him frequently. As soon as he's old enough, make sure he knows how to summon aid from the fire department. Young children sometimes try to hide under beds and tables or in closets. Make certain they understand that they cannot hide from a fire, but they can escape it.

- Have an escape plan and practice it frequently with your household. Also figure out alternative escape routes. Your youngsters should know two safe routes out of every room, especially their bedrooms. Establish a meeting place outside the home where your family can gather and be counted. Emphasize that no one should ever return to a burning building for any reason.
- Teach children to crawl low in smoke, keeping their heads down. Smoke and heat rise, while the cleaner air stays closer to the floor.
- If their clothing catches on fire, they should stop, drop and roll. Make sure they understand that the fire will only burn faster if they run.
- If you live in an apartment building, make certain everyone in your family knows the proper evacuation procedures. Always use the stairs, not the elevator.
- Equip upper-story rooms of your house with rope or chain ladders or outside fire escapes.
- Put fire extinguishers in your kitchen and on each floor of your house.
- Be sure the electrical wiring in your home is sound.
- Never overload the circuits. Be cautious about using extension cords and multiple sockets.
- Buy only electrical equipment and cords with the Underwriters Laboratory (UL) label.
- Frequently examine electric heaters, cooking equipment and other appliances to make sure they are still in good operating condition. Replace frayed cords and broken or loose plugs.
- If an electrical fire does occur, don't try to put it out with water. Pull the main switch to cut off the electrical current, then use a dry chemical fire extinguisher and call the fire department immediately.
- Oily cloths and flammable liquids should be stored outdoors away from heat in closed metal containers. Rubbish should be discarded promptly.
- If you smoke, be careful, and keep household matches and lighters out of sight and reach. Never smoke in bed.
- Use a fire screen in front of your fireplace. Wood stoves and space heaters should be surrounded by a protective screen. Children shouldn't be left alone in the room when they are being used.

You can also protect your child against fire and burns by giving her the supervision her age requires,

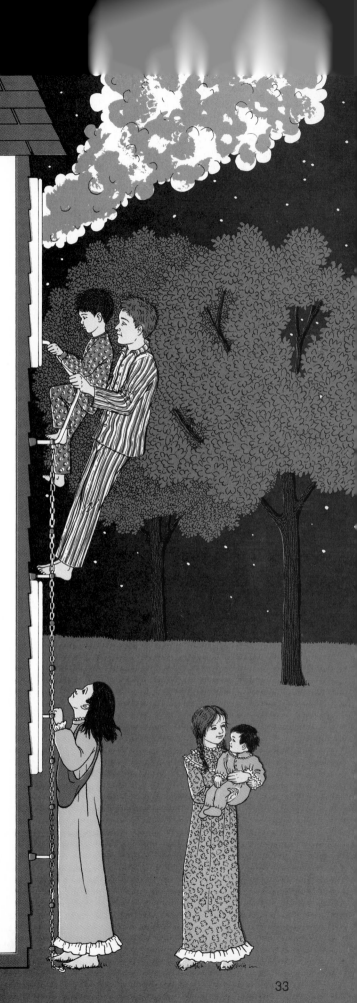

teaching her to avoid foreseeable hazards, and taking care not to imperil her through your own carelessness:

- Make sure she understands that fires can burn and that she is to stay away from stoves, heaters, open flames, hot liquids, matches and cigarettes.
- Be particularly careful when you are cooking. Use the back burners whenever possible, and always turn pot handles to the rear so your youngster can't brush up against them or grab them. Keep high-chairs away from the stove, and never hold your child while you are cooking.
- Keep children a safe distance away from outdoor barbecues.
- At mealtime, keep hot food and drink near the center of the table where a youngster can't get at them. Never pass hot food over a child's head. And don't hold your child while you are eating or drinking anything hot.
- All placemats and tablecloths should be kept out of reach of small children.
- Teach your child to take extreme care when turning on a hot-water faucet, particularly in the shower or bath.
- Younger children sometimes get scalded when left in the care of an older brother or sister. Don't leave your little one with an older sibling around hot water or in the kitchen or bathroom.
- Food and drink heated in a microwave oven can become burning hot while the container remains cool enough to touch. Be sure to test the temperature before giving them to your child. Don't heat your baby's bottle in a microwave; it can split.
- Keep appliance cords out of reach, especially for coffee makers, so young children can't chew them or pull them down on themselves.
- Block off unused electrical outlets with childproof covers or heavy electrical tape. Teach your youngster never to stick keys, pins or other metal objects into an outlet.
- Unplug electric appliances when they're not being used.
- When you disconnect an extension cord from an appliance, don't leave it plugged into the wall. Your child could burn or shock himself badly if he puts it in his mouth or touches it with wet hands.
- Be careful not to leave small appliances, such as radios or hair dryers, plugged in near a water source. And never let your child use a radio, television set, hair dryer or other appliance around water.
- Check that all electrical toys are approved by the UL and inspect them frequently for frayed wires and loose or broken plugs.

Because children have thinner skin than adults, they can sustain more severe burns at lower temperatures from hot liquids, grease or bath water. To prevent scalding injuries:

- Set the thermostat on your hot water heater no higher than 125° F.
- Install a safety valve, called a scald-protector, on bathtub faucets.
- Always test the bath water before putting your child in the tub.

GUNS

Guns are now the fourth leading cause of unintentional injury death to children in the United States, and the majority of firearm deaths occur inside the home. It has been documented that a gun in the home is six times more likely to result in the death of a household member than some unknown intruder it is meant to protect against.

If you have a child in your home, it is far better not to have a gun. Children are extremely resourceful, especially the preteens and teenagers who are at the greatest risk of injury. Keeping a gun unloaded with the ammuni-

tion locked away does not guarantee their safety.

If you do have guns in your home, you must certainly keep them unloaded and locked up out of reach. Ammunition should be locked away in a separate place. Always treat guns as if they are loaded, and never point them at anyone.

Gun injuries and deaths can also take place in other people's homes. When your child is visiting someone, try to make sure no firearms are left around for him to play with and that safe firearm practices are maintained.

ENVIRONMENTAL HAZARDS

Knowledge is increasing about the dangerous levels of indoor pollutants present in many homes. These pollutants are often more dangerous to children, especially infants and younger children, than they are to adults. Here are the more common indoor environ-

mental hazards and some suggestions what to do about them:

LEAD – The Environmental Defense Fund reports that one child out of every six in the United States has some form of lead poisoning. Because some youngsters show no symptoms until it is too late to avoid permanent damage, you must check for the presence of lead as soon as possible. If you suspect your child may be contaminated, have him tested immediately. Lead poisoning must be treated early to be cured.

Lead paint was banned in 1970, but any house built before then probably contains some. Simply painting over it does not remove the problem. Walls have to be covered with sheetrock or paneling to be made safe. If you choose to remove lead paint, it must be done by a certified deleading contractor, and everyone must be out of the house during the procedure. Lead dust or particles of lead in the air are dangerous if inhaled.

There is also a risk of lead in drinking water, especially in older homes with lead water pipes or copper pipes with lead solder. If you are in doubt about lead levels in your water, have it tested by a qualified laboratory.

Some pottery is glazed with lead-containing substances that can leach into food. Do not use any questionably glazed pottery for acidic foods like lemonade or fruit.

RADON DETECTORS

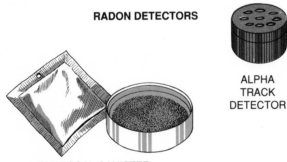

ALPHA TRACK DETECTOR

CHARCOAL CANISTER

RADON – Radon is a colorless, odorless radioactive gas found in rocks and soil. When trapped in buildings and concentrations build up, it can cause lung cancer and other lung damage.

The only way to determine if there is a radon problem in your home is by measuring the levels with inexpensive and easy-to-use passive monitors. If you find the radon levels exceed the safety level set by the Environmental Protection Agency (EPA), you can rectify the situation by sealing foundation cracks, keeping your house better ventilated and making various other changes.

ASBESTOS – When asbestos fibers are inhaled, they accumulate in the lungs, causing asbestosis and cancer. Symptoms do not appear until many years after exposure. Asbestos was commonly used in many building materials like roofing and flooring, pipe and wall insulation and spackling compounds. There is a great deal of controversy about how dangerous it actually is and how it should be treated. There is usu-

ally no health risk from intact, undisturbed asbestos. The danger arises if it becomes dry and crumbly, or if it is disturbed or removed by someone without the proper training. If you don't know exactly what to do about the asbestos in your home, get advice from a knowledgeable source before you act.

FORMALDEHYDE – Formaldehyde is the principal ingredient in UFFI (urea formaldehyde foam insulation), a popular type of building insulation primarily used during the 1970s. It is also present in some building materials and textiles. The concentrations of formaldehyde are not usually high enough to pose a health risk. Consult your local department of health or regional EPA office for information about testing and removal.

Formaldehyde gas is also released in tobacco smoke and by poorly vented gas and wood stoves. These are easily controlled by proper ventilation and not smoking.

CARBON MONOXIDE – This is a colorless, odorless gas that is a by-product of burning fuel, unvented gas and kerosene stoves, tobacco smoke, auto exhaust, and down-drafting from wood stoves and fireplaces. Be careful running your car in a garage, especially if the garage is attached to the house. Make sure to ventilate your house properly if you have a fireplace or a wood or kerosene stove.

TOBACCO SMOKE – Secondhand smoke, or passive smoking, is especially dangerous to children. Children in homes where adults smoke are at a greater risk of respiratory and ear infections, bronchitis and pneumonia, and have a greater likelihood of heart disease and lung cancer later in life. Asthmatic children are particularly at risk. If you smoke, strongly consider stopping. If you do not stop, try to confine smoking to outside your home and car and away from all children.

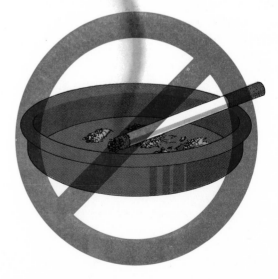

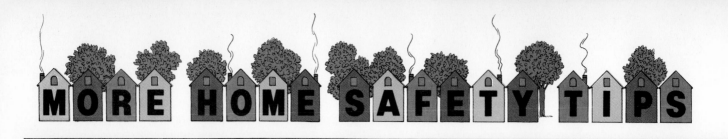

CHILD'S ROOM

- Remove all small objects an infant might put in her mouth.
- Never use plastic bags for toys or waterproof sheets.
- Only use stable furniture, stable or firmly mounted lamps and flame retardant curtains.
- Place the crib safely away from electrical outlets, lamps and hanging pictures.

- Remove large toys and boxes from the playpen. Your youngster could use them to climb out.
- Make sure all the paint in the room is nontoxic.
- Tie back long cords on window shades.
- Don't leave soft toys or pillows in the crib with your baby.
- Any furniture a child can climb upon should be kept away from a window.

STAIRS

- Keep them well lit and free of clutter.
- Make sure the child's head can't fit through banister supports. They shouldn't be spaced more than 4" apart.
- Install safety gates at the top and bottom to bar small children.
- Have handrails on both sides.
- Remove all tripping hazards.
- Don't let children run, play or sit on the stairs.

GARAGE, BASEMENT, LAUNDRY AREA & WORKSHOP

- Teach your children to stay away from these areas. If possible, keep them locked. Certainly, never leave your youngsters alone in them.
- Paints, solvents, insecticides and chemicals should be sealed tightly in their original containers, and kept out of a child's sight and reach, preferably in a locked storage area.

- Make sure everything is stored so it can't fall down.
- Remove the doors from stored refrigerators and freezers.
- Potentially dangerous tools should be kept where children can't get to them. Power tools should always be disconnected when not in use. Don't operate any power tools, including lawn mowers, around children.
- Automatic garage-door openers can crush children and animals. Install switches high up and use the kind that reverses if it meets any resistance.

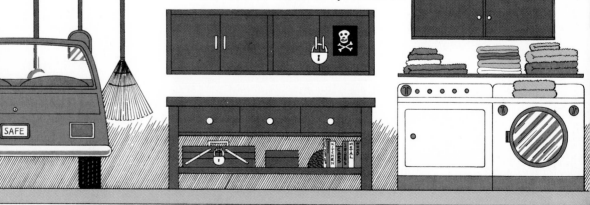

BATHROOM

- Never leave infants or young children in a tub without adult supervision. Don't just leave them alone with an older sibling.
- Drain the water from the bathtub immediately after the bath is over.
- Lock medicine and toiletry cabinets. Open shelves should be high enough so your child can't reach them. Store towels and linens under the sink, and use the high shelves in the linen closet to store medicines, small appliances and the like.
- Get rid of medications you're no longer using.
- Keep the toilet cover closed. It can be sealed down with a safety fastener.
- Keep electrical appliances away from water.
- Install rubber mats or abrasive treads inside the tub and shower. Use non-skid bath mats.
- Don't toss used razor blades or other hazardous or poisonous items into the wastebasket.
- Keep the door closed so your toddler won't wander in.

SOME GENERAL TIPS

- Keep electrical appliances out of reach, away from water and unplugged when not in use.
- Cover unused electrical outlets with heavy electrical tape or special plugs.
- Keep children from leaning against window screens or playing on windowsills and other high places.
- Make sure to unplug an extension cord from the outlet when you remove it from the appliance.
- Never leave an infant or young child home by herself.

KITCHEN

- Turn pot handles toward the back of the stove.
- Household cleaners, chemicals, bleaches and other dangerous substances should be stored high up, and preferably locked away.
- Make sure knives and other dangerous utensils stay out of reach.
- Get unbreakable plates and mugs for your youngsters.
- Don't place a highchair near the stove or around such busy areas as doorways and refrigerators.
- Don't store cookies or other sweets in cabinets over the stove.
- Keep the trash container out of reach.
- Never leave a child alone in the kitchen.

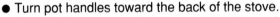

INFANT EQUIPMENT

The old adage "buyer beware" is of particular relevance when buying cribs, carriers and other infant equipment. Because a piece of equipment is manufactured or sold by a company with a familiar name does not necessarily mean it is safely designed and constructed. The American Academy of Pediatrics (AAP) notes that more than 40,000 infants and young children in the United States are treated in emergency rooms each year for injuries related to the use of nursery equipment, and that many of these deaths and injuries could have been avoided if the proper equipment had been employed.

The most important thing to remember is that cribs and playpens are not a substitute for adult supervision. There is frequently an implicit sense of safety when our infants or toddlers are "protected" by these enclosures. A large number of child safety products have become available in recent years that are intended to keep your child from harm. While many are helpful, there are others that are of dubious value, or may be dangerous in themselves. Worst of all, they can give parents a false sense of security. There is no child safety device as effective as constant vigilance and supervision.

You have to be as thorough as possible when deciding what to purchase for your child. Here's what to look for when you shop for a crib, carriage and other infant equipment, along with some pointers about how to use them safely.

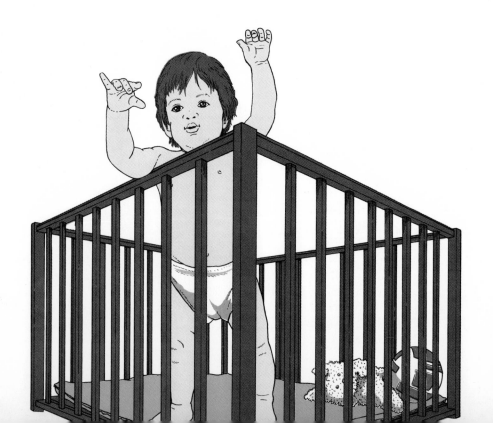

USED EQUIPMENT

When purchasing used infant equipment it is essential to make certain it has not been painted with lead paint. Children chew on the most unlikely things, and the ingestion of lead can cause permanent brain damage. Used equipment should also be carefully checked to be sure it is free of any sharp edges, cracks or breaks, and that it has all essential parts, including restraining straps.

CAR SEATS

The most important piece of infant equipment you will need is a child safety seat, or car seat. Only use seats manufactured after January 1, 1981 that meet Department of Transportation requirements. Be sure the seat is installed in your car properly, that your child is securely buckled in, and that you use it **every time** you take a child in the car, including that first ride home from the hospital. See the section on **CAR SAFETY,** pages 56-58, for more detailed information.

CRIBS

Crib injuries are one of the most frequent mishaps from birth to six months. The AAP says that more than 11,200 infants under the age of one suffered serious crib injuries in a single year.

- The slats should be no more than 2 3/8 inches apart, so your child cannot possibly slip her head or body through the spaces.
- The surfaces should be free of cracks and splinters and be painted with lead-free paint. If you have an old crib, make sure only lead-free paint has been used.
- The mattress should be firm and the same size as the crib, fitting snugly with no space for the head and limbs to get caught. An infant's face can get stuck if there is too much space, leading to strangulation.
- Avoid cribs with high cornerposts, knobs, cut out designs and decals.
- Look for a substantial distance between the top of the side rail and the mattress support. When your child is able to stand, lower the mattress to the bottom position and lock the side rail at maximum height. If the side is less than 3/4 of the child's height, the crib is too small for her, and should no longer be used. Remove bumper pads, large toys and anything else she might be able to use as steps. When she can climb out of the crib, it is time to stop using it.
- Never cover the mattress with plastic bags; they can cause suffocation. Bumper pads should extend around the entire crib and fit securely. The cords should be short and tied tightly, so as not to pose a strangulation hazard.
- The crib should be kept away from window-shade cords and other strings and at a safe distance from any windows.

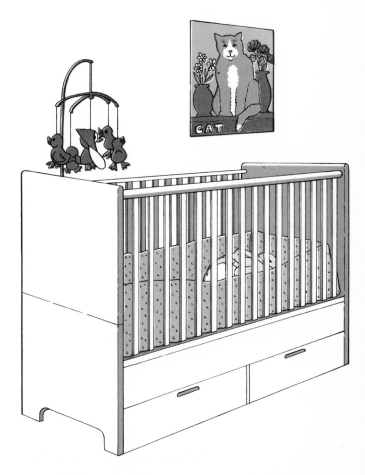

- All hanging toys should be well out of reach. Keep the crib free of diaper pins, buttons, baby powder and the like.
- Always keep the crib sides locked in the up position when the child is in the crib.

HIGHCHAIRS

- The chair should have a wide base to keep it stable, and come equipped with a safety belt that attaches to the frame, not the tray. Be sure to fasten the belt whenever you put your child in the chair. Most highchair injuries occur when youngsters aren't strapped in securely.
- Always make sure the tray is properly latched on both sides. Don't use it as a restraining device; that's what the safety belt is for.
- Check that the locking device on a folding highchair is secure whenever you open it.
- Never leave the room when your infant is in a highchair. Keep an eye on other children, especially toddlers, who may tip the chair over when the baby is in it, and never leave your child alone on the floor where he might try to climb into the chair and tip it over on himself. Falls from highchairs are one of the most frequent injuries to children from six to twelve months old.

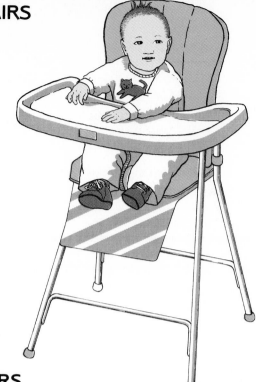

STROLLERS

- Check that there are restraining belts to keep your child from falling out, and **always** use them.
- Brakes on both wheels provide extra safety; make sure they lock securely.
- Avoid strollers with points, sharp edges or scissor-like folding mechanisms.
- Look for a stroller with a wide base to prevent tipping. If it adjusts to a reclining position, make certain it won't tip over backward when the baby lies down. Don't hang bags on the handles; the weight can cause the stroller to tip over.

- Remember that strollers reach traffic and other dangerous situations before you do; push extra carefully in traffic and crowded places.
- Never allow younger children to push the stroller without your guiding hand.
- Don't let older children ride in or play with it; this can weaken the frame or damage the brakes.
- Never leave a child unattended in a stroller. Stroller accidents are also a frequent cause of injury from six to twelve months of age.

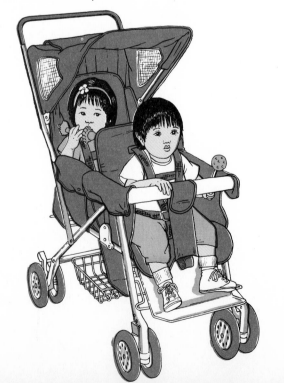

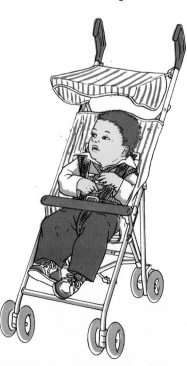

INFANT CARRIERS AND BACKPACKS

- Select the carrier appropriate to your child's size and weight. Use front carriers for infants. They need head and neck support.
- Make sure the carrier is deep enough to support the child's back and comes equipped with safety belts.
- Leg openings should be small enough to keep the child from slipping out but large enough not to chafe her legs.
- Check for sturdy materials, strong stitching and large, heavy-duty snaps. The metal frame near her face should be cushioned with soft padding.
- Be sure to keep your child's head lower than your own, and be particularly careful in revolving doors. Never ride a bike with your child in a backpack. Remember to bend from the knees rather than leaning over to protect her from falling out. Always use the restraining straps. Never use a pack in an automobile; the baby could be crushed between you and the dashboard.

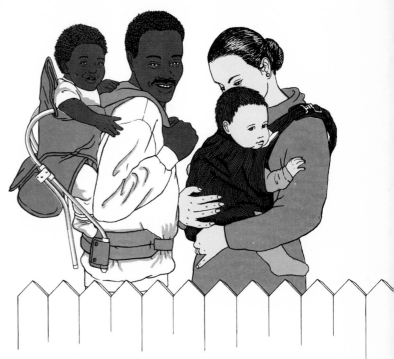

BABY WALKERS

Most authorities consider baby walkers extremely dangerous and without significant benefit. We strongly recommend not using them. It is estimated that between 16,000 and 20,000 children are treated each year for walker-related injuries. Canada has banned their sale.

INFANT SEATS

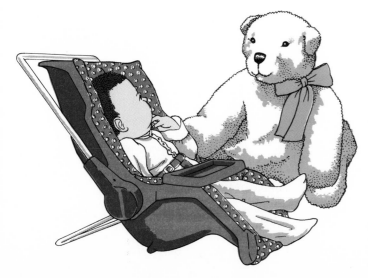

- The base should be wide and sturdy to prevent tipping. Supporting devices must fasten securely to keep the seat from collapsing. Check them regularly to make sure they haven't popped out.
- Be sure that the seat has both crotch and waist safety belts to hold the child in place, and **always** use them.
- Attach rough surface adhesive strips to the bottom of the seat to help keep it from slipping when you set it down.
- Never leave a child unattended in an infant seat; he could roll out of it.
- Keep the seat away from the edge of any elevated surface.
- DO NOT USE AS A CAR SEAT. An infant seat is not designed to protect your child in an accident.

PLAYPENS

- Make sure the slats are no more than 2 3/8 inches apart. The weave of mesh-sided playpens should be small enough not to catch buttons on the baby's clothes. Check the mesh frequently for holes; even small ones can stretch enough to trap a baby's head. Holes also provide toeholds for climbing.
- Playpen sides should lock into place. Check that hinges and latches are fastened securely and won't pinch little fingers.
- Be sure the floor support is sturdy enough to support a jumping child. Install a foam pad on the bottom for comfort.
- Check for torn vinyl, exposed metal, rough or sharp edges or any small, loose pieces that could cause choking.
- Toys or anything else tied across a playpen create strangulation hazards.

- Never leave an infant in a mesh playpen with the side down; if she rolls into the space between the mattress and the loose mesh, she could suffocate.

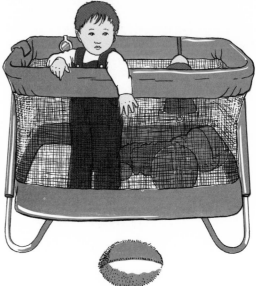

BABY GATES

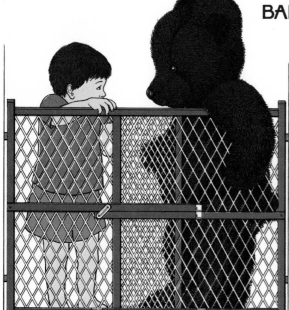

- Only use safety gates with a straight top edge and rigid mesh screening. "V" style gates and accordion gates that form a large diamond-shaped pattern can trap a baby's neck, causing strangulation. Expandable circular enclosures present the same danger and should also be avoided.
- Gates at the top of stairs should be permanently attached to the wall; pressure-type gates can be hazardous on stairways.
- If you use a gate elsewhere that is held in place by an expanding pressure bar, be sure to install the bar away from the side approached by the child so she cannot use it to climb over.
- Never leave a child alone assuming that the gate is an adequate restraint.

CHANGING TABLES

- Look for a table with a wide base.
- Make sure there's a safety strap, and **always** use it.
- Never leave your baby alone on the changing table, not even long enough just to turn your back and get a diaper pin. Always keep at least one hand on him.
- Store the things you use when changing the baby's diaper out of reach of both the infant and any toddlers or young children.

TOY SAFETY

All children love toys, and the playthings we give our sons and daughters benefit them in a number of important ways. Toys teach children to focus their attention, aid their intellectual, psychological and aesthetic growth, help them develop adult skills and provide them with fun and entertainment. Unfortunately, not all toys are safe, nor are the ways they are sometimes used.

Parents could prevent toy-related injuries more effectively if they were caused by unsafe toys alone.

There is no question that entirely too many toys are unsafe and account for a large portion of childhood injuries, yet other factors are usually also involved. Reputable toy manufacturers try to make their products as safe as possible, but they have to assume that parents will choose the appropriate toys for their children and give them adequate supervision. What determines the risk during play is a combination of the particular toy, child and circumstances, and what you do (or fail to do) to protect your child from harm.

A toy is inherently unsafe if its design or materials are defective or if there are flaws in its manufacture. Before buying a toy for your child, examine it carefully for its injury potential, looking for quality design, materials and construction throughout. Test the strength of the toy. Will the rattle come apart? Will buttons, bells, squeakers pull off? Toys with small detachable parts are particularly dangerous for younger children.

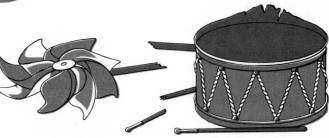

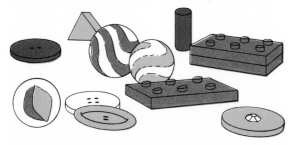

Marbles, small construction-type toys, tiny wheels, buttons and the like present choking hazards for small children.

Look for sharp edges, points and splinters, which can cut, scratch or puncture.

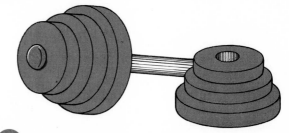

Check that the toy isn't too heavy for your child.

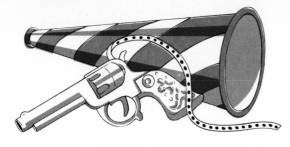

 Overly loud toys may damage your child's hearing. Caps should never be fired close to an ear.

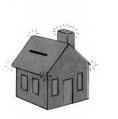

 Make sure that riding equipment is stable and well-balanced.

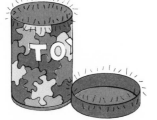

Metal toys with unfinished slots, holes and edges can cause razor-sharp cuts.

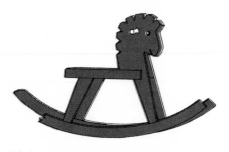

Don't let your child play with lead soldiers or other toys made with lead.

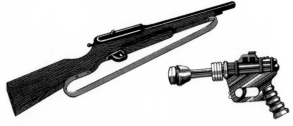

 Air rifles and guns and BB guns are unsafe; children should never play with them.

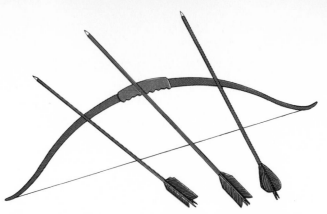

Projectile toys can cause severe eye injuries. It's best to avoid them entirely, but their use should certainly be limited to responsible children over the age of 8. Make sure there is adequate space and that the projectiles have soft, non-removable rubber or cork tips.

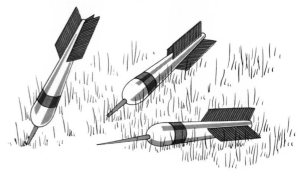

Lawn darts are much too dangerous for children.

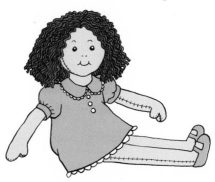

Cloth toys should be labeled "Flame Resistant," "Flame Retardant" or "Nonflammable." Don't buy dolls with cellulose hair or other cellulose toys.

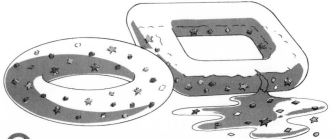

Teethers filled with fluid often break and leak.

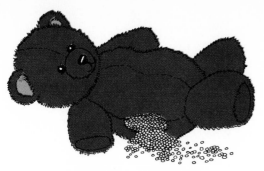

 Unsafe: Poorly constructed dolls and animals stuffed with small loose pellets that will fall out when the seams tear open.

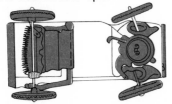

 The driving springs in mechanical toys should be adequately cased. Exposed gears and mechanisms can catch fingers and clothing.

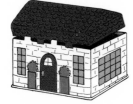

 Hinged playthings should be designed to avoid crushing fingers and hands.

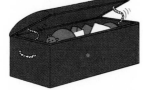

 The lids of toy chests can crash down on heads or necks and may also trap small children inside. Either remove the lids or make sure they have reliable, durable supports and holes for ventilation.

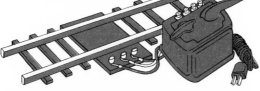

 Don't buy electrical toys operating on house current for children under 8. Limit younger children to electrical toys that use batteries. All electrical toys should be certified safe by the Underwriters Laboratory (UL). Kids can be burned or shocked by electrical toys that are poorly constructed.

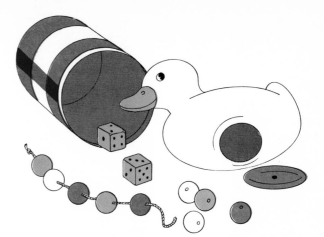

 Toys with small parts that might be swallowed, inhaled or lodged in the ear are particularly dangerous for children under 3. The noise-makers in squeak toys pose a serious choking hazard if they can be removed or fall out; make sure they are molded in.

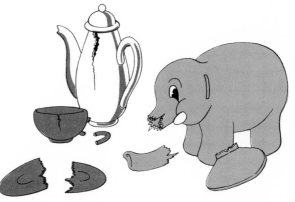

 Cheap plastic is likely to break easily, leaving sharp or jagged edges. Avoid toys with glass or brittle plastic.

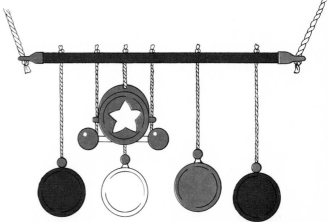

 Remove crib gyms as soon as a child can sit up or get up onto her hands or knees. Older babies can catch their necks on toys that stretch across a crib and may pull hanging toys down on themselves.

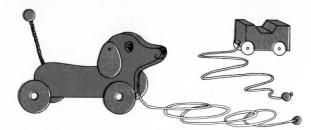

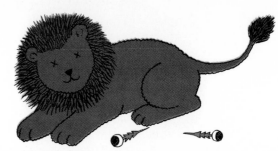

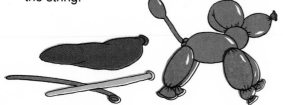

 Toys with strings longer than 12 inches are dangerous for children under 2, and should never be hung over a crib. Infants can get tangled up and have their breathing cut off by the string.

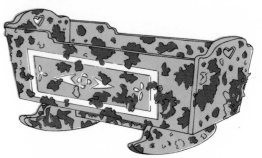

Unsafe: Toys made with straight pins, easily removable nails, or wires that are or could easily become exposed.

Balloons cause more deaths by suffocation than any other toy. Never allow kids to inflate balloons or chew on them. Adults should supervise the use of balloons by children under 6. A young child can choke on an uninflated balloon or a piece of a broken balloon.

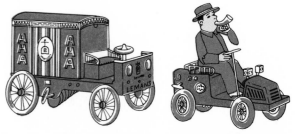

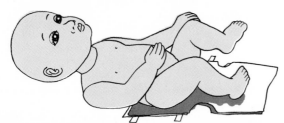

All painted toys and paints should be labeled "Nontoxic." Make sure old toys and nursery furniture haven't been refinished with a lead base paint; chewing on lead paint can cause serious brain damage.

Toy disposable plastic diapers for dolls also can be inhaled and are as dangerous as balloon pieces.

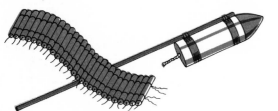

Toys using explosive materials are dangerous. Never let your child play with fireworks.

Be careful when buying or using old toys. Many older toys were made before there were safety standards. Check to be sure there are no missing or loose parts, rough or sharp edges, chipped or lead paint.

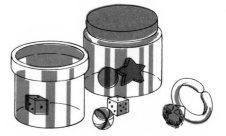

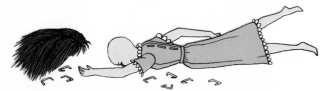

Unsafe: Dolls with clothing, hair and accessories flimsily attached with pins or staples.

Toys found in party favors, gumball machines, candy, cereal or fast food boxes may have small parts and be unsafe.

TOYS TOO OLD FOR YOUR CHILD

Toys appropriate for older children may be hazardous and frustrating for younger ones because of their inability to use them properly. Children themselves purchase 1/3 of all toys sold, so it's particularly important to teach them which playthings are, and are not, suitable for their age.

● When selecting a toy for your child, keep in mind his age, abilities, interests and limitations. Make a point of checking the manufacturer's age recommendations. Such warnings as "Not Suitable for Children Under 3 Years" are generally sound and intended to protect younger children from toys that either have small parts they could choke on, break relatively easily, or for some other reason are not safe for youngsters under the given age.

● When buying toys for older children, consider the risks to their younger brothers and sisters. Young children are always curious about the toys of their older siblings, and since they are usually unaware of the dangers, they can be seriously hurt if allowed to play with them. Teach your older children to keep their toys away from the younger kids in the house. Store toys separately for children of different ages, with the older children's toys kept out of reach and sight of the junior members of the family.

BROKEN TOYS

Even reasonably well-made toys may break eventually, leaving jagged or sharp edges and points. Some toys that appear safe have sharp parts inside that become exposed when the toy is broken.

● Select durable toys likely to withstand being frequently pushed, pulled at and dropped. Children like to explore how their toys are put together, and a toy should be sturdy enough to withstand their probing. Even when it breaks, it should still remain safe. Tug gently at attached parts to test their strength. Flex plastic toys slightly to see if they are brittle and likely to break easily.

● To minimize breaking (and to lessen tripping hazards), make sure that toys are put away soon after your kids finish playing with them. Indoor toys should not be left outdoors, where they may be damaged by moisture and rust.

● Check your child's toys regularly to make sure they are still safe for continued use. Repair broken toys and children's furniture promptly. Use only lead-free paints to restore the finish. If a toy cannot be fixed, discard it.

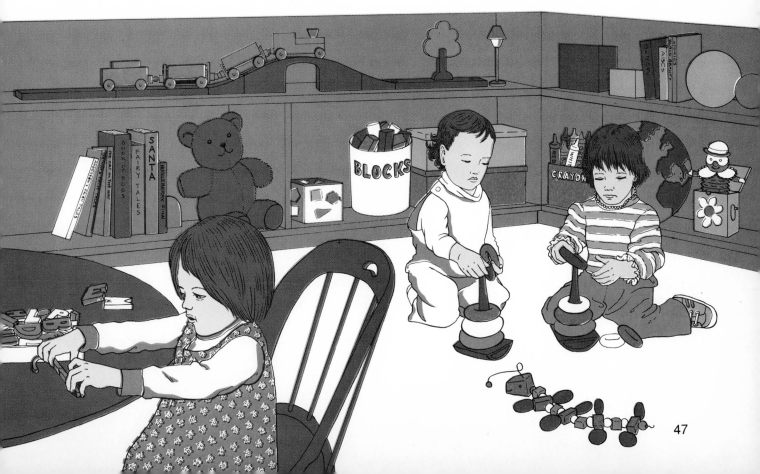

PLAYING SAFELY

Some toy-related injuries have less to do with any defect in the toy itself than with the way it is used. Parents sometimes forget their children's inexperience and neglect the preventive measures that would keep them out of harm's way. We have to remember that children are children and don't behave like adults.

● Give your youngsters the supervision and guidance their age requires. Make the time to play with them. That's the best way to show them how to use their toys correctly.

Infants need protection 100 percent of the time, as they are basically helpless the first few months of their lives and unable to manage on their own when they begin to become mobile.

1 to 2 year olds are curious investigators who like to take everything apart. They have no sense of danger and require extremely close – almost constant – supervision. By the time they are toddlers they can be taught not to walk or run with things in their mouths.

2 to 4 year olds are most susceptible to toy-related injuries and continue to require close supervision. This is particularly the case with boys. From this age on, boys are statistically more likely than girls to have accidents. Safety training in the proper use of toys should be actively undertaken throughout these years.

4 to 6 year olds should be able to demonstrate more of an understanding of possible toy hazards and exhibit good safety practices at play. Safety training should continue.

6 to 8 year olds are now in school and playing further away from the direct supervision of their parents. Make sure your child has internalized the principles of safe play.

8 to 12 year olds may be mature enough to play with toys that require good judgment. Before letting your child play with chemistry sets, projectile toys, sharp tools and other potentially dangerous playthings, be certain she knows how to use them safely. Parental supervision may still be required.

● Keep an eye on your child's playmates and the way they play together. Injuries may occur because a friend has not yet learned the potential dangers of a toy even though your child is well aware of them.

● When your youngster gets a new toy, read over the instructions together and make sure you both understand them. Teach him the proper use of the toy, explaining any hazards that may result from its misuse. Take the time to help him develop the necessary skills.

● Never leave a child unattended for a moment around a bathtub, swimming pool, play pool or water bucket. Children can drown in only an inch of water in a matter of seconds.

● A toy must be given the play space it requires. Outdoor toys should only be used outdoors.

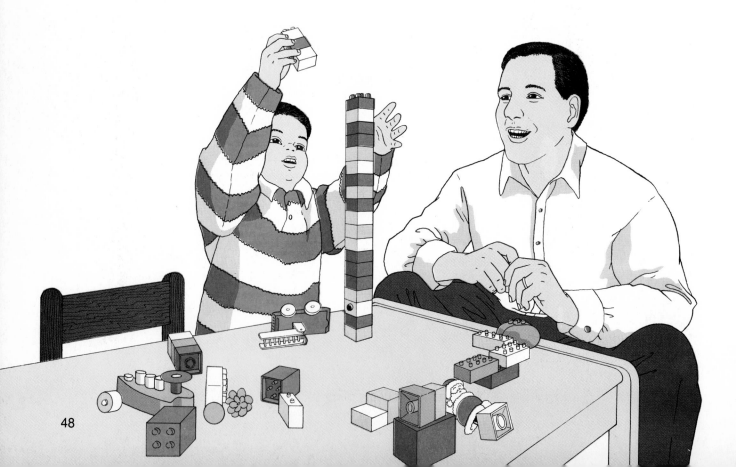

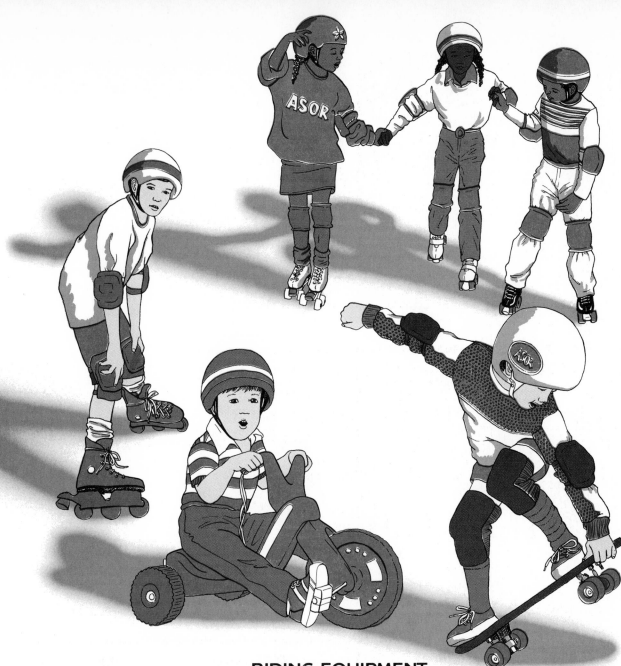

RIDING EQUIPMENT

So-called "riding toys" are the most frequent cause of serious childhood injuries. They are not really toys at all and should never be regarded as such. Children on wheels are always at greater risk.

Skateboards should not be used by children under 5. No child should be allowed to skateboard on highways, streets or near traffic. If your youngster does use a skateboard, make sure he wears a helmet and protective padding on his knees and elbows.

Roller blades and scooters also call for helmets and protective padding.

Do not allow children on any kind of riding equipment to play near the street. Children riding around in driveways cannot be seen by motorists backing up. Make sure small children are supervised by an adult when a car is backing into the driveway from the garage or the street. Check the chapter on **BICYCLE SAFETY** for the proper use of two-wheeled bikes. Your child should know the following basic safety rules for such sidewalk vehicles as coaster wagons, skateboards, roller skates, roller blades, scooters and tricycles:

● Always be careful of other people, and go slowly enough to stop suddenly if you have to.
● Never fool around or show off.
● Only play on sidewalks that aren't crowded.
● Don't hold packages in your arms while you ride. Leave your arms free for balancing.
● Look carefully both ways before crossing a driveway.

TOYS FOR YOUR KIDS

UNDER 1 YEAR

Awareness of sound, motion, touch and color. Hand to mouth curiosity. Toys should be simple, large, light in weight and brightly colored. Crib toys should be washable. The major dangers at this age are choking, suffocation, and the inhalation and ingestion of foreign objects.

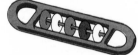
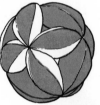

Squeak toys with noisemakers molded in
Sturdy, nonflammable rattles
Brightly colored objects hanging in view (mobiles, etc.)
Washable dolls and stuffed animals with embroidered features
Brightly colored cloth or rubber balls with textured surfaces
Unbreakable cups and other smooth objects that can be chewed
Unbreakable teethers that can be sterilized
Play boards
Blocks with rounded corners
Floating bath toys

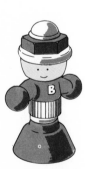

1 TO 2 YEARS

Age of mobility. Hand to mouth exploration. Very curious.
Toys must be able to withstand the need for investigation.

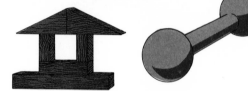

Cloth blocks
Books with large pictures on stiff pasteboard, plastic or cloth pages
Nesting and stacking toys (sets of blocks, etc.)
Sturdy dolls and stuffed animals
Push and pull toys (If the strings are longer than 12",
cut them down; long strings are a choking hazard.)
Non-glass mirrors
Take-apart toys with large pieces
Pots and pans

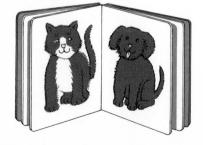
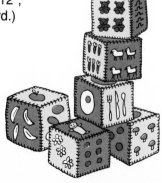

50

2 TO 3 YEARS

Development of language. Very curious. Small parts and sharp edges are still dangerous.

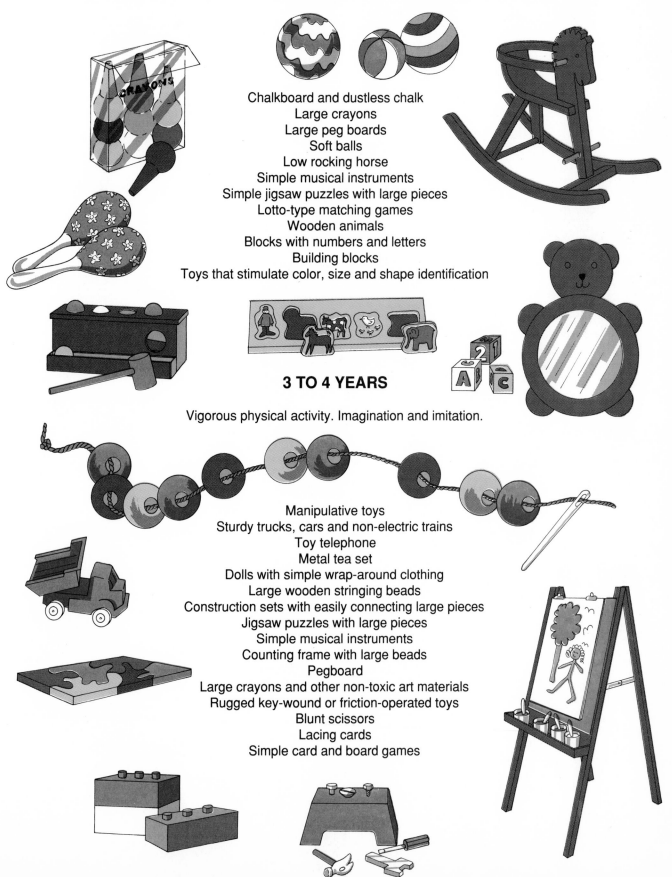

Chalkboard and dustless chalk
Large crayons
Large peg boards
Soft balls
Low rocking horse
Simple musical instruments
Simple jigsaw puzzles with large pieces
Lotto-type matching games
Wooden animals
Blocks with numbers and letters
Building blocks
Toys that stimulate color, size and shape identification

3 TO 4 YEARS

Vigorous physical activity. Imagination and imitation.

Manipulative toys
Sturdy trucks, cars and non-electric trains
Toy telephone
Metal tea set
Dolls with simple wrap-around clothing
Large wooden stringing beads
Construction sets with easily connecting large pieces
Jigsaw puzzles with large pieces
Simple musical instruments
Counting frame with large beads
Pegboard
Large crayons and other non-toxic art materials
Rugged key-wound or friction-operated toys
Blunt scissors
Lacing cards
Simple card and board games

4 TO 6 YEARS

Cooperative social play. Physical coordination.

Blocks of various geometric shapes
Picture books
Pail and shovel
Hand and finger puppets
Non-toxic watercolor paints
Modeling clay
Simple kaleidoscope
Key-wound or friction-operated toys
Cut-out paper dolls
Magnetic numbers and letters
Felt board
More advanced construction toys
Kites
Stencils
Activity books
More demanding board and card games
Simple musical instruments
Dress-up clothes
Tape players and tapes

6 TO 8 YEARS

Independent play. Physical and intellectual interests.

Kites
Boats and planes not driven by gasoline engines
Puppets and puppet theater
More complicated jigsaw puzzles
Games requiring some reading
Well-constructed, lightweight tool sets
Dolls and doll equipment
Equipment for playing store, bank, filling station, etc.
Magnets, magnifiers and sets demonstrating simple principles of science
Flower press
Simple musical instruments
Craft-making supplies
Story tapes

8 TO 12 YEARS

Arts, crafts, building and science interests.

Construction models of boats, planes and cars
Hobby material for coin and stamp collecting, etc.
Arts and crafts kits and materials
Electric trains and other electrical toys certified safe by the Underwriters Laboratory (UL)
Chemistry and other science sets
Bikes and sidewalk vehicles (Buy a helmet when you buy a bike!)

SCHOOL SAFETY

By the time your child goes off to school he is feeling a new independence and is no longer as subject to your direct supervision. The school will take on some of the responsibility for overseeing his safety, but it is crucial that you reinforce the safety lessons he learns there and show him how to protect himself from potential dangers between school and home.

GETTING TO AND FROM SCHOOL

If your child walks all or part of the way to school, map out the safest possible route, the one that exposes her to the least traffic, fewest intersections and avoids such hazards as construction sites. Emphasize that she is to follow this route and this route only, explaining why it is the safest and pointing out the dangers that do exist along the way. Make sure she understands never to hitchhike or accept rides from strangers. She should also understand the rules of pedestrian safety given below. They are probably the best single protection against injury.

If your youngster uses the school bus, make sure

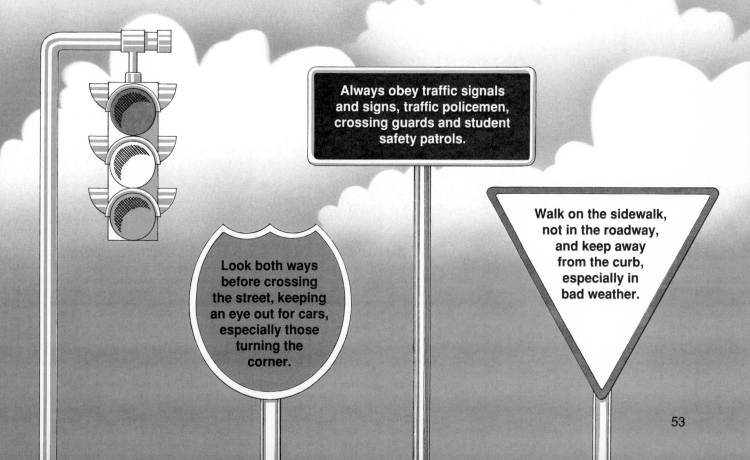

Always obey traffic signals and signs, traffic policemen, crossing guards and student safety patrols.

Look both ways before crossing the street, keeping an eye out for cars, especially those turning the corner.

Walk on the sidewalk, not in the roadway, and keep away from the curb, especially in bad weather.

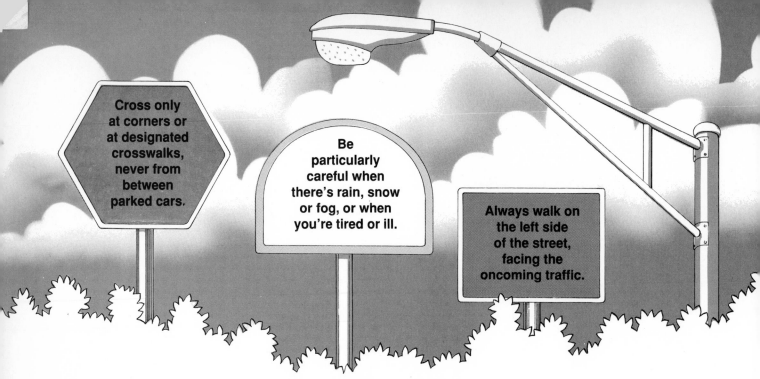

Cross only at corners or at designated crosswalks, never from between parked cars.

Be particularly careful when there's rain, snow or fog, or when you're tired or ill.

Always walk on the left side of the street, facing the oncoming traffic.

he allows himself enough time to get to the bus stop without rushing. Waiting for the bus to arrive probably poses the biggest potential danger he will face all day. Make sure he knows that he should stay away from the edge of the road. If he has to cross the road to enter the bus, tell him to wait until the driver or crossing guard signals that the way is clear.

Here are some other precautions he should follow once he has gotten on board:

- Take your seat promptly and stay there until you reach your destination.
- Always obey the driver, student monitor or school safety patrolman.
- Never distract the driver. Try not to be too noisy or rambunctious. No horseplay.
- Never stick your head or hands out the window or throw anything into the street.
- Make sure you know how to use the emergency exit.

Parents should follow the school bus once or twice to assure themselves of the driver's competence. Bus drivers are said to be responsible for 90% of school bus injuries. If your child talks about fighting or wild behavior on the bus, or dangerous driving, take her seriously and report it to the school authorities. If you have doubts about her safety, make other arrangements until the school has corrected the problem.

If your child uses public transportation, go along with her the first few times to make certain she knows the way. She should always carry some form of personal identification, and enough money to call home in case she gets lost.

If you drive her to school yourself, make a point of dropping her off directly in front of the entrance so she doesn't have to cross the street. Stopping on the other side of the street needlessly exposes her to traffic and may encourage her to cross in the middle of the block.

IN SCHOOL

The classroom is probably the safest place in the school because of the teacher's presence, but much of the school day may be spent moving from classroom to classroom to gymnasium to cafeteria. Every school sets up safety rules to ensure the safe movement of large numbers of children, and you should encourage your child to learn and obey them. It's likely that many of these precautions will be the same ones you use at home, so he will already be familiar with them. But make sure he is also aware of the following basics that apply specifically to the school situation:

- Walk, do not run, in the school corridors.
- Never engage in horseplay.
- When using busy stairways, keep to the right and hold onto the handrails. Take one step at a time. Never jump down the stairs or slide down the railings.

Tell your child to pay particular attention to the teacher's directions in woodwork and metal shop, science and photography labs, and the art and home economics rooms. Hand and power tools, kilns, stoves, chemicals and other specialized equipment can be extremely dangerous if not used in accordance with established safety procedures. Make sure

she learns these rules and follows them carefully:
- Always wear safety glasses when using such equipment as power saws, grinders and lathes.
- Remove rings, wristwatches, bracelets and cumbersome buckles when working around machinery. Make sure to keep neckties, scarves, loose clothing and long hair away from moving parts.
- Never remove or tamper with the safety features of a machine.
- Keep work areas and aisles free of tripping hazards.
- Running and wild play are particularly dangerous in labs and work areas.
- Know the location and use of cutoff switches, fire extinguishers, fire blankets and other emergency devices.
- Stay away from machines you do not understand.

Schools are particularly concerned about fire prevention. Make sure your child has a good understanding of the following safety measures:
- Never bring matches to school.
- Only use stoves, Bunsen burners and the like under a teacher's supervision.
- Always follow the teacher's directions during fire drills.
- Know how to respond quickly and correctly to the fire alarm.
- Report fires immediately to a teacher or other adult.
- Know how to use fire alarm boxes and how to telephone the fire department.

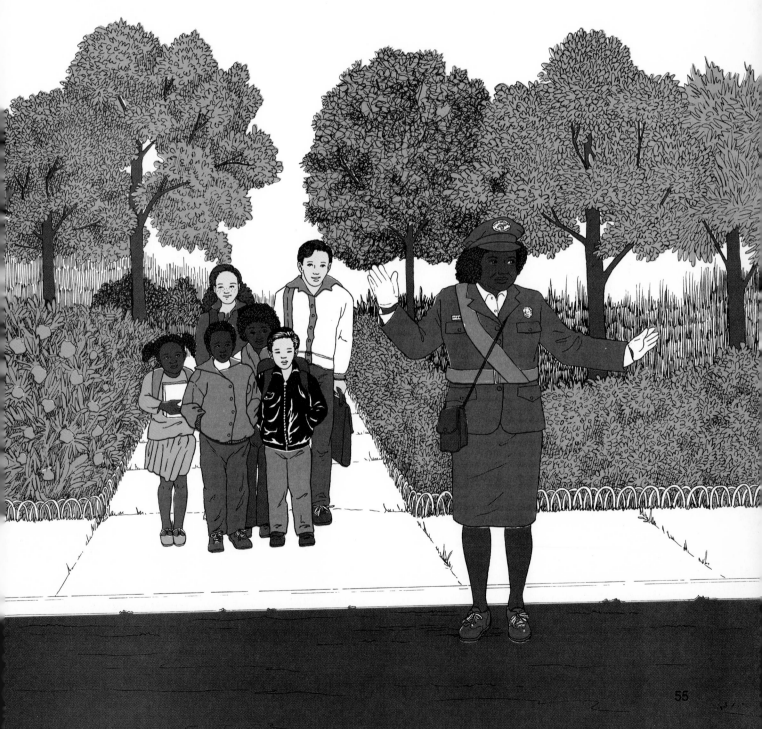

CAR SAFETY

Automobile injuries pose the single most serious threat to our children's safety. According to the National Coalition to Prevent Childhood Injury, they kill and disable more youngsters than all childhood diseases combined. The following preventive measures will offer a great deal of protection:

- Make sure your car stays in good operating condition.
- Drive safely and carefully, taking all the necessary precautions. Obey the rules of the road, and stay alert for any unexpected emergencies.
- Always wear a seat belt — for your own safety and as a constant example to your child.
- Always keep the doors locked, when you're parked as well as when you're in motion. Install childproof locks on the rear doors.
- Teach your youngster to enter and leave the car on the passenger side only, and to be careful not to catch her fingers when the door is being closed.
- Make sure she never sticks her head, hands or anything else outside the window.
- Don't allow loud noises or other distractions when you drive. If your child needs attention, pull safely off the road and attend to him.
- Never allow her to play with the car controls, even when the car is parked.
- Be sure to have a first-aid kit, a flashlight with fresh batteries, and emergency flares in your car at all times.
- Keep all heavy or sharp objects out of the passenger areas, especially off the dashboard and rear shelf. A sudden stop can send them flying.
- On long trips bring along quiet games to keep your youngster occupied, and stop at least every two hours so he can move around and stretch his legs. Try not to travel too far in one day.
- Don't allow your child to play with sharp objects, such as pens, pencils or scissors, when the car is in motion.

- Never leave children alone in a car for even a few minutes.
- Child car seats can get hot enough to burn a baby's skin, especially the metal and vinyl parts. Always test the temperature before you set her down. On a hot, sunny day cover the seat with a light-colored cloth or blanket. Keep infant car seats inside the house in very cold weather.
- The cargo area of a station wagon is not a safe place for a child to ride. No one should ever ride in the back of an open truck.
- Have the right kind of safety restraint system for your child. Make sure it is properly installed. And always remember to use it.

This last point about safety restraints requires some further discussion, because they are crucially important to your youngster's safety. It's been estimated that they reduce the risk of injury by 70%. Household infant seats and travel beds are no substitute for safety restraints and should never be used to transport your child in a moving vehicle. Nor can you offer adequate protection by holding her in your lap or arms. That's probably the most dangerous place for her to be, since any sudden stop will tear her away from you and subject her to the full force of a collision. Some parents wrongly assume this won't happen if they fasten their seat belts around the child while they're holding her. But in the event of a sudden stop or collision, both their weight and the child's weight would be forced into the belt, crushing the youngster and causing serious injury. The only real way to protect your youngster is with the right kind of child restraint that has been correctly installed and is used in the proper way.

Not all safety devices on the market protect children adequately. When purchasing a safety restraint, check that it meets or exceeds current government standards. Look for the label that certifies it conforms to all applicable federal motor vehicle safety standards. Also make sure it is the appropriate model for your child's size and weight and for the vehicle in which it will be installed.

We strongly suggest that you do not buy a used child restraint system. It may be obsolete, be missing some necessary parts or have been involved in an accident. If you should decide to buy one, make certain it is an approved model, comes with an instruction manual and all the parts are intact.

No safety device can offer protection if it isn't used, so make sure to place your child in the restraint for even the shortest trips. Remember that most automobile accidents happen within 25 miles of home. Teach him to request this protection when he's driving with someone else.

There are a number of other important points to keep in mind about the proper use of a safety seat or restraint:

● The back seat of your car is safer than the front seat, and the center of the back seat is the safest place of all. If a toddler must be placed in the front seat in a forward-facing restraint, adjust the seat to its farthest back position to keep her as far away from the dashboard as possible.

● Make sure your child is facing in the right direction: backward for children up to 1 year old or 20 pounds (an infant seat should **always** face backward); forward for youngsters over 20 pounds if they are able to sit up easily. Make sure the harness fits snugly over her shoulders.

● An infant in a rear-facing restraint should always be kept in the back seat **if your car is equipped with a passenger-side airbag.** Recent tests have shown that an infant riding up front in a rear-facing restraint could be seriously injured by the airbag when it inflates in a crash. An older child in a forward-facing restraint can ride in the front seat of a car with a passenger-side airbag, but the seat should be moved as far back as possible.

● An auto booster seat should always be used with either a lap and shoulder belt, a tethered harness with a lap belt, or a shield with a safety belt. The belts should be securely fastened in the proper place. The tether strap should be installed if that's what's required.

● All straps should fit snugly.

● Check that the car safety belt is properly routed through the frame or slots of the child safety seat.

● Don't bundle an infant in blankets before putting him in a safety seat; they will prevent you from positioning the shoulder harness properly. Place the blankets around him after he is already buckled in.

● Never allow a child to lie down or stretch out on the back seat of the car when she wants to sleep. To be protected by her safety belt she must be sitting upright.

● Lap seat belts are potentially dangerous for older children. Lap-shoulder belts are much safer.

● If you are using a child safety restraint in combination with lap-shoulder belts that lock only when the car suddenly stops, follow the safety restraint manufacturer's instructions regarding the use of locking clips to hold the restraint tightly in place at all times.

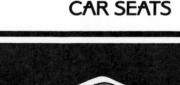

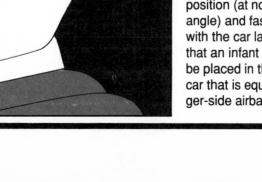

INFANT SEATS

From birth to about 20 pounds. Must always face the rear of the car so as to spread the force of a crash over the infant's back and shoulders — the strongest part of her body. The harness must fasten over her shoulders to a strap coming through the crotch. The seat should be kept in a semi-reclined position (at no more than a 45° angle) and fastened into the car with the car lap belt. Remember that an infant seat should always be placed in the back seat of any car that is equipped with a passenger-side airbag.

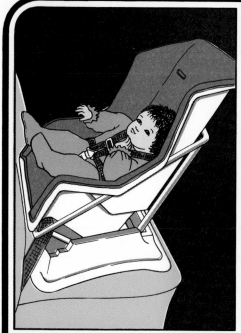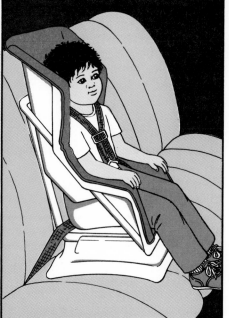

CONVERTIBLE SEATS

From birth to about 40 pounds. Faces the rear of the car and is used in the most reclined position until the child is about 1 year old. The seat then faces forward and he sits upright, secured by a five-point harness or a partial shield. Check that you are using the correct belt routes — they are different when the seat is facing forward than when it is facing backward.

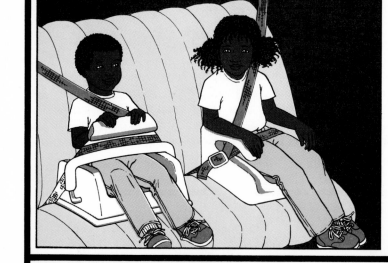

BOOSTER SEATS

For children over about 40 pounds who have outgrown convertible seats but are still too small for adult safety belts. These seats raise the child so that the lap and shoulder belts fit properly, with the lap belt across the child's hips and the shoulder belt away from her face and neck. If the booster seat is going to be used with a lap belt alone, purchase a model that has a large shield across the front to provide some upper body protection. When the eye level of your child becomes higher than the back of the seat, he has outgrown it.

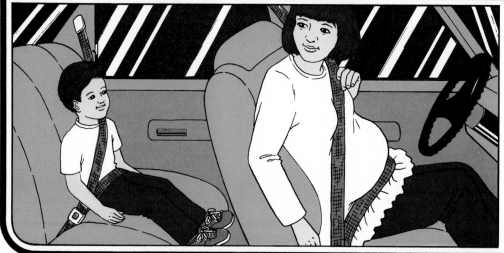

ADULT SEAT BELTS

The back seat is preferable to the front seat, and a lap-shoulder belt is preferable to a lap belt alone. The seat belt must fit snugly over the child's hip bones, not his abdomen.

BICYCLE SAFETY

Bicycles are a wonderful source of exercise and fun, but they are vehicles, not toys, and should always be treated as such. Too many children are injured and killed in collisions and falls that could have been prevented through proper education in bicycle safety. This chapter discusses the most common causes of childhood bike injuries and shows you how to work with your youngster to keep her safe from harm.

BUYING THE RIGHT BIKE

Buy a bike according to your child's size, not his age, and be sure to get the right size. Bicycles are expensive, and parents sometimes buy them too large so their children can use them longer. But a youngster cannot properly control a bike that is too large for him, a potentially dangerous situation that can lead to serious injuries. Nor should you get your child a two-wheeler until he is ready for one, which will usually be around the age of 5 or 6.

Bikes for beginners and younger drivers should be equipped with coaster brakes rather than hand brakes. Younger children don't yet have the strength that hand brakes require. Before buying a bike with hand brakes for an older child, make sure she can grasp the brakes comfortably and apply enough pressure to stop the bike with ease.

Don't buy a beginner a high-rise bike; they are hard to handle.

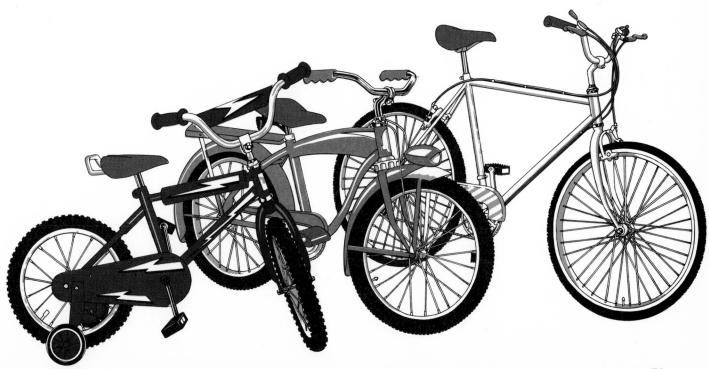

For children up to about age 10, a single-speed bike is the best choice. After 10, a more sophisticated 10-speed or all-terrain bike may be appropriate.

Take your child with you when you shop for a bike; proper fit is far more important than giving her a surprise. Here's how to make sure the bike fits her properly: She should be able to straddle the bike with both feet flat on the ground, with about an inch of clearance between her crotch and the horizontal bar between the seat and the handlebars. With a bike that has a sloping top tube, a yardstick or something similar can be used to simulate a horizontal bar. Once the right size bike is found, the seat and handlebars can be adjusted for a comfortable riding position. The seat should be adjusted so your youngster can place the balls of both feet on the ground while holding the handlebars.

BUY A BIKE HELMET WHEN YOU BUY A BIKE. Consider it standard equipment.

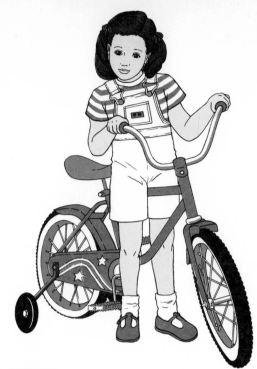

BICYCLE HELMETS

Head injuries from bicycle accidents are often extremely serious, sometimes causing permanent brain damage and even death. Helmets absorb the force of a fall or crash and also protect the head against abrasions and damage from sharp objects. They reduce the risk of head injury by 85% and of brain injury even more.

Helmets should be worn on every ride, no matter how short or close to home. Children should begin wearing them when they start riding tricycles. Helmets will protect them then and get them used to wearing them by the time they graduate to bikes. Adults should wear them too, for their own safety and as an example for their kids.

Only buy helmets that meet the standards set by the American National Standards Institute (ANSI) or Snell Memorial Foundation, which has even more rigorous standards. Look for the ANSI or Snell sticker on the inside.

Take your child along when you go shopping for a helmet so he will be sure to get a proper fit. Involving him in the selection will also help encourage him to wear it. The helmet should fit snugly, but not too tightly, and should not rock back and forth or from side to side. Check that the straps fasten properly and the helmet covers the top of his forehead.

The helmet should have a hard outer shell and an inner liner of shock-absorbent material. There should also be adjustable pads inside to ensure a proper fit.

Helmets with ventilation holes or slots are cooler and much more comfortable in hot weather.

Explain to your child why wearing a helmet is important. She should also understand that throwing or kicking the helmet around can damage it and diminish its ability to protect her.

If a helmet is in a crash, discard it. Crashes decrease the protection a helmet offers, even if there is no visible damage. All helmets should be replaced every five years.

If it is necessary to clean a helmet, use only mild soap and water. Solvents and cleaners can cause damage.

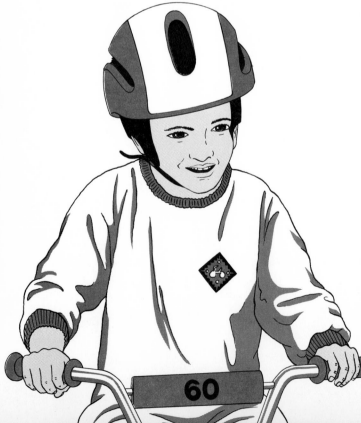

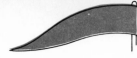

EQUIPMENT AND OPERATING CONDITION

Make sure your child's bike has all the equipment it needs to be driven safely, and periodically inspect it to be certain it is still in good condition. The chances of injuries are greater on a bike that is not well-maintained. Here are some things to look for:

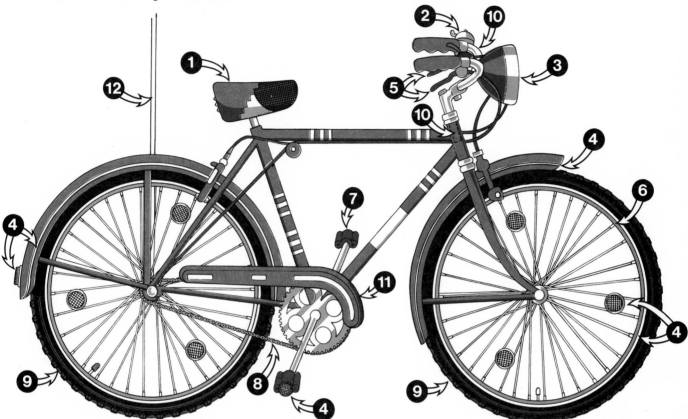

❶ SEAT: Must be tight enough to keep its position when struck on the nose with your fist. Should be adjusted as needed for comfort. Make sure after each adjustment that the seat post is at least 2" down in the frame, and that the nuts and seat clamp bolt are tightened securely.

❷ BELL OR HORN: Must be heard up to 100 feet. If battery-operated, periodically check the batteries.

❸ HEADLIGHT: Should be visible at night from 500 feet. Replace damaged headlights immediately.

❹ REFLECTORS: For added night safety protection. Red reflectors should be visible at night from 200 feet. White reflectors on spokes or pedals and reflectorized tape add additional safety protection. Keep them clean. Reflectorized tires are also available.

❺ BRAKES: Must be able to stop the bike quickly and smoothly. Check frequently.

❻ WHEELS: Should spin without significant wobble (1/16" or less). Replace any missing spokes. Wheel rims should be free of dents. Especially for bikes with caliper brakes, sides of rims should be clean and free of oil and grease. Check to be sure all nuts and bolts are tight.

❼ PEDALS: Should turn freely and be firmly secured in the crank arms. Must be complete and undamaged.

❽ CHAIN: Replace or clean if noisy or rusty; keep well lubricated. When chain is in highest position, it should have only 1/2" play. If more, have dealer adjust.

❾ TIRES: Should be inflated to recommended pressure, usually stamped on side of tire. Valve stems should be straight. Check frequently for any leaks or excessive wear. Clean out stones or glass that have become embedded. Replace worn or damaged tires.

❿ HANDLEBARS: Should be tight and properly aligned. Handlebar stem should have at least 2" remaining in the fork stem and be securely tightened. The grips should always fit tightly.

⓫ CHAIN GUARD: Protects pants and skirts from getting tangled in the chain. Have dealer install one if bike comes without it.

⓬ RED SAFETY FLAG: For added visibility.

BICYCLE SKILLS

It may not take your son or daughter more than a few hours to learn how to remain upright, steer and stop, but there is much more to driving a bike than hopping on and driving away. And the cyclist is always a driver, not just a rider. "Rider" suggests the passive role of someone only "along for the ride" and perpetuates the attitude that the bicycle is a toy. It isn't.

Most injuries to beginning cyclists come from falls. As your youngster gains experience and confidence, she'll fall a lot less, but kids who have been biking less than two years — typically, children about 6 to 8 — are subject to a great many falling injuries. They can be kept to a minimum by enrolling your child in one of the bicycle training programs designed to teach basic driving skills. In many communities these courses are offered by the police, the "Y" and other such organizations as part of their youth activities programs.

Basic biking skills can be taught in a few hours. If you want to do it on your own, all that's required is some patience, some chalk and a paved surface away from traffic, such as a playground or empty parking lot. It will give your child needed protection and provide an enjoyable afternoon or two as well. Youngsters are always eager to demonstrate their mastery of new skills, so it shouldn't be hard to get him involved. And by all means, have some fun with it. Make it a game to be enjoyed rather than an ordeal to be endured.

The most important skills your child has to master are: balance, braking without skidding or swerving, turning both right and left using the proper hand signals, and stopping without swerving, skidding or falling.

Here are six exercises or games that will check out your child's progress. Space has been provided to mark off each skill as it is demonstrated. Keep in mind that these games indicate the child's control of the bike, but do not prepare him to drive in traffic. Study the next section on Driving in Traffic before you allow him to bike on a street or road.

NEEDED: AN OPEN PAVED AREA. CHALK.
ONE CHILD. ONE ADULT. A SUNNY DAY OR TWO. A LITTLE PATIENCE.

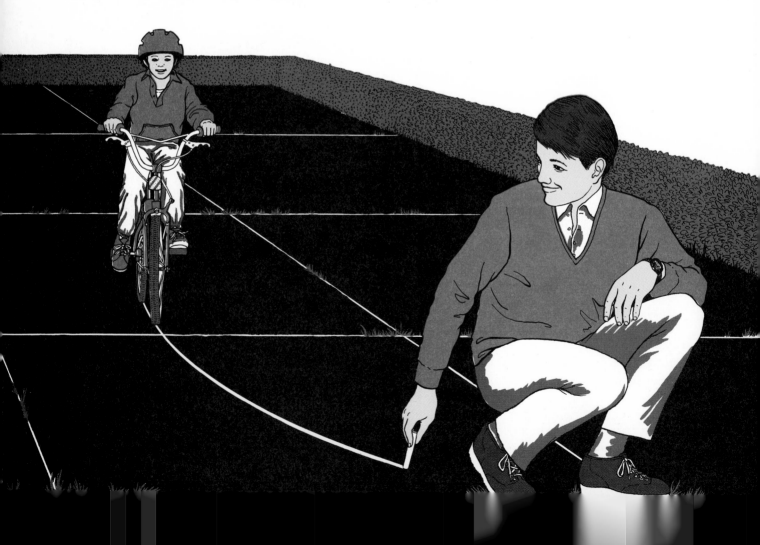

BALANCE

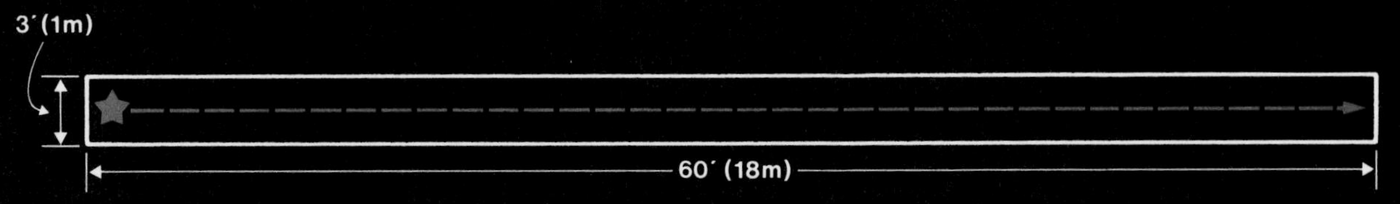

3´(1m)

60´ (18m)

THE CHILD DRIVES VERY SLOWLY THROUGH THE LANE:

☐ Taking more than 30 seconds
☐ Without touching the lines

☐ Without touching either foot to the ground
☐ Without using the brakes excessively

PEDALING & BRAKING

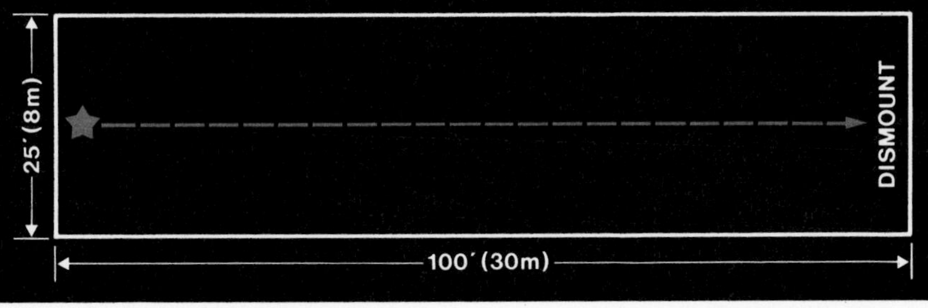

25´ (8m)

DISMOUNT

100´ (30m)

THE CHILD DRIVES THROUGH THE LANE AT AVERAGE SPEED:

☐ Keeping the balls of his feet on the pedals

☐ Keeping his feet parallel to the ground

AS HE APPROACHES THE END OF THE LANE, HE BRAKES THE BIKE TO A STOP:

☐ Without skidding
☐ Keeping the pedal cranks about parallel to the ground

☐ Exerting back pressure on the rear wheel
☐ Stopping about 10' from where he first applied the brake

☐ HE THEN DISMOUNTS ON THE RIGHT SIDE OF THE BIKE

STRAIGHT LINE

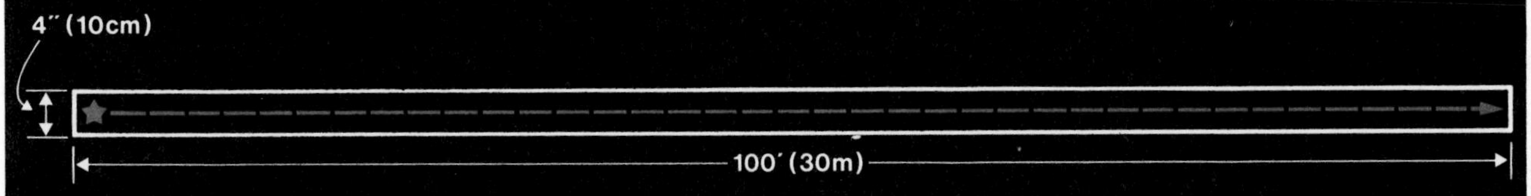

4´´ (10cm)

100´ (30m)

THE CHILD DRIVES THROUGH THE LANE:

☐ Without undue exertion
☐ Without touching the lines

☐ Without touching either foot to the ground
☐ Without skidding when he stops

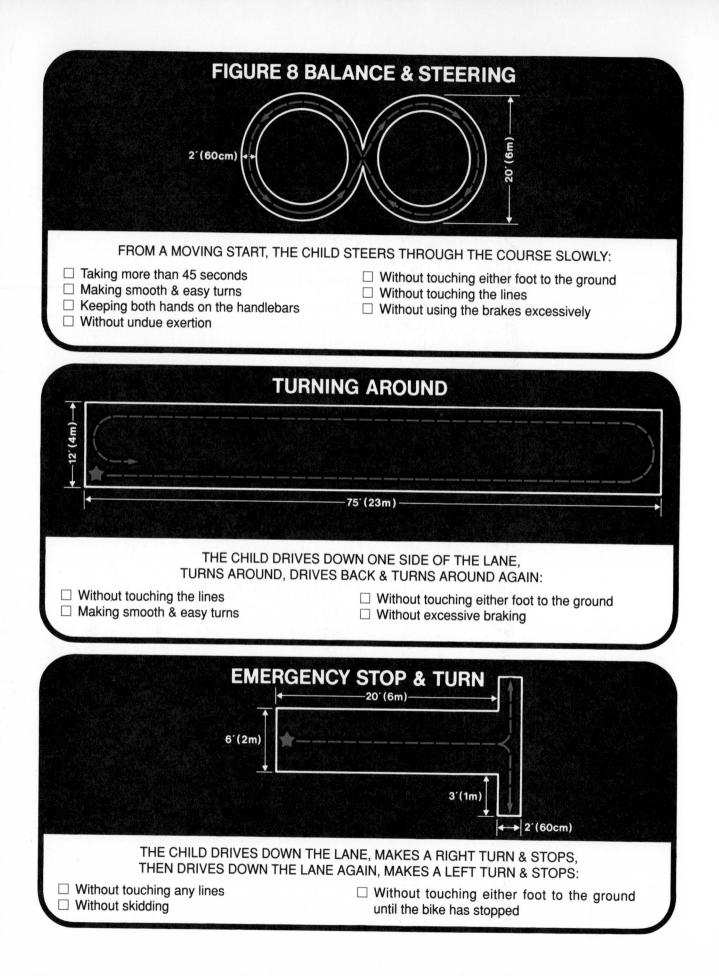

FIGURE 8 BALANCE & STEERING

2' (60cm)   20' (6m)

FROM A MOVING START, THE CHILD STEERS THROUGH THE COURSE SLOWLY:

☐ Taking more than 45 seconds
☐ Making smooth & easy turns
☐ Keeping both hands on the handlebars
☐ Without undue exertion

☐ Without touching either foot to the ground
☐ Without touching the lines
☐ Without using the brakes excessively

TURNING AROUND

12' (4m)   75' (23m)

THE CHILD DRIVES DOWN ONE SIDE OF THE LANE,
TURNS AROUND, DRIVES BACK & TURNS AROUND AGAIN:

☐ Without touching the lines
☐ Making smooth & easy turns

☐ Without touching either foot to the ground
☐ Without excessive braking

EMERGENCY STOP & TURN

20' (6m)   6' (2m)   3' (1m)   2' (60cm)

THE CHILD DRIVES DOWN THE LANE, MAKES A RIGHT TURN & STOPS,
THEN DRIVES DOWN THE LANE AGAIN, MAKES A LEFT TURN & STOPS:

☐ Without touching any lines
☐ Without skidding

☐ Without touching either foot to the ground
until the bike has stopped

DRIVING IN TRAFFIC

Children six years old and younger should always have adult supervision, even on sidewalks. Every driveway crossing is an intersection, and motorists are not always on the alert for kids on bikes. Young bikers must learn to drive defensively and watch out for cars. By the time he is 7 or 8 your youngster may be ready to drive unsupervised, but not out in the street. Before allowing him in the street by himself, you will have to take into account his personal maturity, local traffic patterns and his ability to follow the rules of the road. Around the age of 9 he'll probably be about ready to start.

For the older child, a bicycle is an important means of transportation that may be used to visit friends, go to school or run errands. As she moves from the sidewalk and driveway out into the traffic of the street or road, there is a dramatically increased risk of injury from collisions with fixed objects, other bicycles and automobiles and trucks. Since a bicycle offers no protection at all, and cannot move as quickly as a motorized vehicle, the cyclist is the most exposed and vulnerable element in the traffic flow. Even a minor collision can have serious results.

Before allowing your child to use his bike on the street, make certain he has developed a sensible attitude about driving in traffic and has a good understanding of the rules of the road. A bicycle is considered a vehicle by law and is subject to all the traffic regulations that apply to cars and other motor vehicles. Every cyclist is expected to know these laws as well as the special regulations for bikes. You can obtain a copy of these rules at the Registry of Motor Vehicles in your community. The importance of sticking to these rules may be judged by the fact that over 90% of bicycle deaths are a result of collisions with automobiles, and studies of auto-bike collisions indicate that more than 90% of the collisions occurred because younger bike riders were violating traffic laws at the time.

Make sure your child understands the reasoning behind these laws. Once she grasps the rationale for a sensible safety regulation she is much more likely to follow it. Here are the basics she needs to know:

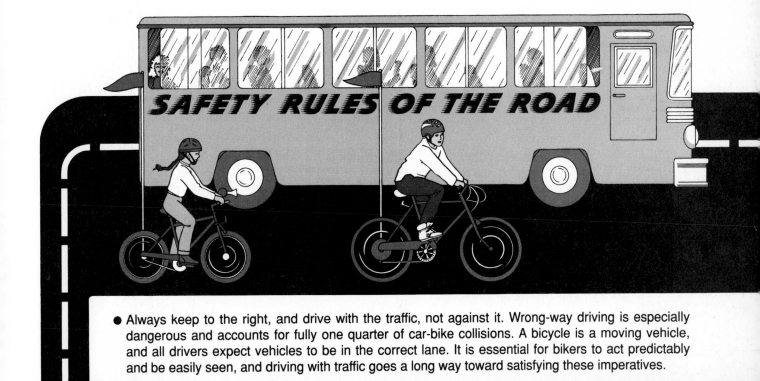

- Always keep to the right, and drive with the traffic, not against it. Wrong-way driving is especially dangerous and accounts for fully one quarter of car-bike collisions. A bicycle is a moving vehicle, and all drivers expect vehicles to be in the correct lane. It is essential for bikers to act predictably and be easily seen, and driving with traffic goes a long way toward satisfying these imperatives.

DRIVE SAFELY

- Stop and look carefully before entering a street. Look to the left, the right and then again to the left. "Rideouts" result in one third of serious bike injuries.
- Stop at all stop signs, red lights and intersections.
- Watch out for potholes, sand, gravel, stones and other surface hazards, as well as other cyclists, pedestrians and any other obstructions that may be in the road. More than 90% of all bike injuries occur as a result of the cyclist running into something or someone or taking a fall. Children need to learn how to avoid road hazards.
- Look back and wait for overtaking traffic before turning left; check for oncoming traffic at the same time. Children have less-developed peripheral vision than adults and more trouble judging where sound is coming from.
- Drive defensively and avoid heavily traveled routes whenever possible.
- Use the proper arm signals to indicate stops and turns. Start indicating turns a half block ahead.
- When turning left at a busy intersection, walk your bike fully across the street, then to the left after the light changes. Then remount and enter traffic again from the right.
- Drive single file, keeping a safe distance from the vehicle ahead.
- Never hitch a ride from another vehicle.
- Carry packages in a basket or carrier, keeping both hands free to control the bike.
- Be on the alert for car doors opening and for parked cars pulling out into traffic.
- To increase visibility, wear brightly colored clothing.
- Avoid driving in snow or on ice.
- Don't drive fast downhill.
- Never turn or apply brakes on unstable or slippery surfaces. Coast through them in a straight line.
- In heavy traffic, dismount and walk the bike across intersections, using the pedestrian crosswalk.
- Never stunt-ride, show off or engage in horseplay on the road.
- Avoid driving at night. It is 20 times more dangerous than driving during daylight. If you must drive at night, be particularly careful and use special precautions: light or white clothing, front bike light, reflectors and reflective tape.
- Always wear a helmet.
- Never listen to headphones when you drive. Not being able to hear other vehicles is extremely dangerous.
- Never ride double, except on adult bikes fitted with special passenger seats.
- Wear clip guards on trouser cuffs.

Closely check your child's awareness of traffic safety before allowing him to venture out into the street or travel in traffic. Here is another game to help you determine his preparedness:

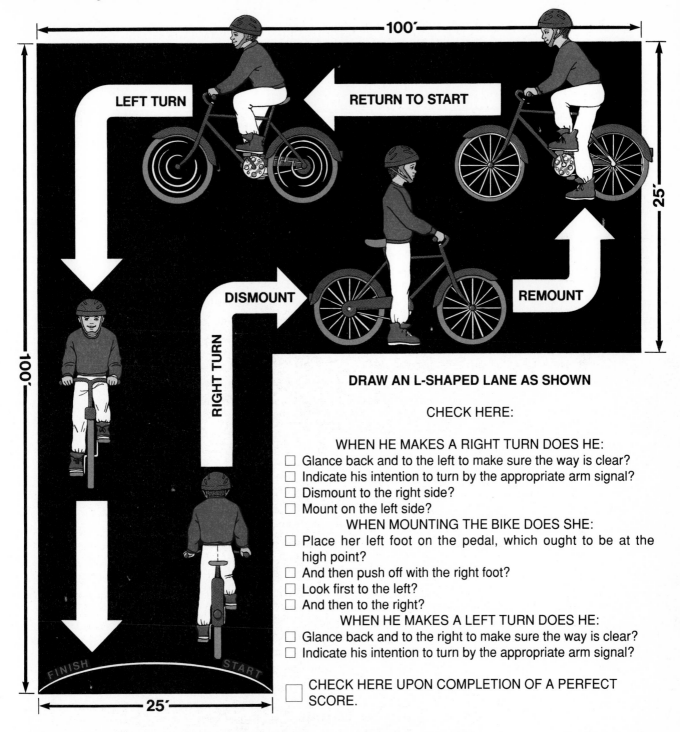

DRAW AN L-SHAPED LANE AS SHOWN

CHECK HERE:

WHEN HE MAKES A RIGHT TURN DOES HE:
☐ Glance back and to the left to make sure the way is clear?
☐ Indicate his intention to turn by the appropriate arm signal?
☐ Dismount to the right side?
☐ Mount on the left side?
WHEN MOUNTING THE BIKE DOES SHE:
☐ Place her left foot on the pedal, which ought to be at the high point?
☐ And then push off with the right foot?
☐ Look first to the left?
☐ And then to the right?
WHEN HE MAKES A LEFT TURN DOES HE:
☐ Glance back and to the right to make sure the way is clear?
☐ Indicate his intention to turn by the appropriate arm signal?

☐ CHECK HERE UPON COMPLETION OF A PERFECT SCORE.

When you are satisfied with your child's driving skill and her knowledge of traffic regulations, it's time to test how well she performs in normal traffic.

Pick out a route about one mile long that requires your youngster to turn, stop, cross intersections and, if possible, ride up and down a hill. Follow her at a safe distance on your bike, or in your car. Observe how well she demonstrates her understanding of traffic safety and how well she performs under actual driving conditions. After completing the drive, discuss her performance with her, calling attention to any errors you noticed and praising all successfully executed actions.

PLAYGROUND & SPORTS SAFETY

Particularly in cities, playgrounds are among the few spaces set aside for the vigorous play of childhood. Although not without their hazards, they are far less dangerous than open streets, abandoned buildings and other improvised play areas. Most playground injuries are of the minor cut, scrape and bump variety, yet more serious injuries can also occur. Not all playgrounds have the right physical environment, nor are they always safely equipped and supervised. And even in the best playgrounds, whenever a group of children are actively climbing, swinging, jumping and running, there is always the possibility that someone will get hurt.

The vast majority of playground injuries happen when children are using equipment in inappropriate and unintended ways. Since playgrounds should encourage exploration and imaginative play, it is important to try to anticipate some of these unexpected uses and to provide equipment that minimizes the risks. Careful supervision is also crucially important. Without it, even the safest equipment can be hazardous.

This chapter sums up the most common playground dangers and the best ways to keep them to a minimum. The recommended preventions apply equally to school and public playgrounds and the play equipment you may have set up in your own backyard. We end with some further recommendations about sports safety, since when a child outgrows the playground she usually moves on to the athletic field and court.

THE PHYSICAL ENVIRONMENT

Before letting your child spend time in a playground, check it out yourself to make sure the play area is safe and adequately supervised at all times. Here's what to look for:

● The playground should be surrounded by fences to prevent younger children from wandering in and out and to allow the area to be closed off when no supervisor is present. Fences also ensure that the equipment will be approached only from the proper direction.

● The equipment should be arranged according to the age group for which it is intended. Facilities for younger children should be separated from facilities for older children. This will keep the younger child away from equipment that requires a strength and skill she may not yet have, and will protect her from being caught up in the more vigorous, potentially dangerous activities of older kids.

● Adequate space should be marked off for each activity to protect both participants and the passer-by from bumps and collisions. There should be room for arms and legs to swing without getting in the way of people walking by. Boundaries must be clearly indicated by painted lines or physical barriers like bushes and hedges. Make sure your child understands the importance of staying outside them when he's not actively playing.

● The most common cause of playground injuries is falls, so the surface of the playground should consist of relatively soft materials, particularly around equipment. Grass and earth are not recommended because they quickly become packed and hard. A better alternative is mulch, shredded bark or chips. Concrete, asphalt and other hard, unyielding surfaces greatly increase the chances of serious injuries. Check that the surface is given the necessary maintenance to keep it safe.

● Make sure the playground is kept clear of broken glass, bottles, cans, metal tabs from cans and other debris, especially around slides, sandboxes and swings. Poisonous or thorny plants are obvious hazards.

PLAYGROUND EQUIPMENT

Broken-down, dilapidated structures are obviously dangerous and should never be used. However, every piece of equipment used in the playground must be examined to make sure it is in good repair and safe for your child's play.

● The equipment must be firmly anchored into the ground. Backyard equipment anchored with pegs must be checked regularly to make sure they haven't worked their way loose. All anchoring devices should be buried well below ground where they won't be tripped over. If the equipment is set in concrete, the concrete should be covered by 8-10 inches of absorbent material.

● Check that the equipment hasn't shifted with use. Structural components designed to be horizontal or vertical must be maintained that way. Shifts in position can impose a strain on the structure that may eventually lead to its breaking or collapsing.

● Screws and bolts holding the equipment together must not be loose or missing. Exposed screws and bolts should fit flush or be capped and any protrud-

ing parts covered with tape. Bolts with round heads are advisable. Fittings must be examined frequently to make sure they remain securely in place.

● Bars and chains should be secure. Split-link chains, S-hooks and similar fittings separate easily and are extremely dangerous.

● Hanging rings should either be much smaller than a child's head or much larger — under 5 inches or over 10 inches. There should be no equipment that can trap a child's body or head.

● Metal structures should be kept free of rust, and chipped paint should be scraped away. All playground paint and preservatives should be lead-free.

● Wooden structures should be protected against deterioration and restored or replaced as needed. Check for splinters.

● Playground equipment should be installed at least 6 feet away from fences.

For a more detailed look at individual pieces of equipment, take a tour of our Ideal Playground on pages 70-71.

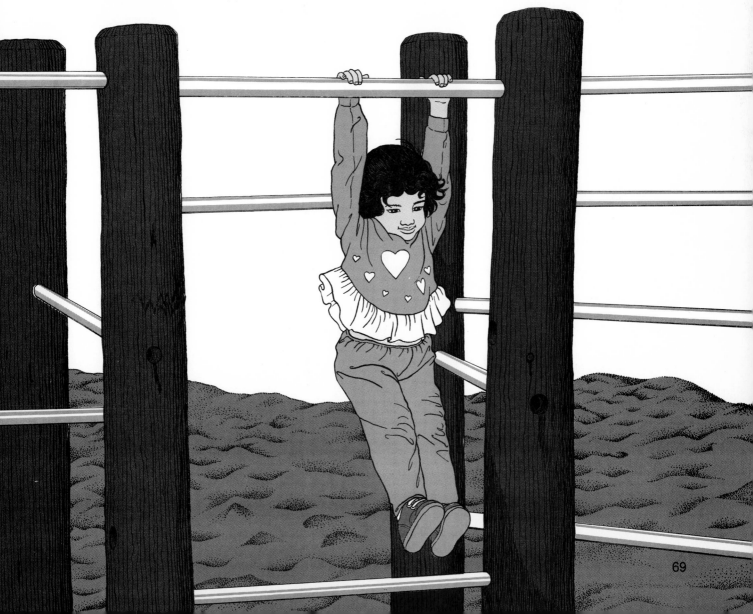

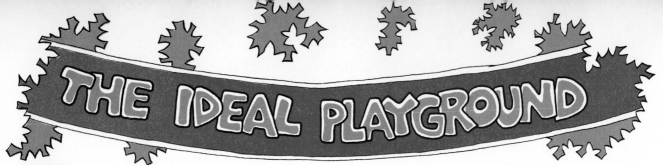

THE IDEAL PLAYGROUND

LADDERS
- Different heights for children of different ages.
- Sand or other soft materials are placed underneath to cushion falls.
- Protective siding around platform heights to keep children from falling off.
- The bars do not turn when grasped.
- Spaces between railings are less than 5 inches or more than 10 inches so children won't get their heads caught.
- Ladders aren't placed near swings so children won't try to leap from one to the other.

SWINGS
- Chair swings for kids under 5.
- Seats set at different heights for children of different sizes.
- All seats have rubber bumpers. Sling and saddle seats are the safest because they discourage children from standing up. Seats made of canvas, rubber or other soft materials are preferable to wood or metal. Tire swings have the lowest incidence of injury.
- There is 6 feet of clearance from walls, other equipment and playground traffic.
- Ropes are checked frequently for fraying.
- Chain links are 1/3 inch or less so fingers won't get caught.
- No S-hooks.
- Worn spots and holes under the swings are filled in with appropriate surfacing materials.
- No spaces small enough to catch a child's foot. Hanging rings are either too small or too big to trap a child's head. (They should be less than 5 or more than 10 inches.)
- No sharp edges.

SANDBOXES
- Should be shaded from the sun.
- No glass or other debris.
- The frame is free of splinters.
- The sand is raked often to keep it clean and expose it to the sun and air.
- The box is covered at night to protect it from moisture, dogs and cats.
- The sand itself is safe. Some manufactured play sand made from crushed marble or limestone contains hazardous levels of asbestos. (Sand that looks especially white or chalky is suspect.)

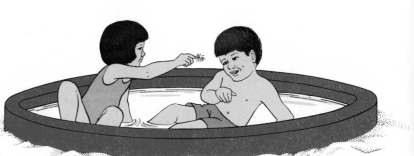

WADING POOLS
- Kept closely supervised. Accidental drownings can occur quickly and easily in as little as 1 inch of water.
- Kept clean by frequent emptying.
- Emptied and turned over so as not to accumulate rain water when not in use.

DRINKING FOUNTAINS
- Free of paper, stones and rubbish.

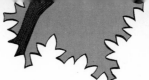

SLIDES

- No higher than 6 feet for children under 8, no higher than 8 feet for older children.
- Should be shaded from the sun, particularly if made of metal, and be free of rust.
- Ten inches of mulch or shredded bark placed under the bottom of the slide.
- Steps, braces and handrails are secure. Both the bed and the sides are free of slivers, screws, nails and rough spots.
- Wooden slides are frequently waxed or oiled with raw linseed oil to keep them smooth, not washed with soap and water.
- A platform with rails between the ladder and the slide allows for a safer transition between climbing and sliding.
- Railings along the ladder make climbing easier and prevent falling off to either side.
- There should be no structures on a slide that might entangle scarves, sashes or ropes.
- The incline near the bottom should decrease to slow the child down.

MONKEY BARS

- To be used only by children around 5 to 12 years old. Younger children should be provided with a simpler structure of interconnected bars.
- The surface underneath is soft and resilient to cushion falls.
- The bars do not rotate when grasped.
- Not placed next to equipment like slides that might encourage leaping from one to the other.

SEESAWS

- To be used only by youngsters under 12. Older children often attempt unsafe stunts.
- The fulcrum and other parts are enclosed or otherwise protected against catching fingers.
- Rubber tires sunk halfway into the ground beneath the seats cushion the impact of the seats striking the ground.
- No splinters.

If you are building or renovating a playground, we recommend getting a copy of the Handbook for Public Playground Safety, Volume I, from the U.S. Consumer Product Safety Commission, Washington, DC 20207.

PLAYGROUND SAFETY RULES

Even in our Ideal Playground, a child can be seriously injured if he doesn't use the equipment safely. Talk over these playground safety rules with your youngster and be sure he understands them.

SWINGS
- No kneeling or standing on the swings.
- Hold on tightly with both hands.
- Wait for the swing to come to a full stop before getting off. Never jump off.
- Don't twist the swings or swing empty seats.
- Don't hold anyone on your lap or ride double.
- Never climb the supports.
- Don't ever walk in front of a moving swing.

SEESAWS
- Hold on tightly with both hands, and sit facing each other.
- Keep your hands and feet out from under the board as it nears the ground.
- Don't stand or run on the board.
- Never bump the board on the ground.
- Warn the other person before getting off.
- To get off, hold the board tightly and let it rise gradually until the other child has her feet on the ground.

SLIDES
- Climb one step at a time, keeping a safe distance from the child in front of you.
- Only one person should slide down at a time. Slide sitting up with your feet in front of you. Don't hold onto the sides.
- Quickly move away from the bottom of the slide.
- Don't try to crawl or run up the slide or slide down backwards.
- Never go sliding in a wet bathing suit.

DRINKING FOUNTAINS
- Fooling around at the fountain can cause broken teeth.

WADING POOLS
- Never go wading if you're overheated, sick or have a skin infection.

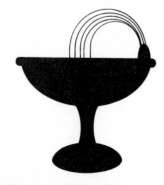
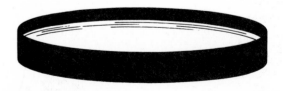

SANDBOXES

- For younger children only.
- Don't take food into the sandbox.
- No sharp or pointed playthings should be brought into the sand.

CLIMBING EQUIPMENT

- Don't try to use a ladder if you can't reach it by yourself.
- Climb in one direction only, either up or down.
- Don't put your head or feet between the rungs.
- Never climb when it is slippery or wet.
- Watch out for swinging feet.

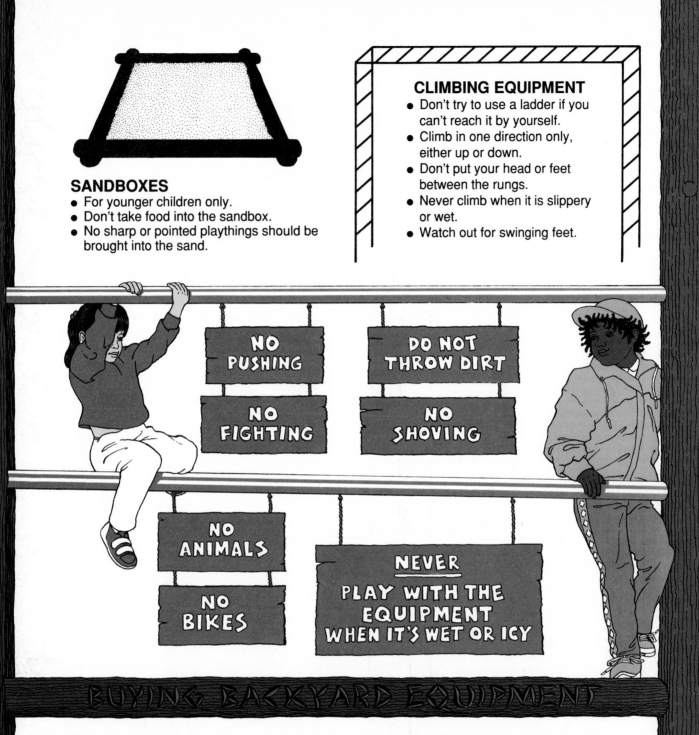

NO PUSHING

DO NOT THROW DIRT

NO FIGHTING

NO SHOVING

NO ANIMALS

NO BIKES

NEVER PLAY WITH THE EQUIPMENT WHEN IT'S WET OR ICY

BUYING BACKYARD EQUIPMENT

- Only buy equipment that matches your child's age, size and physical abilities.
- The more versatile the pieces, the better; children like variety.
- If the equipment doesn't come fully assembled, be sure there are clear, detailed instructions on how to set it up.
- Place the equipment at least 6 feet away from fences, walls and other obstructions.

- Install it over soft material, such as mulch or pine bark chips, never over concrete or other hard surfaces.
- Make sure the equipment is stable. It should come with anchoring devices to hold it firmly to the ground.
- Don't buy structures with sharp edges, rough surfaces or open-ended hooks.
- Check that all nuts, bolts and clamps are tight.

SPORTS

When a youngster outgrows the playground, she usually turns to sports to satisfy her need for excitement and challenging physical activity. Every sport has its own special hazards and benefits, but the principles of accident prevention are essentially the same for all of them:

- The playing area should be large enough to keep children from running into walls and other obstacles, with sufficient space around it to let other people pass by safely. Goal supports and other obstructions that can't be removed must be well padded to reduce injuries from accidental collisions. Playing surfaces should be smooth and even.
- The child should be provided with the equipment the game requires: body padding, cleated shoes and a helmet for tackle football; basketball sneakers for basketball, etc. If your youngster wears eyeglasses, make sure she has unbreakable lenses or eyeglass guards.
- The child should be in the proper physical condition and have practiced the basic skills the sport requires. When he is prepared for the demands of the game, he is less likely to suffer accidental injury and will also enjoy himself more. The greater the inherent risk of injury in a sport, the more time should be given to preparation. Remember that youngsters often attempt things beyond their strength and skill and that every athletic activity makes its own unique demands on coordination, stamina and judgment.

- Don't let your child play when she has a sore arm or leg, and encourage her to play different positions over the course of an afternoon, particularly if she likes to catch or pitch. Children's bones are soft and vulnerable and can be damaged by constant strain. For the same reason, never push a child beyond her capabilities or endurance.
- Competitive sports should always involve children of about the same age, size and physical skill. This will minimize the risk of injury and allow everyone to develop a sound attitude about competition by enjoying at least some success.
- Your child should have a good general awareness of sports safety as well as an understanding of the hazards of a particular activity. Before allowing him out on the playing field, make sure he appreciates the importance of placing the safety of all the players above everything else. Ask him to identify the potential dangers in a given sport and call his attention to any he may have overlooked.
- The chance of injury rises with the degree of contact in a sport — football produces many more injuries than basketball, track or soccer. Youngsters should never engage in boxing; it carries too high a risk of brain damage.

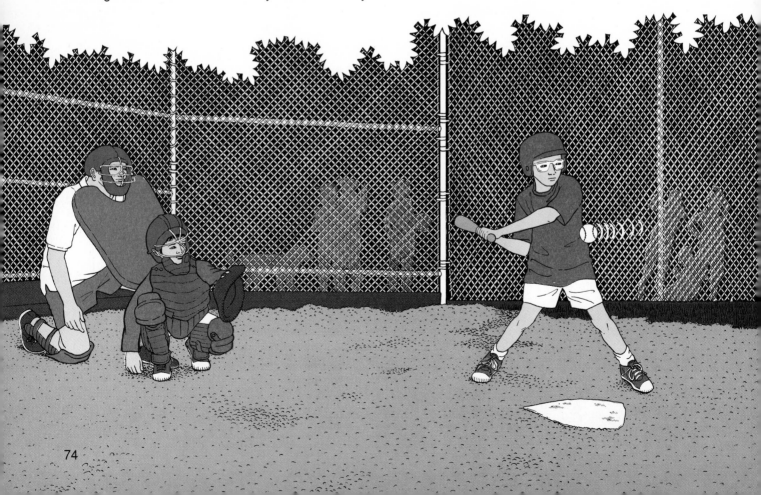

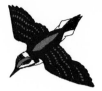

HIKING & CAMPING SAFETY

HIKING

Hiking is a simple, enjoyable recreation that provides excellent exercise and gets your youngster outdoors into the world of nature. The following precautions will keep her hiking experiences safe as well as pleasurable:

- The length and difficulty of the hike should always match the child's age and ability. Young or new hikers should start off with short walks along a road or clearly marked trail. Long hikes over unmarked, rough terrain are best left to older, more experienced children.

- Make sure your child has the necessary supervision or companionship. Solo hikes should be reserved for older children who have demonstrated their mastery of hiking skills. Until then it is best to have at least three people on an outing. The companionship adds to the fun, and in case of an accident someone can stay with the injured person while the third person goes for help. Check that your youngster knows the location of the nearest telephone and ranger station.

- All hikes should be planned and prepared for in advance. The longer the hike and the rougher the terrain, the more planning and preparation that are required. Guidebooks are a valuable resource. The hiker should be aware that there may be seasonal changes in trail conditions, like streams that are swollen in spring and become difficult to cross. Before leaving home she should find out if there are any routes that easily lead to help, in case she needs it. For even short outings, you should know where your child is going and when to expect her back. Be sure she understands never to set out on a hike without your knowledge and approval.

- See to it that your child is properly outfitted and has what he needs to protect himself from sun and insects and unexpected changes in weather. Clothing that can be layered is always the most useful.

He should have a comfortable pack that is the right size for him and can hold whatever he needs to take with him. On all but the shortest walks he should bring along a water-repellent jacket or poncho in case of rain, a wool jacket or sweater, and a handkerchief or bandanna. Brightly colored clothing will make him easily visible.

- Footwear should be appropriate to the length of the hike and the terrain to be traveled. Rubber and other flexible soles provide good footing in the woods, but leather soles are too slippery. Boots are essential for rough ground. Sneakers and other low-laced shoes are satisfactory for roads or improved trails.

- Shoes or boots should fit comfortably and already be broken in. Treat new boots with one of the various waterproofing products specifically designed to make them water repellent. To prevent blisters, check that the child's heels don't slip when she walks. Two pair of socks are preferable.

- A peaked cap will help keep the rain and sun out of your child's eyes. Sunglasses also add comfort and protection.

- Your youngster should bring with him all the food and drink he'll need. For a short outing, a canteen (not a glass jug) of water and a moderate amount of nourishing, not-too-perishable food should suffice.

Many different varieties of trail food are available, and it is a good idea to take some along in case the hike lasts longer than expected. Unless he is extremely knowledgeable about wood lore, he should **never** eat fruit, nuts, berries or other vegetation found along the way. They might well be poisonous.

- Even on a short hike, your child should always take along a first-aid kit to deal with cuts, scrapes and blisters, as well as more serious injuries. Check that the kit contains: gauze pads, elastic and adhesive bandages and sterile dressings, scissors, sunscreen, and moleskin to treat blisters. Photocopy the emergency treatment for **BLISTERS** on pages 178-180 and put it in his first-aid kit.

- He should also carry a compass and a map of the area and know how to use them. Emphasize that until he learns these skills he is never to hike alone or leave a marked path or road. A flashlight is helpful for reading road signs and avoiding bad footing when it gets dark. He should also have a knife, a whistle, waterproof matches, insect repellent, water purification tablets, a portable radio and a pocket mirror to use as a signaling device.

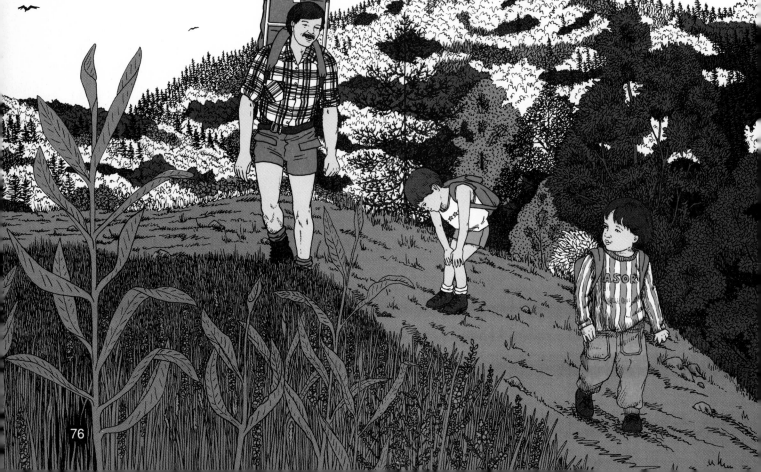

● Teach your youngster not to panic or wander about aimlessly if he gets lost but to stay where he is until help arrives. Explain that if he doesn't get back when expected, a search party will look for him along the route he originally projected. He should always carry a whistle among his emergency supplies and know the universal distress signal — three short blasts repeated frequently. The signal will help rescuers find him, even in the dark.

● Make sure she understands the dangers of lightning and never to seek shelter under a tall tree, especially if it stands alone in a clearing or is higher than the trees around it. If she is caught in the woods during a storm and can't find any other protection, the safest spot is under a group of young trees about the same height. In open countryside, she should look for a protected spot away from anything tall. She should never stay in or near water, and should try to avoid wet ground.

● Your youngster should never approach a strange dog or other animal he might encounter in the woods or along a country road. If a dog comes up to him, he should stand still with his hands at his sides, let the dog sniff him to get his scent, and speak to it in a calm, low voice. Sudden movements, yelling or running away will only increase the chance of an attack.

77

CAMPING

After gaining some experience in hiking, many children want to camp out overnight. Camping requires greater preparation, more elaborate equipment and specialized knowledge and skills. Initial trips should be made with parents or other adults or as part of organized youth activities. Before letting your child camp out, make sure she is in good physical condition and doesn't have a cold or other ailment that might be aggravated by sleeping outdoors. If she has any special medical problems, consult her doctor to see what safeguards are required. Here are some other basic precautions that will ensure her comfort and safety:

● Find out as much as you can in advance about the camping area. Talk with people who have camped there and get their suggestions and warnings. Obtain a detailed map of the area so your youngster can familiarize herself with such major features of the countryside as mountains, valleys, swamps, rivers and streams. The map will also help her choose the best route and campsites and steer her away from natural or man-made hazards. Superior inexpensive maps of the United States are available from the United States Geological Survey, Room 2650, U.S. Department of the Interior, 1849 C Street N.W., Washington, DC 20240. (Road maps are made for drivers and don't usually show the details a camper needs.)

● Work out a timetable with your child so you will know where he will be at various times and when he will return. Stress the importance of sticking to this schedule if he possibly can. He should also have an alternate plan in case the weather becomes unsuitable for camping.

● While your youngster shouldn't be overloaded with equipment, she should certainly take along everything she will need for her enjoyment and safety. This will vary according to the length of the outing, the character of the countryside and the weather likely to be encountered, but the basics include:

☐ Food and water.

☐ A change of clothes, a warm wool sweater, extra socks, a cap and a waterproof jacket or poncho. It's always safest to assume that it will be cold and damp at night and rainy during the day. Clothes that can be layered provide the greatest versatility.

☐ Sleeping and cooking equipment, including a tent or tarp, a warm, lightweight sleeping bag, an insulated pad or ground cloth, a canteen, eating and cooking utensils, a good folding saw and several waterproof containers of matches to be carried in different pockets.

☐ A first-aid kit, insect repellent, soap, a toothbrush and other toilet equipment, a pocketknife, a whistle, a compass and a map.

● A campsite should always be selected well before nightfall. Tell your child to look for a level spot out in the open, preferably not too far from good water and firewood. It should be somewhat higher than its surroundings so water will drain away if it rains. Teach your children about ecologically safe, low-impact camping and respect for our increasingly fragile environment.

● See to it your child knows how to build a campfire safely. The area 10 feet around the fire should be cleared of grass, brush and anything else that might accidentally ignite, and the fire should be no larger than necessary for cooking and warmth. If she builds it in a shallow pit she has dug in the ground, the wind won't scatter the embers. Tents should be set up a safe distance from the fire and one or two buckets of water kept nearby as a safety measure.

● Check that your youngster's tent is light in weight, easily assembled and fire retardant. No tent is truly fireproof, so he should never light a campfire or camp stove inside it. Nor should he use paraffin or kerosene to make it water repellent since this will make it more flammable. Show him how to use it properly and keep it in good repair. The fine netting provided to keep out mosquitoes and other insects will work well if it is kept tightly closed and free of holes.

● A camper shouldn't attempt to feed or play with any animals she may come across. In the woods, all animals are wild, and no matter how cute or friendly they seem they can inflict nasty bites and scratches. Large animals usually avoid humans, but raccoons, skunks, porcupines and the like may visit the camp, particularly if food or garbage is left in the open. If the camp is kept clean at all times, animals will have little reason to come around.

● Make sure your youngster can recognize poisonous snakes and knows to stay away from them. (See **POISONOUS SNAKE IDENTIFICATION,** pages 151-152.) Photocopy the emergency treatment for **SNAKEBITE** on pages 153-155 and put it in his first-aid kit.

WATER SAFETY

The principal danger from water is, of course, drowning, a tragic mishap that claims thousands of young lives each year. Many, perhaps all, of these children might have been saved if their parents had provided constant supervision and taught them how to stay out of harm's way. This chapter details the most common causes of childhood drownings and the recommended preventions. After reading it yourself, we suggest that you review it with your youngster, your baby-sitter and anyone else who shares responsibility for your children's safety.

AROUND THE HOME

Around the home, as everywhere else, the best protection against drowning is close adult supervision. NEVER leave a baby alone near water for even the briefest moment. She can drown in only a few seconds. If you're bathing your child and the telephone or doorbell rings, wrap her in a towel and bring her with you while you tend to it. If the phone rings while you are supervising at the pool, get all the kids out of the water before you leave to answer it. When your child becomes old enough not to need constant watching, continue to stay nearby, keeping an ear tuned to the sounds of her talk and play. Tragically, pool drownings often occur when several adults are present but everyone has assumed that someone else has his eyes on the kids. Always make sure there is a designated adult to watch the children.

Full bathtubs and wading pools are obvious hazards, but even an open toilet, diaper pail, ice chest or vaporizer can be dangerous. If there is enough water to cover an infant's or toddler's nose and mouth, there is enough to drown him. Your child may be attracted to the light shimmering on the surface, the sound of water running or by something floating on top. His curiosity aroused, he may tumble in headlong and not have the strength or coordination to pull himself out. To prevent this from ever happening, never draw water until you are ready to use it, never leave it within your child's reach, and discard it as soon as you are done with it.

Always keep the lids on diaper pails. Drain scrub buckets and store them away promptly. Empty bathtubs when they are not being used. And make it a habit to close the cover on all toilets.

Hot tubs and spas pose the danger of entrapment and overheating as well as drowning. Young children should not be allowed to use them unattended.

Outdoors, don't let your child play around cesspools, puddles and ditches without close supervision. Empty small wading pools after each use and turn them over or deflate them to keep rain water from collecting.

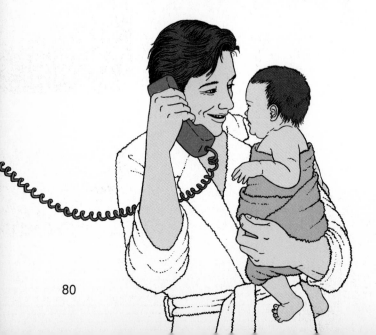

SWIMMING

One of the best protections against drowning is knowing how to swim. Good programs are offered by the Red Cross, the Boy and Girl Scouts, the "Y" and other community organizations. If your child does not know how to swim, he can still learn to float.

Most children are ready for swimming lessons around the age of four or five. Despite the popularity of swimming lessons for very young children, infants and toddlers do not have the coordination to swim and breathe at the same time. There is also the risk that they may swallow too much water, which can cause convulsions, infection and hypothermia. If you do decide to teach your toddler to swim, be aware of these dangers, and do not be lulled into a false sense of security that now she is able to take care of herself in the water.

Though swimming lessons are very important, they do not guarantee a child's safety. Fully 25% of children who drown have had swimming lessons. Parents should understand that their youngsters require constant supervision in and around water even if they know how to swim.

Even good swimmers under the age of 12 or so still need adult supervision. Infants, toddlers and young non-swimmers require it constantly. Don't let a lifeguard do all your watching for you, particularly in a crowded pool or on a large beach. Make sure you are not responsible for so many small children that you cannot keep track of all of them all the time. Never let a toddler run loose near a pool. Pool decks are often slippery, and she could easily fall in. It is best not to let a non-swimmer enter the water without you, and you should certainly always keep her within immediate reach.

Non-swimmers should not be allowed to use inflated tubes, rafts or water wings. They deflate very easily and build a false sense of confidence, allowing the child to drift into deep water. They also inhibit learning how to swim.

Know the water you are letting your child play in. Before entering the water with a non-swimmer, make certain it really is shallow enough for her to stand in comfortably, without unexpected sharp drop-offs or an irregular or slippery bottom. A non-swimmer should never go out over her head.

Swimming in cold water can be extremely dangerous. It's been estimated it is the cause of death in half of all drownings. Sudden immersion in cold water is especially perilous. Water only has to be colder than you are to be a potential danger.

Your child should know the rules for playing safely in the water by the time she is old enough to go off to a pool or beach without you. Make sure she learns and understands the following precautions:

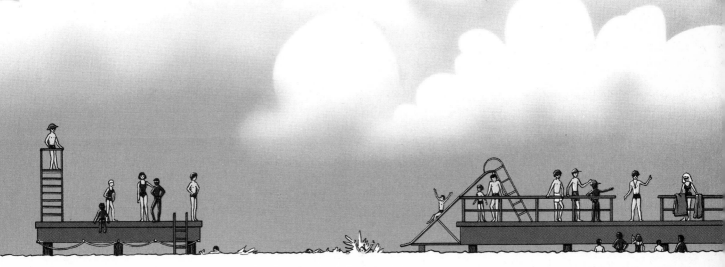

- Never go swimming alone. Always use the "buddy system."
- When swimming with a group, choose someone as lookout to oversee everyone's safety, even if a lifeguard is present.
- Swim only in protected areas. Obey the posted rules and the lifeguard's instructions. Never swim at a public beach if there isn't a lifeguard present.
- Don't swim near anchored boats, in boat lanes, or where people are water-skiing or actively engaged in other water sports.
- Before wading, swimming or diving in an unfamiliar place, find out the depth of the water and whether there are any strong currents, sudden drop-offs or

hidden rocks, branches or roots. Stay out of very cold or fast-moving water, and watch out for undertows.

● Never dive or jump into shallow, murky or unfamiliar water. Always go in feet first. Never dive from rocks or under buoys or boats.

● Check that diving boards and pool slides are sturdy and not slippery, and make sure the water underneath them isn't too shallow. Never run on diving boards or dive off the sides. Learn how to dive properly.

● Don't engage in horseplay, roughhousing or showing off. And never scream for help as a game or joke.

● Always pay attention to the weather. Stay out of the water if it's going to storm. Never swim or go near the water during an electrical storm.

● Know your limitations and never push yourself beyond them.

● Never swim when you are tired, overheated or chilled.

● Wait at least an hour after eating before you enter the water.

● Before swimming in the ocean, find out about changes in the tides and whether there is any danger of sharks or poisonous marine life. Remember that ocean swimming is more difficult and tiring than fresh-water swimming.

● Be careful about hyperventilating before swimming underwater. Excessive deep breathing can inactivate the body's warning signals that you need a fresh breath, and you may black out before you can surface.

● If you find yourself in trouble in deep water, try to stay calm and think out the best plan of action.

● Don't panic if you get entangled in underwater weeds. Move arms and legs gently to free yourself; thrashing around will only tangle you up worse.

● Use a sunscreen even on cloudy days.

● Wear shoes with treads if wading in rocky areas, and watch out for sea urchins and sharp coral.

● Home swimming pools need to be fenced on all four sides to keep youngsters from wandering in alone. The house should not be one of the sides, and there should be no direct access to the pool area from the house.

● Construct the fences at least 5 feet high. Use vertical posts with the supports on the pool side, so a child can't climb over easily and enter the pool area.

● Don't put anything near the fence that a child could use as a step to climb over.

● Access gates should swing shut automatically and be self-latching, with the latch well above a child's reach. Keep the gates locked when the pool isn't being used.

● Give your neighbors spare keys or the lock combination so they can get in quickly if you are away.

● Install an alarm on the pool gate and a pool alarm in the water.

● Install artificial lighting for emergencies and nighttime swimming. Use wiring approved by the Underwriters Laboratory (UL). Installation should be made by a competent electrician.

● No electrical equipment or appliances should be allowed near a pool.

● Make sure there is a non-slip surface around the edge of the pool.

● Remove the steps from an above-ground pool when it isn't being used.

● Tell your child never to dive in an above-ground pool.

3 FEET

POOL SAFETY

Most drownings around the home take place in larger backyard swimming pools, so the following precautions are particularly important:

● Keep the pool covered during the months it isn't in use. Rigid covers are preferable to flexible models because they won't collect rain. Translucent solar pool covers, which float on top of the water and are not attached to the pool sides, present a special hazard. This sort of cover appears solid to a child, and she may venture out on it, then slip under the edge, where she will be hidden from rescuers.

● Make sure your pool slides and diving boards are well-constructed and kept in good shape. Pool ladders and stairs should be equipped with handrails on both sides.

● Keep all riding equipment and toys with wheels away from the pool area.

● Use plastic glasses or cans instead of glass bottles or glasses.

● Teach your child never to play in any pool away from home without your knowledge and approval. Many childhood drownings occur in the pools of neighbors.

● If there is a pond near your home, make sure the safe swimming areas are marked off and the danger points indicated with warning signs. The pond should be equipped with the same rescue devices shown below for pools.

It's a good idea for pool owners, as well as anyone else responsible for supervising children in and around water, to be certified in cardiopulmonary resuscitation (CPR).

Post the location of the nearest telephone, the numbers to call in an emergency (the local rescue or emergency squad, ambulance, doctor) and instructions for water rescue, drowning first aid and artificial respiration. Photocopy pages 384, 256-258, 259-260 and 201-215, and hang them inside a shed or keep them in a waterproof can at poolside.

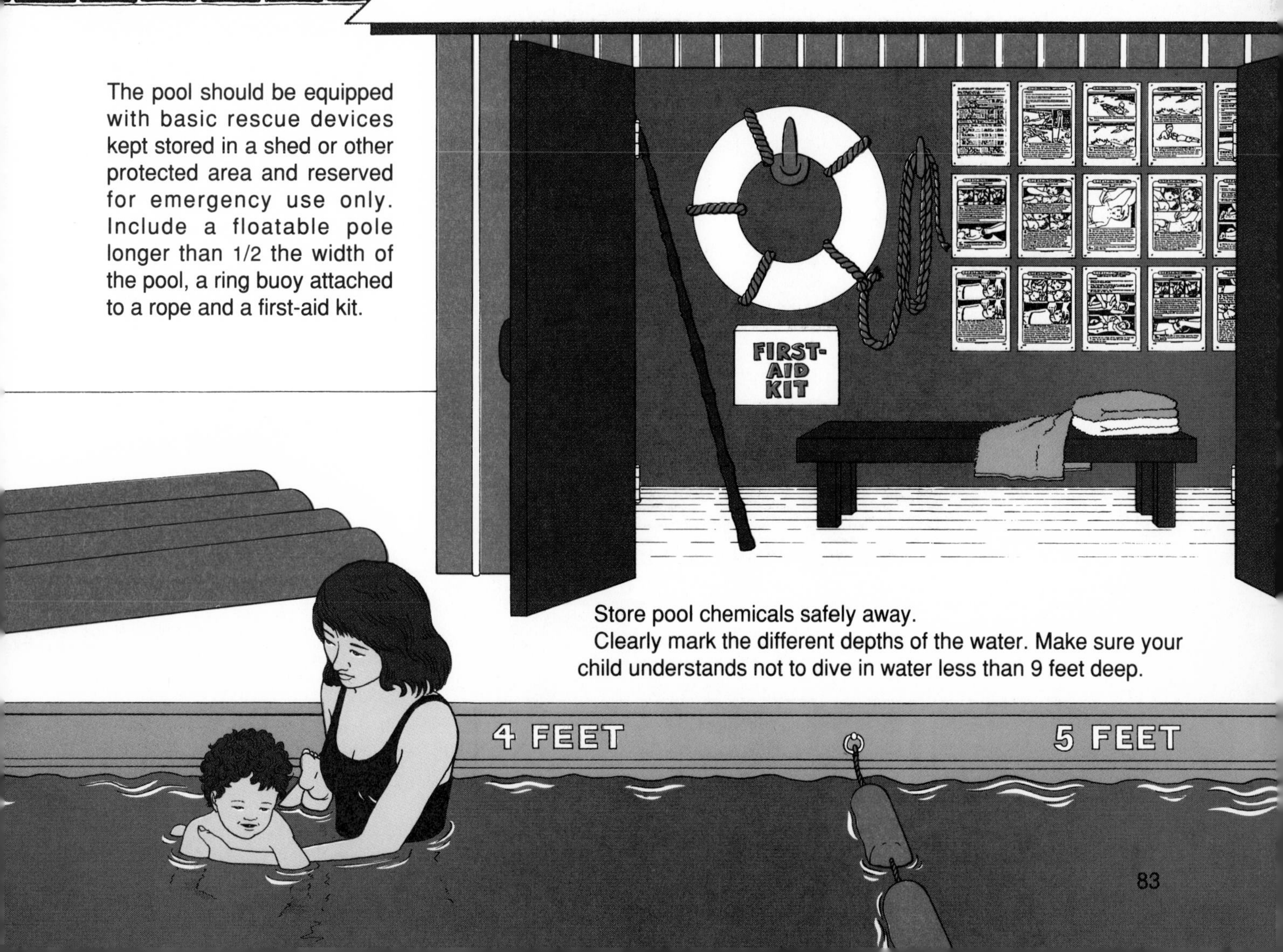

The pool should be equipped with basic rescue devices kept stored in a shed or other protected area and reserved for emergency use only. Include a floatable pole longer than 1/2 the width of the pool, a ring buoy attached to a rope and a first-aid kit.

FIRST-AID KIT

Store pool chemicals safely away.
Clearly mark the different depths of the water. Make sure your child understands not to dive in water less than 9 feet deep.

4 FEET

5 FEET

BOATING

Particularly for younger children, the boating environment is filled with hazards — poisons, gas cans, sharp objects, low doorways and ceilings, stairways, ropes, holes, protrusions, etc. Always check it out carefully and watch your child closely to keep him out of trouble.

Know where poisonous substances are kept and make sure they are securely closed and placed where your child can't get to them. Sharp objects should be stored out of a youngster's reach and ropes kept where he can't get tangled up in them. Keep him away from stairways and places where he might trip or fall or bump into protruding objects. Stairways should always be closed off when not in use. Continue to supervise your child carefully when you take her out on a boat, and be sure you are prepared for any emergency.

There should be Coast Guard approved personal floatation devices (PFDs) for everyone on board, and everyone, adults and children alike, should wear them constantly even if they are expert swimmers. In case of an emergency, the PFDs, or life jackets, will keep you afloat until help arrives and help protect you from cold water. Floats, tubes or rafts are no substitutes for PFDs. Obviously, for the PFD to do its job it has to be taken care of so it remains in good operating condition.

Several types of PFDs are on the market, and what kind to get is determined by the type and size of the boat, where you will be boating, and the sizes of the people on board.

Your child's PFD should fit her snugly enough to keep her from slipping out. Have her practice wearing it in the water so she can learn how it feels and works and acquire some confidence that it will help keep her afloat in an emergency. Children are more likely than adults to float facedown, so they should practice floating faceup while wearing their PFDs.

Make sure that for every child who doesn't swim there is an expert swimmer who will keep an eye on her. Take a first-aid kit with you as well as rescue lines and life preservers. Check that you have bailing cans. A motorboat should be equipped with a fire extinguisher.

Before a child takes out a boat himself, he must be a skilled swimmer and understand all the above precautions. It's equally important that he knows the following basics of safe boating:

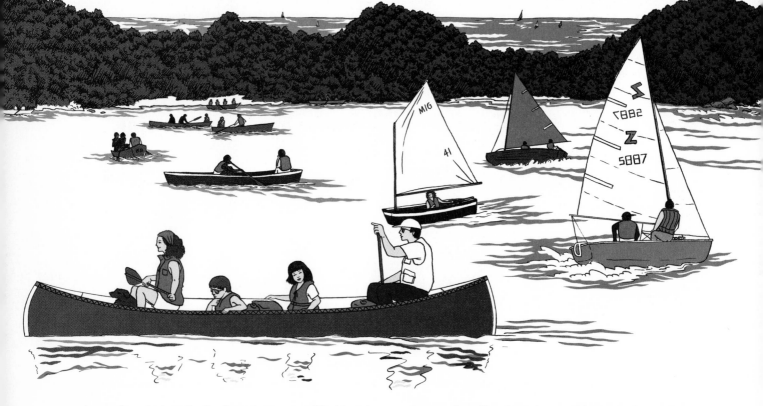

- Learn how to handle the boat from a qualified teacher. Before taking it out in deep water, put in the necessary hours practicing near shore. Know how to right a capsized canoe and climb back into it and how to handle a boat in a sudden squall or storm.
- Be sure the boat is in good repair and properly equipped, especially with PFDs for everyone on board.

- Know the water you are boating in.
- Never overload a boat. Know its correct capacity. Distribute the weight evenly and keep it low.
- Never smoke around fuel. Closed-in fueling areas must be ventilated before a motorboat is started, and all fuel spills wiped up promptly.
- If the boat should capsize or be incapacitated, stay with it until help arrives unless you are certain you can swim to shore and no one is around to help you.
- Know how to conduct yourself safely on board. Never engage in showing off or horseplay. Be careful around slippery decks. Don't stand upright in a canoe or rowboat. A younger child should always sit toward the middle of a rowboat or motorboat, never in the bow where any sudden movement could knock her into the water.
- Know about right-of-way rules, channel markings, anchorages, the correct use of lights and the relevant boating laws.
- Never go out if there is a chance of a storm. Check the weather forecasts in advance.
- Have a plan of travel and leave this information with someone on shore.
- Don't drink alcoholic beverages and boat.
- Be aware of "boater's hypnosis": exposure to sun, glare, wind, noise and constant vibration can slow down reaction time.
- Protective coverings, called propguards, should be installed over exposed motor blades.

WATER-SKIING, SURFING, SNORKELING AND SCUBA DIVING

These water sports involve many of the same dangers as swimming and boating as well as their own special hazards. Before letting your child take part in them, make sure she understands these fundamentals:

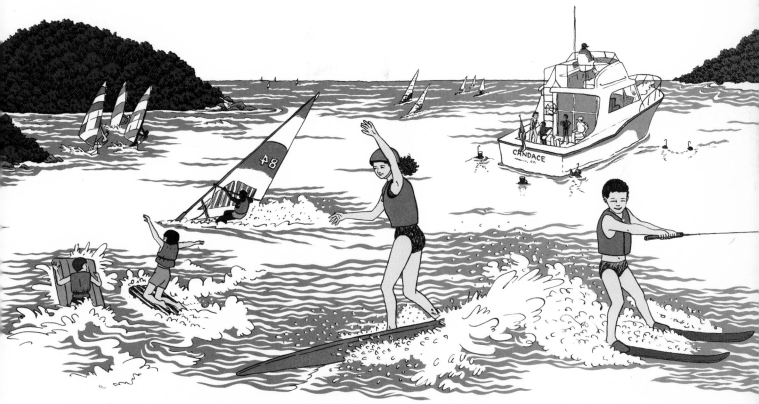

- Know how to swim expertly and be in good physical condition. Don't scuba dive if you have a respiratory ailment.
- Learn the basics of the sport from a qualified teacher. Build up your skills gradually without trying to do too much at once. As with swimming, know your limitations and don't push yourself beyond them.
- Never use restricted areas. Keep away from swimmers and stay conscious of other water-skiers, surfers and divers.
- Make sure your equipment is in good shape.
- When water-skiing, wear a PFD and have a third person along to keep watch and pass your signals to the driver.
- Don't go out in bad weather or rough water.

FISHING

Fishing is much more reposeful than surfing or water-skiing, but it is not without its potential dangers. Your child should pay attention to the following precautions:

- Carry your fishing rod disassembled if possible. Keep hooks and plugs secured to a hook keeper on the rod, or cover the barbs with cork.
- Never wade into a stream, lake or pond by yourself. There may be underwater shelves, holes or other sudden drops into deep water. Test each step in advance, keeping most of your weight on the foot that is already grounded. Be on the alert for stumps, roots and other tripping hazards.

- Maintain plenty of distance between yourself and other people fishing.
- Never fish where people are swimming.
- When baiting a hook, keep a firm grip on the bait. Hold the fish securely when you remove the hook.
- Know what to do if a fishhook becomes impaled. Photocopy pages 169-170 and carry them in your tackle box along with the necessary first-aid supplies.

SURVIVAL TECHNIQUES

Even an experienced swimmer may sometimes find herself in danger and should know how to cope with it beforehand. The following survival techniques can help your child through many emergencies. Talk them over with her and practice them together in a pool until she has them mastered. Knowing in advance what to do will build up her confidence and decrease the chance of panic. Her survival could be affected by her ability to remain calm and bring herself to safety quickly.

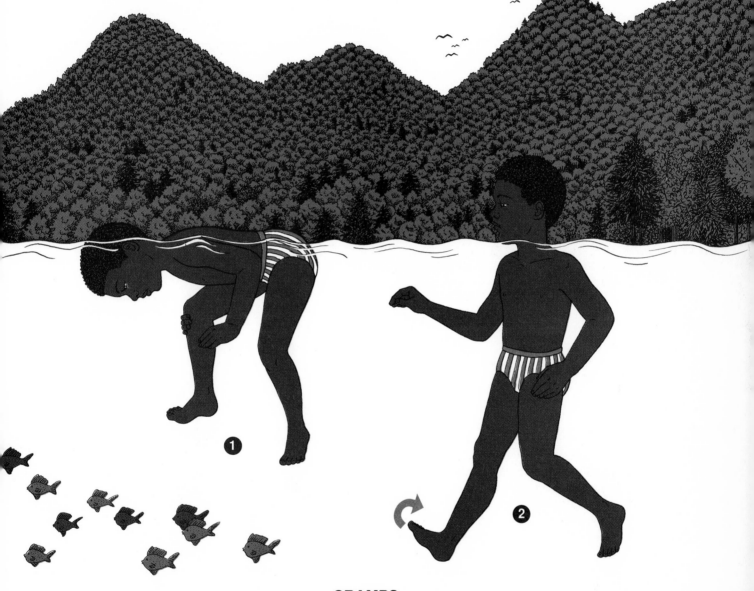

CRAMPS

Every swimmer occasionally experiences a cramp, a painful muscle contraction that greatly impedes the body's movement. Make sure your child understands that a cramp need not be serious if he keeps calm and takes proper action. ❶ When he feels his muscle tighten, he should take a deep breath, roll to a facedown position in the water, and grasp the cramped area firmly with one or both hands. Continued firm pressure will release the cramp. ❷ He can also ease a leg cramp by straightening his leg and forcing his toes upward toward the knee. Cramps are most likely to occur when muscles are tired and the water is particularly cold, good reasons for taking relatively short swims at the start of the summer.

DROWNPROOFING

Should your child ever get caught far from shore or a boat, the following technique will help keep him afloat and conserve his energy until help arrives:

1 Take a breath through your mouth and allow yourself to sink below the surface. Hang there loosely with your arms, legs and head relaxed. The air in your lungs will bring you effortlessly back to the surface.

2 When your head is partly out of water, stretch out your arms and at the same time move one leg forward and the other back, as in a scissors kick.

3 To take a fresh breath, gently pull your arms downward toward your hips and bring your legs together, pressing against the water with your soles and heels. As soon as your arms start downward (not before), begin to exhale through your nose and continue exhaling until your nose rises above the surface. Be sure to keep your eyes open. Then inhale through

your mouth. Your chin should be right on the water, not above it.

4 Just as your head goes under again, give a slight downward push with your arms or legs or with both of them together. This will keep you from sinking too deeply.

5 Rest underwater completely relaxed. Stay under until you would **like** a fresh breath, not until you absolutely **must have** one.

Drownproofing should not be used in cold water unless it is absolutely necessary; you will conserve more life-sustaining body heat by keeping your head above water and staying still. If your child becomes chilled, she should assume the Heat Escape Lessening Position (H.E.L.P.); see **COLD WATER,** page 90.

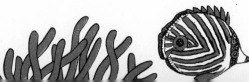

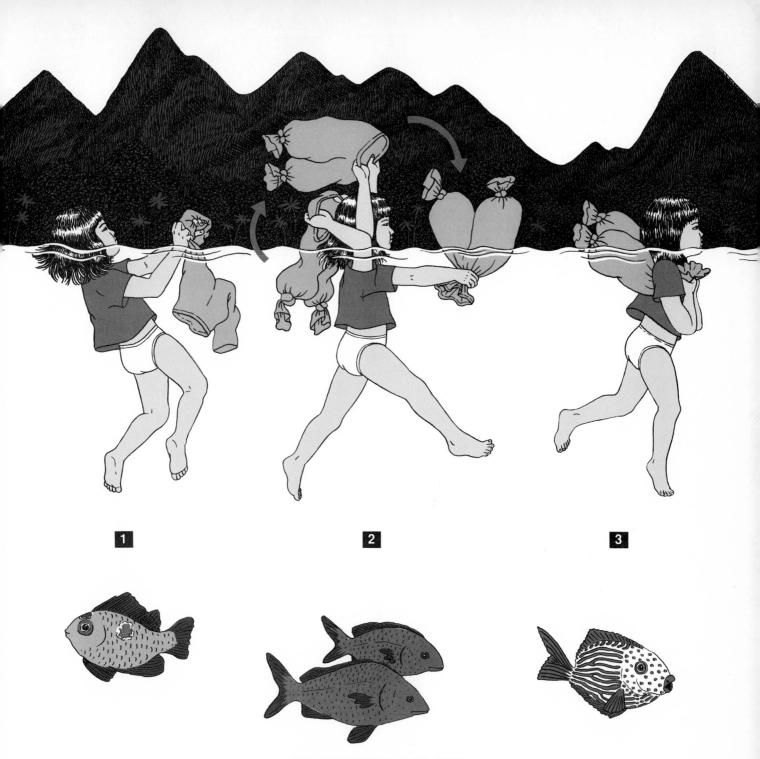

1   **2**   **3**

IMPROVISING A FLOAT

Show your youngster how she can use such clothing as her trousers or shirt to help stay afloat in an emergency. Air forced into wet clothing will form a buoyant air pocket that will last as long as it is kept submerged.

To inflate a shirt or jacket, button it to the neck, hold the lower front out and away from your body with one hand, then cup your other hand and drive it down into the water, letting the air trapped in your palm escape out of the water and into the garment.

Repeat the process until an air pocket forms, and replenish the air as it gradually leaks out.

Trousers work even better because they can hold more air. To inflate a pair of pants: **1** Take them off, close the zipper, and knot each leg at the cuff. **2** As you tread water, hold the pants at the waist, swing the legs behind your head, then quickly whip the waist down into the water, trapping the air in the legs. **3** Take a relaxed floating position and use small underwater strokes.

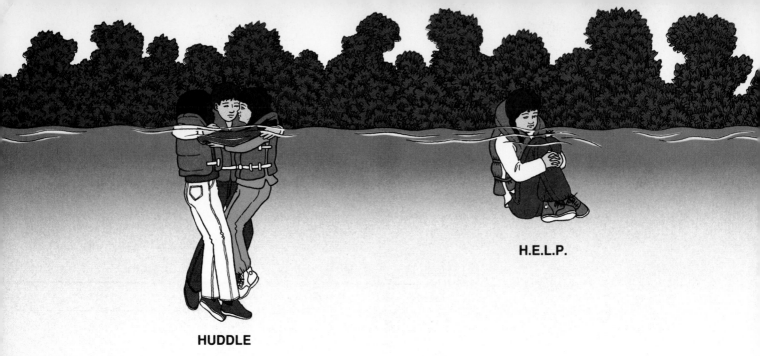

HUDDLE

H.E.L.P.

COLD WATER

Should your child fall into cold water it is essential that she knows how to minimize the loss of body heat. She should not remove her clothing. Obviously, she should try to get out of the water as quickly as possible, but unless she is in danger of drowning, she should not try to swim a long distance, since the energy this requires will lower her body temperature even further. If other people are in the water with her, as in the case of a capsized boat or falling through ice, huddling together will help keep everyone warmer. If she is alone, she should assume the Heat Escape Lessening Position (H.E.L.P.) until help arrives: Hold your knees to your chest, wrap your arms around your legs and clasp your hands together.

Immersion in cold water for even a few minutes can result in hypothermia, a life-threatening emergency caused by the lowering of the core temperature of the body. See **HYPOTHERMIA (COLD EXPOSURE),** pages 332-335.

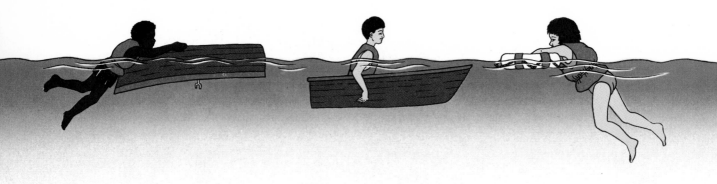

CAPSIZED BOATS

Teach your child to stay near a boat that has capsized or flooded. Even when submerged a few inches under the surface, it will probably continue to float because of its natural buoyancy or the air trapped inside. A youngster can conserve his strength until help arrives by clinging to the bottom of an overturned boat, and by kicking with his feet as he holds on, he may be able to propel himself back to safety. It is also possible to sit in a boat that has filled with water and paddle with your hands. Your PFD will keep you afloat, but floating objects from the capsized boat — a thermos jug, oar, life preserver, etc. — may offer extra support. You can gain additional flotation as you hold on by keeping only your nose above water.

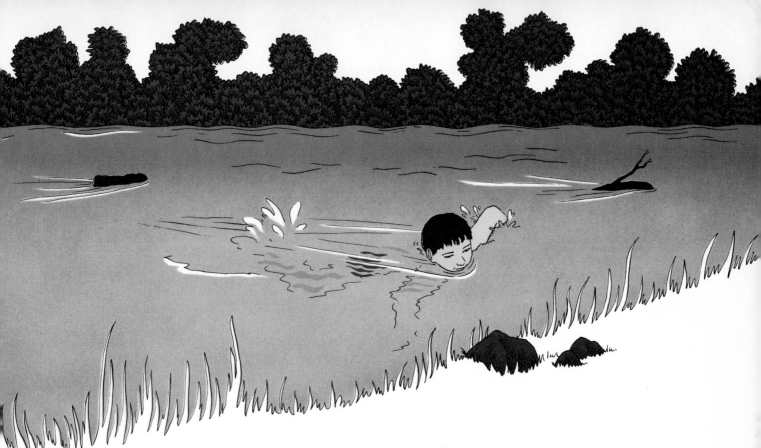

STRONG CURRENTS

A river current can be exceedingly strong and may easily carry a young swimmer away from land. Make sure your child knows that if he is caught in a strong current he will probably exhaust himself if he tries to fight it. Instead, he should swim diagonally across the current with its flow, even though he may come to land some distance away. Most river currents make their way closer to shore eventually.

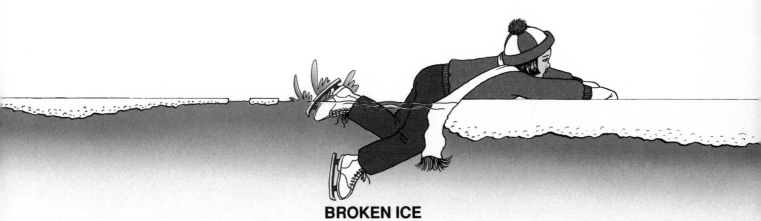

BROKEN ICE

Should your youngster ever break through the ice while skating or playing on the frozen surface, she shouldn't try to climb out immediately. If the ice is thin or weakened, her efforts will only break more of the ice and subject her to repeated dunkings. Rather, she should kick her feet to the surface and to the rear to avoid going under the ice, extend her hands and arms in front of her onto the unbroken ice and slide forward onto the solid surface. If the ice breaks again, then continue to slide forward until the ice is firm enough to give the needed support. To distribute her weight over the widest possible area, she should remain prone as long as the ice is still thin and inch herself along in that position, rather than stand upright and put her full weight on one small area. Anyone who has fallen through ice or into icy water should be seen by a physician for treatment for possible hypothermia.

HELPING SOMEONE IN TROUBLE

Besides knowing how to save himself from drowning, your child should also know how to rescue someone else without jeopardizing his own safety. Unless he is fully trained in lifesaving techniques, he should never try to swim to the aid of a drowning person. Instead, he should use the following methods of assistance, which are also treated on pages 256-258. For helping someone who has fallen through broken ice, see **ICE RESCUE,** pages 336-337.

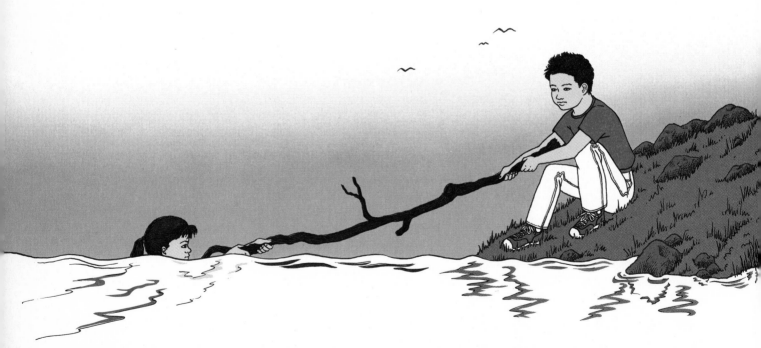

Near shore, use a reaching assist. Drop to the ground, extend your head and chest over the water and reach out a hand to the person in trouble. If you can't reach him without losing your own balance, reverse the position and extend your legs while holding onto a branch or other firm handhold.

If the person is just out of body reach, look around for something else to reach her with — a stick, fishing pole, rope, etc. A shirt or coat held by the sleeve may be long enough to pull her to safety. Even if the person is underwater, as long as she is still conscious, she will instinctively grasp anything thrust into her hands or pushed against her chest.

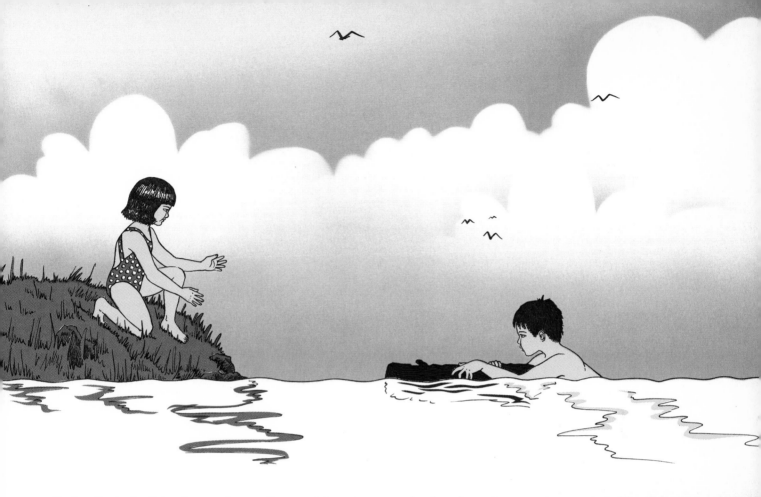

Find a float. Anything buoyant — a thermos, board, log, buoy, oar, boat, etc. — that can be gotten within reach of a drowning person can provide at least momentary relief while you seek further help.

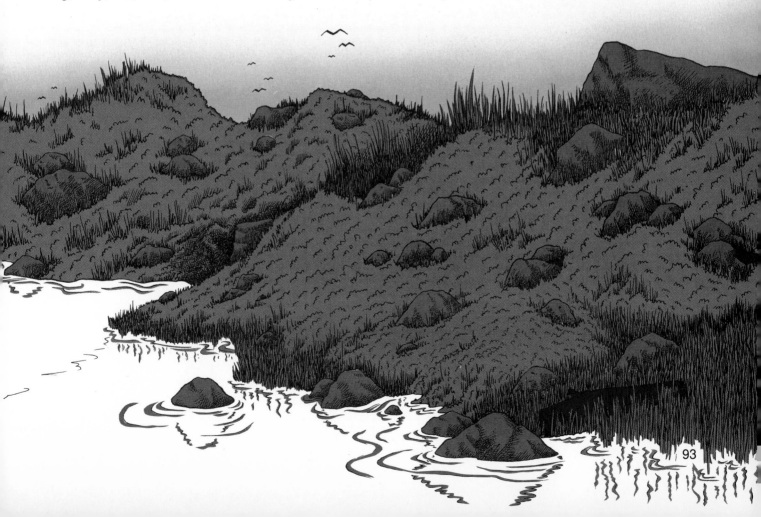

CHILD ABUSE

Child abuse has become a matter of increasing public concern. Approximately 600,000 cases are reported every year in the United States, and the large number of unreported cases brings the total even higher, to as many as four million, according to some estimates.

The abuse of children takes many different forms, ranging from overt physical, emotional or sexual mistreatment to physical neglect and emotional deprivation. Child abusers come from every segment of society, cutting across all social, economic, racial, ethnic and religious boundaries. In the vast majority of cases they are a close relative, most often a parent.

Many abusive parents genuinely love their children, do not deliberately intend to harm them and are filled with remorse about the hurt they have inflicted. Their behavior is commonly caused by misdirected anger or an inappropriate response to stressful situations beyond their immediate control—health problems, money pressures, unhappy working situations, marital difficulties, unsatisfactory living arrangements. They are often emotionally needy people without a network of family and friends to help them cope, and have failed to acquire the basic childrearing information and skills. Frequently they were abused themselves as children and are replaying a pattern of behavior learned from their own parents.

In some cases, the child singled out for abuse reminds his parents of their old childhood selves or someone else they dislike. In other cases, the child was unwanted or was expected to compensate for some deficiency in their lives or is perceived as "different" because of some physical or behavioral characteristic that makes him difficult to care for. Abusive parents also tend to have unrealistically high expectations about their children, and respond to their "bad" behavior by "disciplining" them through physical or emotional punishment, the only sort of discipline they know.

EMOTIONAL ABUSE

Though emotional mistreatment is less obviously injurious than physical abuse, it can be just as damaging. Constantly criticizing or belittling a child, withholding affection and approval, treating him as inferior to the other youngsters in the family, being indifferent to his problems, concerns and fears—all these things undermine his basic human need to feel safe and loved and competent and worthwhile. The result can be devastating. Recent research indicates that emotionally abused children tend to develop physically at a slower rate than other youngsters their age, and have a higher incidence of speech problems, ulcers, asthma and severe allergies. Psychologically, they are often beset with habit disorders like sucking and rocking, and neurotic traits like sleep disorders and a diminished capacity to engage in normal play.

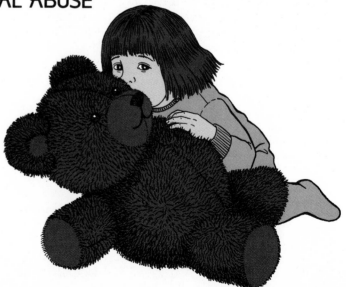

Behaviorally, they may become unpleasant and may be hard to get along with, overly aggressive and frequently in trouble. Or at the other extreme, they may turn out unusually shy and withdrawn, too anxious to please and much too submissive, tolerating hostility from their peers without protest.

Parents who abuse their children emotionally with an ongoing barrage of unkind words and reactions need to take a good look at their own behavior and ask themselves how they would feel if subjected to the same sort of demeaning treatment. They should seriously consider whether their anger is directed at the appropriate source or if the child is serving as a scapegoat for other problems that, once identified, might be corrected. It would probably benefit everyone in the family if parents sought out professional help from a therapist or counselor, or at least found someone to talk to—a teacher, a doctor, a minister or trusted friend—who might be able to offer a better perspective on how to interact with their child and perhaps give them some sound advice about how to break this destructive pattern of abuse before it is too late to avoid permanent harm.

PHYSICAL ABUSE

The most blatant indications of physical abuse are recurrent physical injuries: bruises (in various stages of healing), welts, burns, human bite marks, fractures, lacerations and abrasions. When pressed for an explanation, the child is likely to say they are the result of an "accident," but the injuries tend to be located in parts of the body not commonly affected by normal childhood activities (the back, thighs, buttocks, genital area, etc.) and the account doesn't usually jibe with the nature and seriousness of what happened.

Since the injuries are often not readily visible and the child does his best to conceal them, going so far as to wear long-sleeved, heavy clothing in hot weather to keep his body covered, the physical evidence that he is being abused may not always be that apparent. But the mistreatment he has suffered is also manifested on an emotional and behavioral level. Typically, the physically abused youngster has an unkempt appearance, loses or gains weight suddenly, has nightmares and other sleeping problems, and is subject to irrational fears and psychosomatic illnesses. If he doesn't cling unreasonably to his parents, he is deeply afraid of them and filled with dread about what might happen when they find out about some relatively minor mistake or infraction. Some abused children carry this fear over to other adults, finding it difficult to trust or relate to anyone. Others seek affection from any grownup likely to offer it and are overly eager to please and excessively submissive.

Most physically abused children have trouble with personal relationships and have very few friends. Some are verbally and physically aggressive with other youngsters, provoking their dislike and anger with bragging, criticism and other alienating behavior. At the other extreme, some are too withdrawn and depressed or too demanding of loyalty and affection to make meaningful contact with their schoolmates. Similarly, the victim of physical abuse may be chronically late or absent from school and do poorly in his studies, or he may come to school much too early and hang around long after classes have ended to avoid being home.

The physical abuse of children is considered a crime in all fifty states, and teachers, physicians and other professionals who work with children are required by law to report suspected cases to the proper authority. Every state has at least one statewide agency to receive and investigate instances of child abuse and neglect, usually called the Department of Social Services or Department of Children and Family Services. The telephone number of the local office can be found in the emergency listings in the front of your telephone book.

The primary purpose of the child protection agency is to make sure the abused child receives the necessary medical treatment and is guarded against further harm. In extreme cases, where the youngster's life or health is seen to be in immediate danger, the agency may have the child removed from the home and placed in temporary foster care, but whenever possible, it tries to keep the family together. To ensure the child's future safety, the agency will recommend a program of therapy intended to strengthen the family's positive aspects, heal the harm that has been done, and help abusive parents change their destructive pattern of behavior by teaching them how to cope with stress and face their problems maturely instead of taking out their frustrations on their children.

Since the protection of children is everyone's responsibility, relatives, neighbors and friends also have a moral obligation to make their suspicions of child abuse known. Understandably, you may be extremely reluctant to intervene in another family's "private business," especially if you are not absolutely certain that physical abuse has taken place. But keep in mind that you may be saving a young life.

Abusive parents and parents who fear they may be headed in that direction can reach out for help from a variety of sources. Many communities have child abuse hotlines, cross referral services and mental

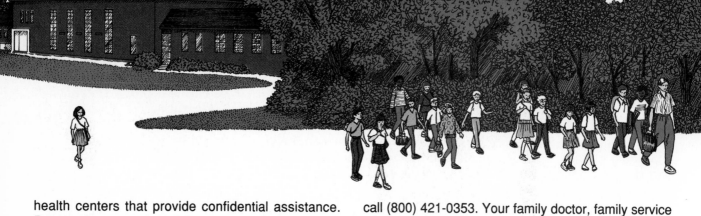

health centers that provide confidential assistance. Parents Anonymous, a national organization of recovering abusive parents, offers valuable mutual support and counseling. To find out the most convenient location of the more than one thousand local chapters, call (800) 421-0353. Your family doctor, family service agency or local health clinic may also be able to guide you toward the best sort of help for your particular situation.

SEXUAL ABUSE

Child sexual abuse has been defined as any sexual contact between a child and an adult or older child perpetrated for the sexual gratification of the older person. It can range from nonphysical contact like harassment, exhibitionism and voyeurism to direct contact offenses like fondling, oral sex and sexual intercourse, and includes victimizing a child through pornography and prostitution. Sometimes the abuse is accompanied by violence, as in the case of rape, but even when it isn't, some kind of force is always involved. Frequently it takes the more subtle psychological forms of bribery, exploiting the child's dependence and lack of knowledge, and threats of physical harm or the withdrawal of love. The abuse may occur as a single incident, but most often it involves a gradual increase of inappropriate behavior, and once it has begun, it may continue for a period of months or even years.

The incidence of sexual abuse is hard to establish because so many cases go unreported, but the increased attention the problem has received in recent years has led to a much fuller disclosure than in the past, when it was often kept secret. Many researchers now conclude that it may be even more common than physical abuse and more pervasive than AIDS. According to some estimates, as many as one in four girls and one in seven boys have been sexually abused before the age of eighteen. Though the old belief persists that the sexual molester is usually a depraved stranger, current studies indicate that 85 percent to 95 percent of the time the abuser is someone the child knows and trusts, usually a relative, often a parent. Some are women; most are men. In a large percentage of cases, molesters were sexually abused themselves as children.

The physical effects of sexual abuse can be extremely serious, and may include physical injury, pregnancy, venereal disease and AIDS. But the psychological effects can be just as destructive, causing long-term personality problems that may follow the child into his adult life. Sexually molested children feel betrayed by the people who molested them, and the closer the relationship, the deeper the sense of betrayal will be and the harder they find it to give anyone their trust. They often come to believe they have lost control over their lives, and when they don't feel chronically victimized, may mistakenly carry a sense of guilt for causing the abuse or not objecting strongly enough when it started. For the wounds to heal before permanent damage has been done, it is essential that the caring parent recognize when sexual molestation has taken place, allow the child to talk about it to vent his feelings, and obtain the appropriate help to ensure a complete recovery. Obviously, it is also important to take the necessary preventive measures beforehand to keep such abuse from ever happening.

The signs of sexual abuse are not always easy to detect. Sexually abused children are often too frightened, ashamed and confused to tell their parents what happened. Or they may volunteer information in such a fragmentary, roundabout way the parents fail to understand what is really being said. Nor do all forms of sexual abuse leave physical traces. Still, in an estimated 30 to 40 percent of cases there will be some form of physical evidence, such as torn or stained underwear; vaginal or rectal bleeding; itching, swelling or redness in the genitals, rectum or mouth; and urinary difficulties and infections. Though most of these symptoms can be caused by other problems, their presence in your child indicates a real possibility that sexual abuse has taken place.

You should also be on the alert for sudden changes in your child's behavior. Extreme mood swings, depression, loss of appetite, sleeping disorders, aggressive or regressive behavior and problems at school are all very generalized responses to stress and may indicate other difficulties, but they are also common reactions to sexual molestation. Other behavioral changes may be more specifically related to what the child has undergone. Sexually abused children sometimes develop a sudden dislike for a particular person or a fear of certain places such as showers or washrooms. They may become overly self-conscious about their genitals, or at the other extreme, unusually interested in sexual matters, playing out sexual acts with toys, pets and other people or exhibiting a newfound sexual sophistication beyond their years.

If you discover your child has been sexually abused, do not deny the problem. Believe what your youngster tells you. Children almost never lie about such matters, and what they need most at this difficult moment is the total support of a parent who doesn't question their truthfulness. Try to remain calm and control your sense of outrage. Outbursts of anger will further frighten the already frightened child and only make things worse. Take the child to a private place so she can discuss the incident without being embarrassed by the presence of other people. Ask her to tell you what happened in her own words, allowing her to express her feelings without pressing her for more details, particularly if she is upset. Let her know that she did the right thing by telling you and that you regret what happened and will protect her from further harm. And don't criticize or rebuke her for any errors in judgment that may have allowed the abuse to take place. Make sure she understands that the full responsibility rests with the abuser and that you still love and respect her as much as ever. Be physically affectionate with her and comfort her with words and gestures.

After you have spoken with your child and established the basic facts, you will need to contact your local child protection services agency and notify the police. Prepare your child for the meetings that follow by letting her know she will be questioned about what happened, and reassure her that you will remain with her as much as possible. Police and caseworkers dealing with child abuse vary greatly in their skill and sensitivity, and you may have to advocate strongly on her behalf. Even if she shows no signs of physical injury, she should have a medical examination to protect her against venereal disease and gather possible evidence. Rather than go to a hospital emergency room, where the atmosphere can be threatening and there is a risk of being treated by inexperienced personnel, take her to a family doctor who has been trained in treating victims of sexual molestation. Call your local child protection services agency or the local branch of the American Academy of Pediatrics or American Medical Association for specific recommendations. Since sexual abuse is one of the most traumatic things that can happen to a child, ongoing counseling or therapy is strongly recommended. Again, look for someone who is trained in the area and has had significant experience working with youngsters.

Though all these steps are necessary, they can be extremely disruptive, and you should do everything you can to maintain a calm environment at home and make your child's life as normal as possible. Give her the special protection she needs, but don't let her feel isolated or "different." Children are wonderfully resilient, and with time, love and the proper attention, this too shall pass.

There is no completely foolproof way to protect your child against sexual abuse, but there are a number of things you can do to minimize the possibility. One of the most important is to establish good communication with your youngsters. Talk to them. Listen to them. Encourage them to express their concerns and problems. Ask them about their daily activities: where they go, what they do and whom they spend their time with. Make your home a place of love, trust

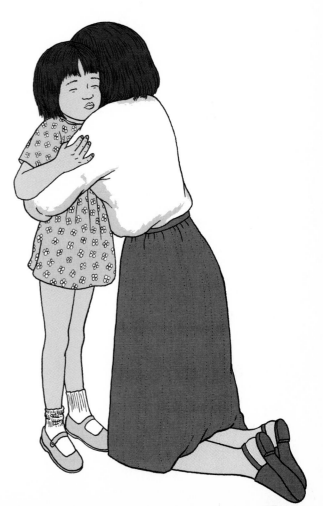

and support, so they won't be vulnerable to someone ready to exploit their need for affection.

Experts agree that it is also important to teach your children about sex at an early age so they will feel free to come to you with their questions and fears. You should also talk to them about sexual abuse in a low-keyed, matter of fact way that doesn't frighten them, imparting the basic information that will help keep them safe from harm. Children need to know that their body belongs to them and they have the right to keep it private when they are dressing, bathing and sleeping. They need to know they have the right to decide who touches them and how. And that if anyone touches them without permission or in a way that makes them feel uncomfortable or "funny," they have a right to tell him to stop, even if he is a member of the family or someone in a position of authority. They need to know that nobody has the right to ask them to keep any behavior that makes them uncomfortable "secret," and that they will never get in trouble for telling you what happened.

Contrary to popular opinion, only a very small percentage of sexual abuse is perpetrated by strangers, but since this does happen sometimes, you should also teach your child the proper precautions. Explain to him that a stranger is anyone he doesn't know and though not all strangers are bad, some of them are, so he should never become involved with one in any way. Teach him to be suspicious of any stranger who asks him for help or tries to engage him in conversation, and never to accept the offer of a ride or gift. And make sure a young child understands that he should avoid going into public restrooms, public swimming pools, playgrounds and parks when he is by himself.

You can further protect your children by carefully screening child care centers, baby-sitters and anyone else who takes care of them while you're away. Ask a prospective baby-sitter for references and check them out thoroughly. Question your child about how she gets along with the people who sit for her and how she feels about them. When choosing a preschool or child care center, check with your local child care community agencies to make certain it is properly licensed and has never been subject to complaints. Question the administrators about how thoroughly they examine the credentials and previous employ-

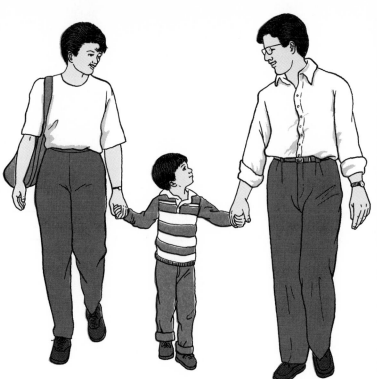

ment records of the people they hire. Talk to some of the other parents about their experiences. You might also make a few unannounced visits to see for yourself how the staff interacts with the children. Once your youngster has been enrolled in a program, ask her how she feels about it—and listen to her opinion.

Child abuse in all its various forms is such a disturbing subject that many parents prefer not to think about it, and would like to pretend it doesn't exist. But this attitude fails to meet the primary responsibility all of us have to keep our youngsters safe from harm. While we shouldn't morbidly dwell on the possible emotional, physical or sexual exploitation of our children, neither can we deny the reality that such dangers do exist. We owe it to our sons and daughters to keep our eyes open to the ever-present possibility of child abuse both inside and outside the home. And we must do everything in our power to keep it from ever happening and stop it immediately should we discover that our children have been subjected to this terrible violation of their fundamental rights as human beings.

PART TWO

BE PREPARED

CHOOSING A DOCTOR

It is essential to find the right doctor for your child, not only to provide the medical attention she will need in case she falls ill, but also to oversee her ongoing health and development through regular checkups, immunizations against infectious diseases and other preventive treatment. In most communities, a wide variety of options are available. Many parents use private medical practitioners, either their regular family doctors or pediatricians, who are specially trained in caring for children. Others choose independent or hospital-based clinics or neighborhood health centers staffed by physicians and other health professionals. Some parents with prepaid medical insurance plans have access to health maintenance organizations that offer pediatric care either through physicians working full time for the organization or private practitioners who participate in the plan. Whichever option you decide upon, it's a good idea to narrow your choice down to a particular doctor even before your baby is born.

Look for a skillful, highly qualified physician who relates well to young children, someone who makes you feel confident he will give your youngster the best possible medical care. You might begin by asking friends and relatives whose opinions you trust for their recommendations. Hospitals in your area or your local, county or state medical society can supply you with the names of qualified candidates. Should you decide you want to use a pediatrician, your family doctor can probably offer some suggestions.

Get as much preliminary information as you can about anyone you are considering. To find out about his training and credentials, consult the **American Medical Dictionary** or the **Dictionary of Medical Specialists** at your local library, or telephone the medical society in your area. A doctor's hospital affiliations are also important, so make sure he has admitting privileges at a children's hospital or a general hospital with a well-regarded pediatric service. If the

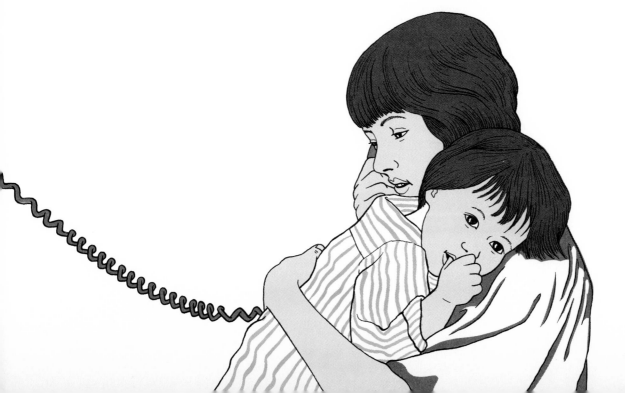

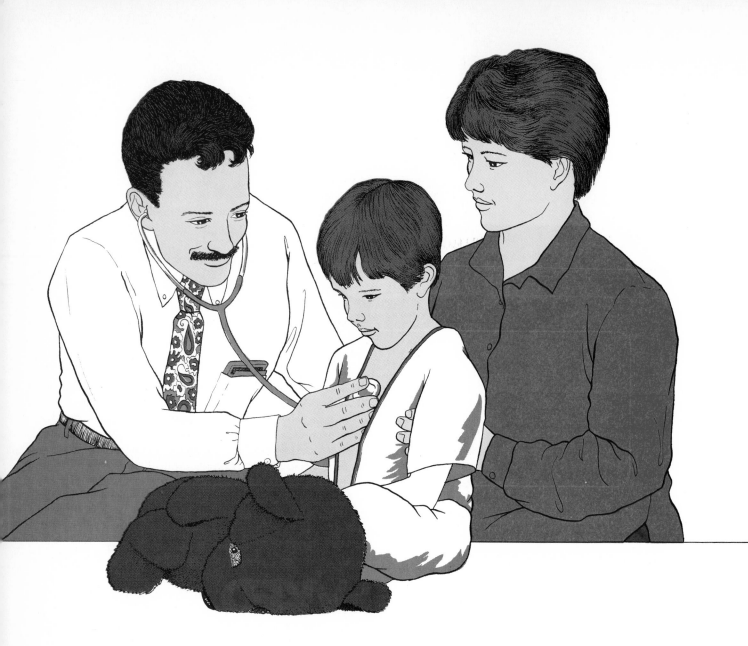

hospital is connected with a medical school, he is likely to have access to expert specialists and the most up-to-date information and equipment.

Telephone the doctor's office and talk with his receptionist or office manager. **Don't be afraid to ask questions.** How difficult is it to get an appointment? How long do you usually have to wait in the waiting room? Does he ever make house calls? Who covers for the doctor when he is away, and what are his credentials? If it is a group practice, will you get the same physician most of the time, and can you choose which of the associates you usually see? Since cost may be a factor, find out his fee schedule in advance and whether or not he accepts payments from your health insurance program. Obviously, you also want to be sure his office is near your home and his regular office hours are convenient.

Before coming to a final decision, meet with the doctor personally to be certain you are making the proper choice. Does he seem to be a thorough sort of person who exhibits sound judgment? Is he interested in preventive care? Do you feel comfortable with him? He should be able to talk easily with you, listen to what you have to say and encourage you to ask questions. You want to come away assured that you will be putting your child in the hands of someone who is caring and perceptive and readily accessible, and will always give you the information you need.

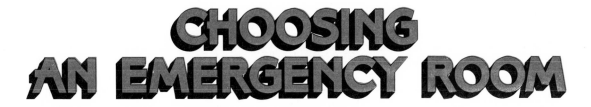

CHOOSING AN EMERGENCY ROOM

You may never need to use one, but it's still a good idea to choose an emergency room in advance so you will immediately know where to go and what to do should you ever have to rush your child to a hospital.

Time is, of course, crucially important in any medical emergency, so you want an emergency room that is close to your home, easy to reach and participates in your local EMS system. But keep in mind that emergency rooms vary greatly in the size and skill of their staffs and the equipment they have available. The hospitals they are attached to often specialize in a particular area of medical care, and this will also have a bearing on the type and quality of emergency treatment they are able to offer. You should make a point of investigating all the emergency facilities in your community to find the one that is most suitable.

Begin by asking your doctor for his recommendations. You might also talk to your friends and neighbors about their experiences. Your local EMS office will be able to give you the names of nearby emergency rooms that meet its requirements by being open to receive patients at all hours of the day and by being adequately staffed and equipped.

Your physician may suggest the emergency room of the hospital he is affiliated with, so if your child needs to be admitted he will be able to take care of her. But he may also advise you to check out some other facilities that offer other advantages.

Some hospitals are trauma centers and have a variety of specialists and advanced equipment that can instantly be brought into play should your child be injured in a way that requires very sophisticated treatment. Other hospitals have special facilities for children or treat children in a separate area, which might make it less upsetting for your youngster and less complicated for you. Some hospital emergency rooms feel it is helpful for parents to stay with a hurt or sick child as long as they remain calm and cooperative; others have a different philosophy. Ask the hospitals you are considering what policy they follow and consider how that fits in with your own personal feelings. Also find out what they would like you to do to help them care for your child quickly and effectively. Do they want you to call ahead? Do they want you to bring any particular information with you? (At the very least, you should always take along your child's Immunization Record and Emergency Medical Information chart on pages 109 and 107 of **A Sigh of Relief**.)

Once you have decided upon where you would take your child in an emergency, map out the shortest or most direct route, along with an alternate route in case that might be necessary, then make a practice run. When you get to the hospital, note where the emergency entrance is located as well as the parking lot. In the event that you will need an ambulance and for some reason EMS isn't immediately available, also find out about the ambulance service in your community: what number to call and how long it should take the ambulance to reach your home.

CHOOSING A BABY-SITTER

When choosing a baby-sitter it's best to use somebody you already know and feel confident will be able to take good care of your youngster while you are away. If you have to depend on recommendations or advertisements, always ask for a full list of references and check them out thoroughly.

Obviously, the younger the child, the greater the responsibility placed on the sitter, but a trustworthy, competent person is essential for any age. Students between 12 and 15 years old are often well qualified and usually most available for baby-sitting jobs, but older people who want part-time work can also be excellent sitters. It is important that the prospective sitter knows first aid. Many Red Cross chapters offer a course in first aid for baby-sitters, and your local chapter may be able to give you the names of people in your neighborhood who have passed it successfully.

When you have found someone who sounds suitable on the telephone, set up a visit at your home so she can meet you and your youngster. You should discuss the job and your expectations, and feel comfortable and secure about the conversation. You want someone who likes children, is responsible and calm, and listens carefully to your instructions. Have her spend some time with your child so you can see how they're getting along.

Before you go out, give the new sitter a tour of your home, pointing out light switches, thermostats, telephones, fuse boxes, smoke alarms, etc., as well as potentially dangerous areas that should be avoided. Show her where you keep your first-aid kit and other emergency supplies, including your copy of **A Sigh of Relief.** Carefully explain what escape routes and plans you have worked out in case of a fire. Make sure

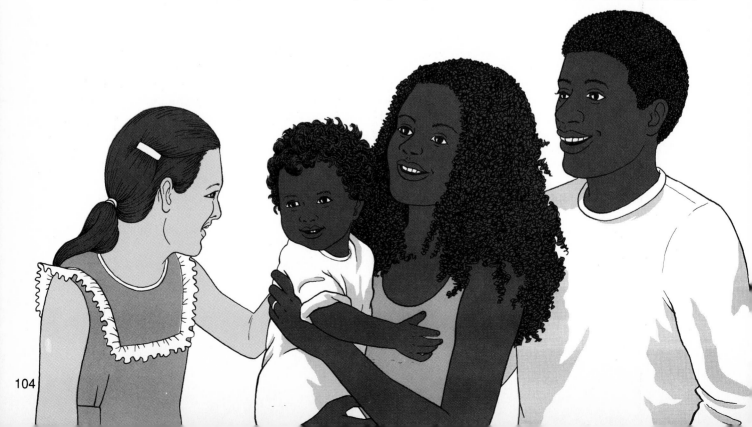

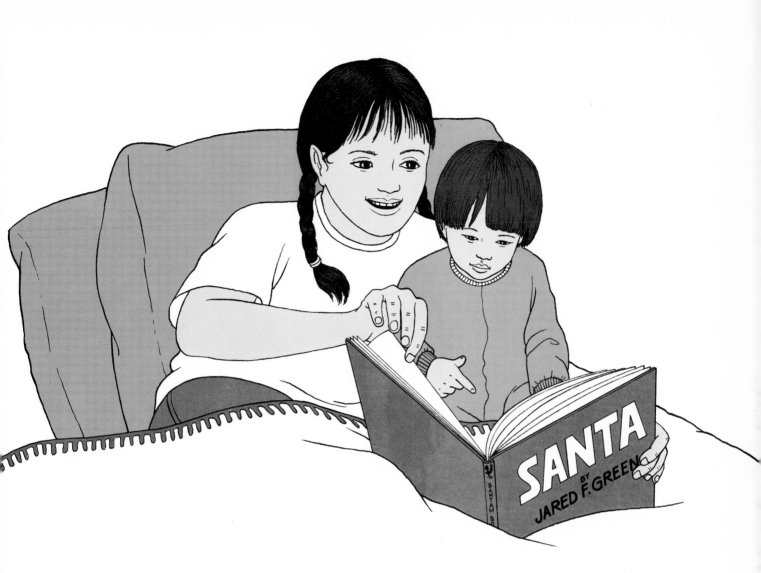

she knows where the fire extinguishers are kept and how to use them, and how to call the fire department.

Be sure to give the sitter all the pertinent information about your child's current health problems, including allergies and any medication to be taken. Leave the medicine out for her, along with clearly written instructions about time and dosage, and show her how it is to be administered. Ask her to keep a written record of what medication your child has taken, how much he took and when he took it.

You should always leave the telephone number where you can be reached in case of a medical or some other emergency, along with the number of someone who can make decisions for you if you aren't available. Emergency numbers, including those for the fire department, police, Emergency Medical Services (EMS) and your child's doctor, should be on all the telephones in the house as well as in the Emergency Telephone Numbers section of this book.

Tell the sitter when you plan to be home and whether you are expecting any telephone calls, visitors or deliveries. Obviously, she should never open the door to strangers. Leave her a pencil and pad so she can write down any messages. If you have installed a security system, show her how to use it, and review whatever procedures you follow to keep your home safe from intruders.

Carefully explain your child's normal routine, so the sitter will know what to expect. If she is to give him a bath, make sure she understands the necessary safety procedures; see page 80. And tell her how you feel about having her friends over, using the phone, raiding the refrigerator, etc. The clearer and more specific you can be, the easier she will find it to take good care of your youngster and give him a pleasant, unstressful time until you return.

Every household should have a first-aid kit stocked with the basic supplies necessary for treating childhood emergencies. You can put your own kit together by purchasing the individual items listed on this page. Check off each item as you place it in the kit. If you prefer to buy a commercial kit that is already assembled, use this list to make sure its contents are complete. Always keep the kit stored in the same place, well out of a youngster's reach, and be sure your family and baby-sitter know where to find it. Keep it fully stocked and replace supplies as they are used.

You should also have first-aid kits for your car or boat and for hiking and camping expeditions. If your child has severe allergic reactions to insect bites and stings, have his doctor prescribe an insect sting kit and keep it with your other emergency supplies.

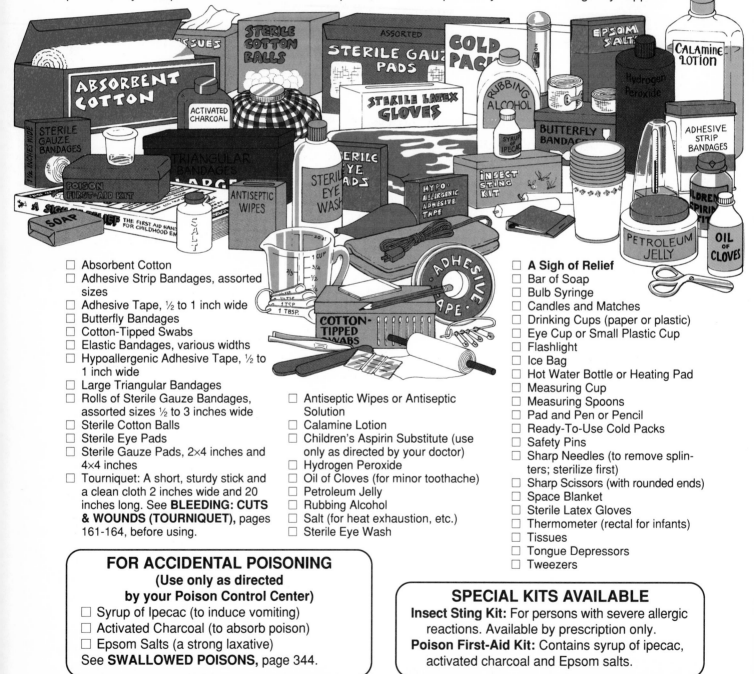

- ☐ Absorbent Cotton
- ☐ Adhesive Strip Bandages, assorted sizes
- ☐ Adhesive Tape, ½ to 1 inch wide
- ☐ Butterfly Bandages
- ☐ Cotton-Tipped Swabs
- ☐ Elastic Bandages, various widths
- ☐ Hypoallergenic Adhesive Tape, ½ to 1 inch wide
- ☐ Large Triangular Bandages
- ☐ Rolls of Sterile Gauze Bandages, assorted sizes ½ to 3 inches wide
- ☐ Sterile Cotton Balls
- ☐ Sterile Eye Pads
- ☐ Sterile Gauze Pads, 2×4 inches and 4×4 inches
- ☐ Tourniquet: A short, sturdy stick and a clean cloth 2 inches wide and 20 inches long. See **BLEEDING: CUTS & WOUNDS (TOURNIQUET)**, pages 161-164, before using.

- ☐ Antiseptic Wipes or Antiseptic Solution
- ☐ Calamine Lotion
- ☐ Children's Aspirin Substitute (use only as directed by your doctor)
- ☐ Hydrogen Peroxide
- ☐ Oil of Cloves (for minor toothache)
- ☐ Petroleum Jelly
- ☐ Rubbing Alcohol
- ☐ Salt (for heat exhaustion, etc.)
- ☐ Sterile Eye Wash

- ☐ **A Sigh of Relief**
- ☐ Bar of Soap
- ☐ Bulb Syringe
- ☐ Candles and Matches
- ☐ Drinking Cups (paper or plastic)
- ☐ Eye Cup or Small Plastic Cup
- ☐ Flashlight
- ☐ Ice Bag
- ☐ Hot Water Bottle or Heating Pad
- ☐ Measuring Cup
- ☐ Measuring Spoons
- ☐ Pad and Pen or Pencil
- ☐ Ready-To-Use Cold Packs
- ☐ Safety Pins
- ☐ Sharp Needles (to remove splinters; sterilize first)
- ☐ Sharp Scissors (with rounded ends)
- ☐ Space Blanket
- ☐ Sterile Latex Gloves
- ☐ Thermometer (rectal for infants)
- ☐ Tissues
- ☐ Tongue Depressors
- ☐ Tweezers

FOR ACCIDENTAL POISONING
(Use only as directed by your Poison Control Center)
- ☐ Syrup of Ipecac (to induce vomiting)
- ☐ Activated Charcoal (to absorb poison)
- ☐ Epsom Salts (a strong laxative)
See **SWALLOWED POISONS**, page 344.

SPECIAL KITS AVAILABLE
Insect Sting Kit: For persons with severe allergic reactions. Available by prescription only.
Poison First-Aid Kit: Contains syrup of ipecac, activated charcoal and Epsom salts.

EMERGENCY MEDICAL INFORMATION

This page provides an immediate overview of your youngster's medical history and can save valuable time in an emergency. If you have more than one child, make as many extra photocopies as you need and tape them into the book. You should also give copies to your children's teachers, camp counselors and the other adults with whom they spend significant time. **Be sure to keep the information current.**

CHILD'S NAME:_____ Date of Birth: _____

Address:_____ Home Phone: _____

Father's Phone at Work:_____ Mother's Phone at Work: _____

PEDIATRICIAN: Name: _____ Office Phone: _____ Home Phone: _____

FAMILY DOCTOR: Name: _____ Office Phone: _____ Home Phone: _____

ALTERNATE DOCTOR: Name:_____ Office Phone: _____ Home Phone: _____

DENTIST: Name: _____ Office Phone: _____ Home Phone: _____

MEDICAL INSURANCE: Company Name: _____ Phone: _____

   Address: _____ Policy Number:_____

DATES OF MOST RECENT IMMUNIZATIONS

Hepatitis B:_____ Combined Diphtheria, Tetanus & Pertussis (DTP): _____

Polio: _____ Haemophilus Influenza Type B: _____

Measles, Mumps & Rubella: _____ Combined Tetanus & Diphtheria: _____

Other: _____

PRESENT MEDICAL PROBLEMS & CHRONIC CONDITIONS (EPILEPSY, ASTHMA, ETC.)
_____   _____

ALLERGIES (DRUGS, INSECT BITES, ETC.)
_____   _____
_____   _____

BLOOD TYPE:_____

RH Factor   RH Negative ☐
(check one)   RH Positive ☐

MEDICINES TAKEN REGULARLY

Name: _____ Reason Taken:_____ Dose & Frequency: _____

Name: _____ Reason Taken:_____ Dose & Frequency: _____

Name: _____ Reason Taken:_____ Dose & Frequency: _____

Name: _____ Reason Taken:_____ Dose & Frequency: _____

	NATURE	DATE	DOCTOR	PHONE
Hospitalizations:				
Surgery:				
Major Injuries:				
Psychiatric Care or Counseling:				

IMMUNIZATION SCHEDULE

Immunization offers your youngster the best possible protection against many childhood diseases. It is extremely important to make sure she receives the necessary vaccines at the recommended ages. If you don't have a pediatrician or family doctor, contact your local public health department. Many such agencies will immunize your child without charge.

The following chart indicates what vaccines are normally required and the times when "peak immunization" can usually be obtained. Your pediatrician may vary the schedule somewhat according to your child's individual circumstance. He may delay giving her a shot, for example, if she has been running a fever, or decide to omit the pertussis vaccine if she has been subject to seizures, has a history of severe vaccine reactions or suffers from suppressed immunity. He may also advise additional booster shots and other vaccines that have been newly recommended, or want to give her additional immunizations if she will be traveling abroad.

It's a good idea to prepare your child before taking her to the doctor for an injection. Let her know it will only hurt for a second. Adverse reactions to vaccines are usually mild but may include headaches, mild fever and some temporary soreness. Occasionally a youngster may develop a slight rash after receiving the measles vaccine.

Though your doctor will maintain a record of your child's immunizations, you should also keep an up-to-date record at home in case information is required in an emergency and the doctor is unavailable. Make sure the accompanying **IMMUNIZATION RECORD** stays current.

BIRTH
● Hepatitis B: 1st shot

1 TO 2 MONTHS
● Hepatitis B: 2nd shot

2 MONTHS
● Combined Diphtheria, Tetanus and Pertussis (Whooping Cough) (DTP): 1st shot
● Oral Polio Vaccine: 1st dose
● Haemophilus Influenza Type B: 1st shot

4 MONTHS
● Combined Diphtheria, Tetanus and Pertussis (DTP): 2nd shot
● Oral Polio Vaccine: 2nd dose
● Haemophilus Influenza Type B: 2nd shot

6 MONTHS
● Combined Diphtheria, Tetanus and Pertussis (DTP): 3rd shot
● Haemophilus Influenza Type B: Depending upon which of the 2 approved vaccines was used earlier, another shot may be required now.

6 TO 18 MONTHS
● Hepatitis B: 3rd shot

12 TO 15 MONTHS
● Haemophilus Influenza Type B: Depending upon which of the 2 approved vaccines was used earlier, another shot may be required now.

15 MONTHS
● Measles, Mumps and Rubella (MMR): Vaccination
● Haemophilus Influenza Type B: Depending upon which of the 2 approved vaccines was used earlier, another shot may be required now.

15 TO 18 MONTHS
● Combined Diphtheria, Tetanus and Pertussis (DTP): 4th shot
● Oral Polio Vaccine: 3rd dose

4 TO 6 YEARS
● Combined Diphtheria, Tetanus and Pertussis (DTP): 5th shot
● Oral Polio Vaccine: 4th dose

11 TO 12 YEARS
● Measles, Mumps and Rubella (MMR): A booster shot should be given if your child has not already had measles. The booster may be required earlier if there is an outbreak of measles in your community or if you live in a high-risk area.

14 TO 16 YEARS
● Combined Tetanus and Diphtheria. (In the event of a deep puncture or severe wound, a tetanus shot should be given immediately if more than 5 years have passed since the last one.)

IMMUNIZATION RECORD

NAME_____DATE OF BIRTH _____

HEPATITIS B

1st DATE _____PHYSICIAN_____

2nd DATE _____PHYSICIAN_____

3rd DATE _____PHYSICIAN_____

COMBINED DIPHTHERIA, TETANUS AND PERTUSSIS

1st DATE _____PHYSICIAN_____

2nd DATE _____PHYSICIAN_____

3rd DATE _____PHYSICIAN_____

4th DATE _____PHYSICIAN_____

5th DATE _____PHYSICIAN_____

ORAL POLIO VACCINE

1st DATE _____PHYSICIAN_____

2nd DATE _____PHYSICIAN_____

3rd DATE _____PHYSICIAN_____

4th DATE _____PHYSICIAN_____

HAEMOPHILUS INFLUENZA TYPE B

1st DATE _____PHYSICIAN_____

2nd DATE _____PHYSICIAN_____

3rd DATE _____PHYSICIAN_____

4th DATE _____PHYSICIAN_____

MEASLES, MUMPS AND RUBELLA

1st DATE _____PHYSICIAN_____

Booster DATE _____PHYSICIAN_____

Booster DATE _____PHYSICIAN_____

COMBINED TETANUS AND DIPHTHERIA

DATE_____PHYSICIAN_____

OTHER VACCINES

Type_____DATE _____PHYSICIAN_____

Type_____DATE _____PHYSICIAN_____

Type_____DATE _____PHYSICIAN_____

Type_____DATE _____PHYSICIAN_____

Type_____DATE _____PHYSICIAN_____

NAME_____DATE OF BIRTH _____

HEPATITIS B

1st DATE _____PHYSICIAN_____

2nd DATE _____PHYSICIAN_____

3rd DATE _____PHYSICIAN_____

COMBINED DIPHTHERIA, TETANUS AND PERTUSSIS

1st DATE _____PHYSICIAN_____

2nd DATE _____PHYSICIAN_____

3rd DATE _____PHYSICIAN_____

4th DATE _____PHYSICIAN_____

5th DATE _____PHYSICIAN_____

ORAL POLIO VACCINE

1st DATE _____PHYSICIAN_____

2nd DATE _____PHYSICIAN_____

3rd DATE _____PHYSICIAN_____

4th DATE _____PHYSICIAN_____

HAEMOPHILUS INFLUENZA TYPE B

1st DATE _____PHYSICIAN_____

2nd DATE _____PHYSICIAN_____

3rd DATE _____PHYSICIAN_____

4th DATE _____PHYSICIAN_____

MEASLES, MUMPS AND RUBELLA

1st DATE _____PHYSICIAN_____

Booster DATE _____PHYSICIAN_____

Booster DATE _____PHYSICIAN_____

COMBINED TETANUS AND DIPHTHERIA

DATE_____PHYSICIAN_____

OTHER VACCINES

Type_____DATE _____PHYSICIAN_____

Type_____DATE _____PHYSICIAN_____

Type_____DATE _____PHYSICIAN_____

Type_____DATE _____PHYSICIAN_____

Type_____DATE _____PHYSICIAN_____

CHILD IDENTIFICATION RECORD

All parents have experienced the occasional stab of fear that one day a precious son or daughter may suddenly disappear. The chances of this ever happening are extremely remote, but it is still a good idea to take the necessary precautions just in case it does. Make sure your youngster knows the first and last names of both his parents, his home address (including the city, state and zip code) and his home telephone number (including the area code). If your child is missing, you will want to contact the police immediately. Before they could begin their investigation they would need a substantial amount of specific information that you would almost certainly have a great deal of difficulty putting together under the stress of the moment. By having this Child Identification Record on hand you would avoid unnecessary confusion and delay, and enable them to start their search without the loss of valuable hours or days.

Make a separate photocopy of these pages for each child in your family, and then fill them in. **As your children grow older and the information changes, photocopy these pages again and bring the information up to date.** It would also be extremely helpful to have a current videotape available of each of your children, along with copies of their birth certificates, current dental records, contact lens or eyeglass prescriptions, and vaccination records. (See **IMMUNIZATION RECORD,** page 109.) Keep these Child Identification Records and other aids to identification in a safe place known to everyone in your household.

CHILD'S NAME: _____   Home Phone: _____

Home Address: _____

Date of Birth: _____

Height: _____ Weight: _____

Hair Color: _____

Eye Color: _____

Description of Eyeglass Frames:

_____

_____

Blood Type: _____

CURRENT COLOR PHOTOGRAPH (PROFILE)

CURRENT COLOR PHOTOGRAPH (FULL FACE)

Birthmarks, Moles or Scars: _____

Physical Handicaps & Other Distinctive Physical Features: _____

_____

Medical Problems That Require Medication & List of Needed Medicines: _____

_____

_____

_____

Unusual Speech Characteristics: _____

LEFT HAND					FINGERPRINTS					RIGHT HAND

CONTINUED ON NEXT PAGE

PARENTS AT WORK

Mother's Name: _____ Phone: _____

Company Name & Address: _____

Father's Name: _____ Phone: _____

Company Name & Address: _____

SCHOOL

Name: _____ Phone: _____

Address: _____

Doctor's Name: _____ Phone: _____

Address: _____

Dentist's Name: _____ Phone: _____

Address: _____

CLOSE RELATIVES, SCHOOL & NEIGHBORHOOD FRIENDS

Name: _____ Phone: _____

Address: _____

Name: _____ Phone: _____

Address: _____

Name: _____ Phone: _____

Address: _____

Name: _____ Phone: _____

Address: _____

Name: _____ Phone: _____

Address: _____

RECREATIONAL HABITS
Names, Addresses & Phone Numbers of Places the Child Frequents When Not in School:

_____

_____

_____

_____

_____

Brand Name, Description & Registration Number of Bicycle or Other Vehicle:

_____

CURRENT DISTRESS WORD (the secret word you and your child have
agreed he will use if he needs to tell you privately that he is in danger): _____

PART THREE
COMMON CHILDHOOD ILLNESSES & DISORDERS

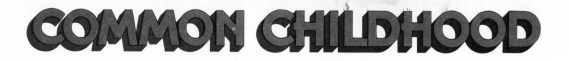

	SIGNS & SYMPTOMS	INCUBATION	DURATION
BRONCHITIS	Runny nose. Sneezing. Frequent coughing. Labored breathing. Possible fever. **In severe cases:** Flaring nostrils. Rattling sounds in the throat and chest. Bluish color around the mouth and under the fingernails. Difficulty sleeping.	1 to 7 days	2 to 4 days
CHICKEN POX	Fever. Discomfort. Headache. Tiredness. Lack of appetite. Itching. Pink or red spots on the chest, stomach and back, which may spread to the scalp and face. Spots change to blisters, which eventually crust.	10 to 21 days, usually 14 to 17 days	7 to 10 days
COMMON COLD	Sneezing. Stuffed or runny nose. Headache. Sore throat. Watery eyes. **May include:** Coughing. Chills. Low fever. Ear pain. Mild swelling of the lymph nodes in the neck.	1 to 7 days	2 to 14 days, usually 5 to 7 days
CROUP	Labored breathing. Hoarseness. Croaking sound when inhaling. Loud hacking cough. **May include:** Difficulty drinking. Restlessness. Crying. Desire to sit or be held upright. **In severe cases:** Paleness. Bluish lips or fingernails. Extreme anxiety. Symptoms often come on at night.	2 to 6 days	4 to 5 days
GERMAN MEASLES (RUBELLA)	Chills. Low, sometimes high fever. Runny nose. Swollen glands in the neck, behind the ears and on the lower back of the head. A rash of tiny flat or slightly raised pink-red spots, which begins on the face, then spreads over the rest of the body. **May include:** Headache. Inflamed eyes. Slight sore throat. Coughing. Decreased appetite. Overall physical discomfort.	14 to 21 days	3 to 6 days
INFLUENZA (VIRUS, FLU)	Chills. Drowsiness. Weakness. Sudden high fever. Headache. Aches and pains. Coughing. Sore throat. No appetite. **May include:** Dizziness. Nausea. Vomiting. Diarrhea. Earache.	1 to 3 days	3 to 14 days

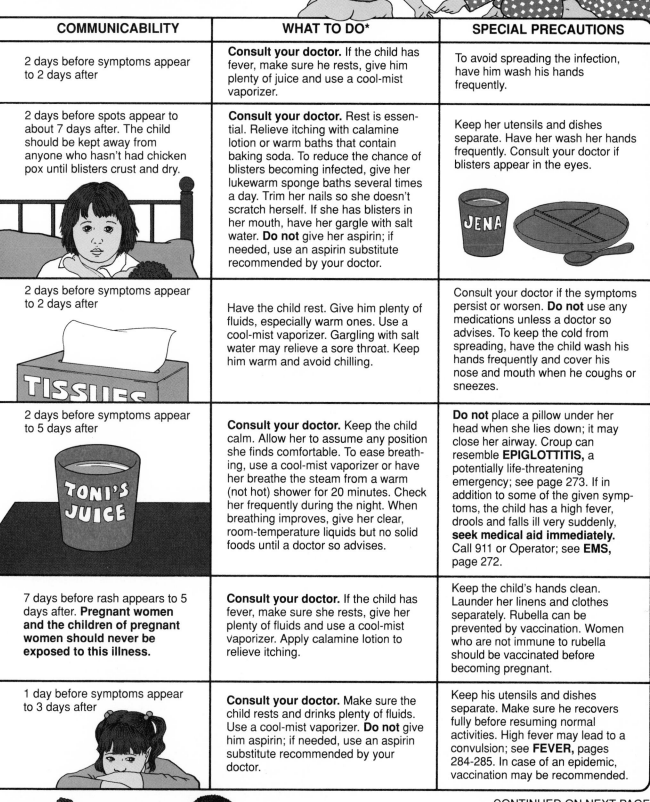

COMMUNICABILITY	WHAT TO DO*	SPECIAL PRECAUTIONS
2 days before symptoms appear to 2 days after	**Consult your doctor.** If the child has fever, make sure he rests, give him plenty of juice and use a cool-mist vaporizer.	To avoid spreading the infection, have him wash his hands frequently.
2 days before spots appear to about 7 days after. The child should be kept away from anyone who hasn't had chicken pox until blisters crust and dry.	**Consult your doctor.** Rest is essential. Relieve itching with calamine lotion or warm baths that contain baking soda. To reduce the chance of blisters becoming infected, give her lukewarm sponge baths several times a day. Trim her nails so she doesn't scratch herself. If she has blisters in her mouth, have her gargle with salt water. **Do not** give her aspirin; if needed, use an aspirin substitute recommended by your doctor.	Keep her utensils and dishes separate. Have her wash her hands frequently. Consult your doctor if blisters appear in the eyes.
2 days before symptoms appear to 2 days after	Have the child rest. Give him plenty of fluids, especially warm ones. Use a cool-mist vaporizer. Gargling with salt water may relieve a sore throat. Keep him warm and avoid chilling.	Consult your doctor if the symptoms persist or worsen. **Do not** use any medications unless a doctor so advises. To keep the cold from spreading, have the child wash his hands frequently and cover his nose and mouth when he coughs or sneezes.
2 days before symptoms appear to 5 days after	**Consult your doctor.** Keep the child calm. Allow her to assume any position she finds comfortable. To ease breathing, use a cool-mist vaporizer or have her breathe the steam from a warm (not hot) shower for 20 minutes. Check her frequently during the night. When breathing improves, give her clear, room-temperature liquids but no solid foods until a doctor so advises.	**Do not** place a pillow under her head when she lies down; it may close her airway. Croup can resemble **EPIGLOTTITIS,** a potentially life-threatening emergency; see page 273. If in addition to some of the given symptoms, the child has a high fever, drools and falls ill very suddenly, **seek medical aid immediately.** Call 911 or Operator; see **EMS,** page 272.
7 days before rash appears to 5 days after. **Pregnant women and the children of pregnant women should never be exposed to this illness.**	**Consult your doctor.** If the child has fever, make sure she rests, give her plenty of fluids and use a cool-mist vaporizer. Apply calamine lotion to relieve itching.	Keep the child's hands clean. Launder her linens and clothes separately. Rubella can be prevented by vaccination. Women who are not immune to rubella should be vaccinated before becoming pregnant.
1 day before symptoms appear to 3 days after	**Consult your doctor.** Make sure the child rests and drinks plenty of fluids. Use a cool-mist vaporizer. **Do not** give him aspirin; if needed, use an aspirin substitute recommended by your doctor.	Keep his utensils and dishes separate. Make sure he recovers fully before resuming normal activities. High fever may lead to a convulsion; see **FEVER,** pages 284-285. In case of an epidemic, vaccination may be recommended.

CONTINUED ON NEXT PAGE

*If a fever reaches 102° F (38.8° C), see **FEVER,** pages 284-285.

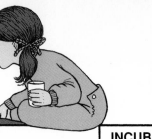
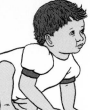

	SIGNS & SYMPTOMS	INCUBATION	DURATION
MEASLES	Early symptoms include: Low fever. Slight hacking cough. Runny nose. Sore throat. Fatigue. Discomfort. Eye irritation. White spots may appear inside the mouth. Around the 4th day, fever and cough worsen, and a rash of faint pink spots appears on the forehead, neck and cheeks and around the ears, then spreads to the rest of the body.	8 to 12 days	7 to 12 days
MUMPS	Painful swollen glands below the ears or under one or both sides of the jaw. Mild headache. Fever. Stomachache. Loss of appetite. Listlessness. Earache.	12 to 24 days	6 to 14 days
PNEUMONIA	Coughing. Rapid, sometimes painful breathing. Wheezing. Chills. Fever. **May include:** Hot, dry skin. Weakness. Abdominal pain. Drowsiness, restlessness or anxiety. Loss of appetite. Nausea and vomiting. Coughing up thick yellow sputum, sometimes tinged with blood.	2 to 14 days	7 to 12 days
ROSEOLA	Sudden high fever lasting several days. After fever is gone, a pink, often itchy rash of flat or raised spots appears on the chest, stomach or back, then may spread to the arms, neck and the rest of the body.	8 to 17 days	5 to 6 days
SCARLET FEVER	Sudden high fever. Painful sore throat. Weakness. Headache. Chills. Discomfort. Stomachache. Nausea and vomiting. **May include:** Abdominal pain. Rapid pulse. Within several days a fine red rash appears on the neck, armpits, groin and inner thighs, then spreads to the rest of the body.	1 to 5 days	5 to 8 days
STREP THROAT	Painful sore throat. Fever. **May include:** Nausea and vomiting. Headache. Listlessness. Swollen glands on the sides of the neck.	2 to 5 days	About 6 days
WHOOPING COUGH	**Begin with:** Sneezing. Runny nose. Sore throat. Red, watery eyes. Mild cough. Mild fever. Infants may have thick mucus in their noses and throats. **After 1 or 2 weeks:** Severe coughing spasms that interfere with breathing. Usually followed by massive whoops of inhaled air. Reddened or purplish face. **May include:** Bulging, watery eyes. Protruding tongue. Enlarged veins in the neck. Increased salivation. Vomiting. Continued fever. Listlessness. Weight loss.	5 to 10 days	Depending upon severity, from less than 2 weeks to as long as 2 months

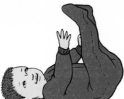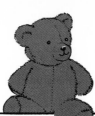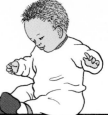

COMMUNICABILITY	WHAT TO DO*	SPECIAL PRECAUTIONS
4 days before rash appears to 5 days after	**Consult your doctor.** If the child's eyes are sensitive to light, keep the room dim. If she has fever, make sure she rests, give her plenty of fluids and use a cool-mist vaporizer.	Keep her utensils and dishes separate. Can be prevented by vaccination.
2 days before symptoms appear to 3 days after they disappear	**Consult your doctor.** Give the child soft food and a lot of liquids. Avoid citrus juices as they may be painful to swallow. Cool compresses applied to the cheeks may help relieve pain. The child may need to rest.	Keep his utensils and dishes separate. Can usually be prevented by vaccination.
Varies	**Consult your doctor.** Make sure the child rests. Give him plenty of juice. Use a cool-mist vaporizer. Keep him on a light, low-fat diet.	Early treatment is essential. **Seek medical aid immediately** if the child coughs up sputum tinged with blood. Avoid smoking around the child.
Varies	**Consult your doctor.**	High fever may lead to a convulsion; see **CONVULSIONS & SEIZURES**, page 253.
1 day before symptoms appear to 6 days after	**Consult your doctor.** Make sure the child rests. Give her plenty of fluids.	Keep her away from other children for at least 48 hours after she begins taking the prescribed antibiotic. Check other family members for symptoms.
1 day before symptoms appear to 6 days after	**Consult your doctor.** Make sure the child rests. Give him plenty of fluids. **Do not** give him aspirin; if needed, use an aspirin substitute recommended by your doctor.	Keep the child at home away from other children for at least 24 hours after he has begun taking the prescribed antibiotic. Check other family members for symptoms.
Highly contagious	**Consult your doctor promptly.** Severe cases often require hospitalization. If treated at home, keep the child comfortable and relaxed to minimize coughing spasms. Make sure she eats properly, especially if she is subject to vomiting. Give her encouragement and reassurance. **Watch breathing closely.** If necessary, see **BREATHING: ARTIFICIAL RESPIRATION,** pages 201-215. When breathing is restored, seek medical aid immediately. If necessary, call 911 or Operator; see **EMS,** page 272.	Can usually be prevented by DPT (diphtheria, pertussis, tetanus) inoculations; see **IMMUNIZATION SCHEDULE,** page 108.

*If a fever reaches 102° F (38.8° C), see **FEVER,** pages 284-285.

COMMON CHILDHOOD DISORDERS

ADENOIDITIS

SIGNS & SYMPTOMS
Inflamed mucous membrane inside the nose. Blocked nasal passages. Fever. Headache. Vomiting. Impaired taste and smell. Snoring. Night coughing. Bad breath. Nasal-sounding or muffled voice. Usually caused by a viral infection. May be accompanied by **TONSILLITIS;** see page 122.

WHAT TO DO
Seek medical aid.

CAR SICKNESS (MOTION SICKNESS)

SIGNS & SYMPTOMS
Nausea. Dizziness. Lightheadedness. Vomiting. Paleness. Sweating. Anxiety.

WHAT TO DO

1 If possible, have the child sit in the center of the vehicle looking straight ahead, not out a side window. If her eyes are below window level, raise her up a little so the passing scenery does not seem to bounce up and down.

2 Give her crackers, flat carbonated beverages and chewing gum to help settle her stomach.

3 Keep good air circulation in the vehicle by opening the windows or turning on the air conditioner. Do not smoke. Drive as steadily as possible.

4 Try to distract the child with word games or songs, but don't allow her to read.

5 Take frequent breaks over the course of a trip.

SPECIAL PRECAUTIONS
- **Do not** give the child any preventive medications unless a doctor so advises.
- **Consult your doctor** if motion sickness is a recurrent problem.

CHILLS

SIGNS & SYMPTOMS
Shivering. Shaking.

WHAT TO DO

1 Take the child to a warm place and make him comfortable.

2 Give him sips of warm non-caffeinated liquids.

3 Consult your doctor.

SPECIAL PRECAUTIONS
- **Seek medical aid immediately** if there are signs of **HYPOTHERMIA;** see pages 332-335, or **POISONING;** see pages 344-352.
- Check for **FEVER;** see pages 284-285.
- Consult your doctor if the chills persist or worsen.
- **Do not** use heating pads or hot-water bottles.

CONJUNCTIVITIS (PINKEYE)

SIGNS & SYMPTOMS
Pink or red eyes. Itching and burning. Yellowish discharge. Wakes up with eyelids stuck together and caked with crusts. **May be accompanied by:** Fever. Sore throat. Diarrhea. Sensitivity to light. An inflammation of the membrane that lines the eyelids and eyes. Can be caused by a virus, bacteria, household chemicals or an allergic reaction.

WHAT TO DO

1 Remove the child from the cause of the conjunctivitis if it is known.

2 If caused by a chemical, immediately flush the eye with water; see **EYE INJURIES: CHEMICALS IN THE EYE,** page 277.

3 Consult your doctor.

CONTINUED ON NEXT PAGE

4 Apply cool compresses for 10 to 15 minutes several times a day to relieve itching.

SPECIAL PRECAUTIONS
● To control the spread of the infection, have the child use disposable towels, wash her hands frequently and refrain from rubbing her eyes. Also wash your hands after any contact.

CONSTIPATION

SIGNS & SYMPTOMS
Unusually infrequent bowel movements. Unusually hard and dry stool. Pain or difficulty defecating. Can be caused by dietary problems, emotional stress, anal fissures and, rarely, an obstruction in the intestine or other serious physical problem.

WHAT TO DO
1 Avoid premature or over-zealous toilet training.

2 Provide a well-balanced diet rich in fruits, vegetables and grains, without an excess of fats and proteins.

3 Encourage the child to go to the toilet as soon as he feels the urge and to stay there as long as necessary.

SPECIAL PRECAUTIONS
● **Do not** give the child enemas or laxatives unless a doctor so advises.
● **Consult your doctor** if constipation persists or if the child has severe pain while trying to defecate, there is blood in his stool or he has cracks or tears in his rectum.

COUGHING

SIGNS & SYMPTOMS
Coughs vary greatly in severity, duration and underlying cause. Can be caused by tension, colds, allergies, infectious diseases, environmental irritants, inhaled foreign objects, etc.

WHAT TO DO
1 Have the child rest until the coughing subsides.

2 Give him plenty of water, and keep him on a light diet that includes warm, clear liquids.

3 If the cough is caused by an environmental irritant, remove him from the source.

4 If the cough is due to a cold, steam or a cool-mist vaporizer may offer some relief.

SPECIAL PRECAUTIONS
● **Seek medical aid immediately** if the child coughs up blood. If necessary, call 911 or Operator; see **EMS,** page 272.
● If the child turns blue, see **CHOKING,** pages 239-252. If necessary, call 911 or Operator; see **EMS,** page 272.
● If the cough sounds like a bark, see **CROUP,** pages 114-115.
● **Do not** give any cough medication to a child under 2 without consulting a doctor. With an older child, cough medicine should be used sparingly, if at all, and preferably only when recommended by a physician.
● **Consult your doctor** if the cough persists or worsens, or is accompanied by a fever, rash or headache.

DIAPER RASH

SIGNS & SYMPTOMS
Rough, red patches on the infant's buttocks, genitals or thighs. May become severely inflamed if bacteria breaks down the urine into ammonia. Usually caused by irritation from wet diapers, but may also result from fungi in the infant's stool.

WHAT TO DO
1 Keep the infant's skin dry and exposed to the open air. If possible, have him go without diapers until the rash clears. If that isn't possible, use very absorbent, completely dry diapers and change them frequently.

CONTINUED ON NEXT PAGE

2 Whenever you change the baby's diapers, wash his buttocks area with water if there is just urine in the diaper or with mild soap and water if the diaper contains stool. Dry thoroughly. A mild, unscented baby powder will help keep him dry.

3 Ask your doctor if he recommends zinc oxide ointment or some other protective skin coating.

SPECIAL PRECAUTIONS
● Diaper rash can be aggravated by disposable plastic-covered diapers and close-fitting plastic pants.
● Use mild soap rather than detergent if you wash the diapers at home, and put them through an extra rinse cycle to make sure all the soap has been removed.
● **Consult your doctor** if you suspect the rash may have some other cause, or if it is very severe, does not begin to clear up after 3 days, or is accompanied by fever, irritability or loss of appetite.

DIARRHEA

SIGNS & SYMPTOMS
Increased bowel movements. Increased liquidity and amount of stool. Stools may be light brown, yellow or green. May contain partially digested food. **May be accompanied by:** Abdominal pain. Nausea. Vomiting. Fever. Frequency, duration and seriousness vary greatly. Usually caused by viral or bacterial infections, but may also result from microscopic animal organisms, fungi, parasitic worms, metabolic and dietary problems, food poisoning, allergies, emotional stress, etc.

WHAT TO DO
1 Have the child rest.

2 Keep her off solid foods but give her frequent small sips of broth, apple juice or other clear liquids (**not** milk) to guard against dehydration, a potentially serious emergency.

3 When the diarrhea eases, begin feeding her small amounts of simple, low-fat, binding foods, and continue giving liquids.

SPECIAL PRECAUTIONS
● **Do not** give the child any medication unless a doctor so advises.
● **Seek medical aid immediately** if she has severe pain in her abdomen that lasts for more than half an hour. If necessary, call 911 or Operator; see **EMS,** page 272.
● **Seek medical aid immediately** if a child, especially an infant, is drowsy, has a dry mouth or sunken eyes, cannot retain liquids, or if the diarrhea persists, recurs frequently, contains blood or is accompanied by vomiting, high fever or decreased urination.
● To help prevent infectious diarrhea from recurring and spreading to other members of the family, make sure the child washes her hands thoroughly after going to the toilet.

EARACHE

SIGNS & SYMPTOMS
Pain in the ear. Itching. Tenderness. Swelling. Discharge of pus. Temporary hearing loss. An infant may cry, pull his ear or turn his head back and forth. Usually caused by a viral or bacterial infection. **May also result from** accumulated ear wax, a foreign object in the ear, irritation of the external ear canal, sore throat, infected tonsils, middle ear infection, disease in the mouth, or high altitudes.

WHAT TO DO
Consult your doctor within 24 hours after the earache begins.

SPECIAL PRECAUTIONS
● **Do not** use any medication, including aspirin, unless your doctor so advises.
● **Do not** put cotton swabs or any other objects in the child's ear.
● Keep the ear dry until the ear infection is completely eliminated.

HEADACHE

SIGNS & SYMPTOMS
Internal head pain. **May be accompanied by a variety of other symptoms including:** Fever. Nausea. Stiff neck. Loss of appetite. Confusion. Headaches vary greatly in severity and duration. Most are minor, short-term and easily relieved, but others may be caused by a chronic migraine condition, infectious disease, injury to the head or central nervous system, or other serious underlying problems.

WHAT TO DO

1 Consult your doctor if you cannot determine the underlying cause from the child's recent activities or health problems.

2 Comfort and reassure him.

3 Have him rest quietly in a dimly lit room and try to nap.

4 To help relieve the pain, apply heat to the back of his neck, gently massage his head and neck, place a cool compress on his forehead or give him a warm bath.

5 Give him a light meal if he feels up to eating.

SPECIAL PRECAUTIONS
● **Seek medical aid immediately** if the headache is severe or sudden; awakens the child from sleep; is accompanied by a stiff neck, high fever, vomiting, blurred vision, confusion or extreme drowsiness; or interferes significantly with normal activities for more than an hour.
● **Consult your doctor** if a headache persists, worsens or recurs frequently.
● **Do not** give the child any medication unless your doctor so advises.
● Be alert for other symptoms.

RASH

SIGNS & SYMPTOMS
Red or purple spots, bumps or blisters anywhere on the body. **May be accompanied by:** Itching and stinging. Bleeding under the skin. Bruises. Fever. Can be caused by excessive perspiration (heat rash); skin irritation; viral, bacterial, parasitic or fungal infections; allergic reactions to foods, medications, plants, insect bites, etc.

WHAT TO DO

1 Consult your doctor if you cannot determine the underlying cause from the child's recent activities or health problems.

2 Relieve the itching and stinging with cool compresses and baths several times a day, or calamine lotion if your doctor so advises.

3 For a heat rash, also use an air conditioner or fan to lower the temperature and humidity of the child's immediate environment, and have him wear lightweight, loose-fitting clothing. For more on **HEAT RASH,** see pages 327-328.

SPECIAL PRECAUTIONS
● **Consult your doctor** if the rash appears after the child has taken medication.
● **Consult your doctor** if the spots are blue or blood red, if the rash persists or worsens, contains red streaks or pus, or is accompanied by fever, very severe itching or other symptoms.
● Try to keep the child from scratching the rash.

SORE THROAT

SIGNS & SYMPTOMS
Pain in the throat. Difficulty swallowing. Inflamed throat tissue. **May be accompanied by:** Fever. Swollen glands. Headache. May come on suddenly or gradually. Vary greatly in duration and seriousness. Can be caused by colds, flu, strep throat and other viral and bacterial infections, laryngitis, tonsillitis, environmental irritants, sleeping with the mouth open, breathing through the mouth, excessive talking and shouting.

WHAT TO DO

1 Have the child rest.

CONTINUED ON NEXT PAGE

2 Have her drink plenty of warm, clear fluids.

3 Gargling with warm salt water may also be soothing.

4 Use a cool-mist vaporizer or humidifier in her bedroom.

SPECIAL PRECAUTIONS
- **Do not** give the child any medications, including aspirin, unless a doctor so advises.
- **Consult your doctor** if the sore throat is accompanied by severe pain, skin rash, pus in the throat or other severe symptoms; or the child has been exposed to strep throat.

STIES

SIGNS & SYMPTOMS
Eyelid becomes red and swollen and feels painful. Eyes may itch or tear. Small bumps on the upper or lower eyelid. Within a few days, a pus-filled head usually forms. Caused by a bacterial infection.

WHAT TO DO

1 Apply hot compresses with a clean washcloth or cotton balls for 10 or 15 minutes several times a day until the sty comes to a head and then drains.

2 Consult your doctor if the sty seems to be getting worse or does not respond to home treatment within a few days.

SPECIAL PRECAUTIONS
- **Do not** try to open the sty.
- To keep sties from recurring, have your child wash his hands frequently and refrain from rubbing his eyes.
- Keep his towel and washcloth separate to prevent sties from spreading to other members of the family.

STOMACHACHE

SIGNS & SYMPTOMS
Pain in the abdominal area. **May be accompanied by:** Fever. Cramps. Nausea. Vomiting. Diarrhea. Constipation. Can be caused by overeating, indigestion, food allergies, fatigue, minor emotional stress, or more seriously, food poisoning, physical injury, pneumonia, strep throat, appendicitis, etc.

WHAT TO DO

1 Give the child clear liquids (but no milk or food) until the stomachache passes.

2 Keep her warm and offer reassurance.

3 Use a warm heating pad to help relieve the pain.

SPECIAL PRECAUTIONS
- **Consult your doctor** if there is extreme pain for more than half an hour or if the stomachache persists, worsens or recurs repeatedly.
- **Do not** give the child an enema or any medication, including aspirin, unless your doctor so advises.

TONSILLITIS

SIGNS & SYMPTOMS
Swollen tonsils. Swollen glands in the neck and jaw. Sore throat. Painful swallowing. Obstructed breathing. Headache. Fever. Lack of energy. Aching arms and legs. Drowsiness. Vomiting. Stomachache. Loss of appetite. Bad breath. Caused by a viral or bacterial infection. Symptoms may develop suddenly. May be accompanied by **ADENOIDITIS;** see page 118.

WHAT TO DO
Seek medical aid.

VOMITING

SIGNS & SYMPTOMS
May be accompanied by: Nausea. Coughing, gagging or choking. Cold, moist skin. Sweating. Rapid heartbeat. Mild fever. Hiccups. Aches. Weakness. Dizziness. Can be caused by overeating, food allergy, car sickness, anxiety and, more seriously, viral and bacterial infections, infections in other parts of the body, poisoning, eating disorders, etc.

WHAT TO DO
1 Give the child comfort and reassurance, and have her rest.

2 After several hours, offer her frequent small sips of sweetened clear liquids (**not** milk) to guard against dehydration.

3 After about 6 hours, feed her some plain crackers if she is hungry, then a few hours later small amounts of soft, easy-to-digest low-fat foods. Encourage her to continue sipping liquids.

SPECIAL PRECAUTIONS
- **Do not** give the child any medications unless a doctor so advises.
- **Consult your doctor** if the vomit contains blood or if vomiting persists, recurs several times within 2 hours or is accompanied by high fever, diarrhea, severe headache, listless behavior or severe abdominal pain that lasts for more than 1 hour.
- **Always consult a doctor** if an infant vomits, or if the vomiting occurs after a head injury or convulsion.

WARTS

SIGNS & SYMPTOMS
Lumps or bumps on the skin. May be white, pink, dirty yellow or dark brown. Most commonly appear on the hands and feet but may also appear on the face and neck or in the genital and anal areas. An abnormal growth of skin cells caused by a viral infection.

WHAT TO DO
It's best to leave warts alone. They usually disappear by themselves, and home treatment is often unsuccessful or leaves scars. Consult your doctor if the warts persist, are large or painful, or change size, shape or color.

SPECIAL PRECAUTIONS
- **Consult your doctor immediately** if the child has genital or anal warts. They are highly contagious and may indicate inappropriate sexual contact.
- **Do not** attempt to treat facial, genital or anal warts yourself.

PART FOUR
EMERGENCIES & MISHAPS: FIRST-AID PROCEDURES

CONTINUED ON NEXT PAGE

124

125

INTRODUCTION

Remember that first aid is not a substitute for professional medical care. If your child becomes seriously injured or ill, you should always try to obtain the immediate assistance of a physician or EMS paramedical team. Unfortunately, this isn't always possible. Emergencies have a way of happening when help isn't available right away, and if they aren't dealt with promptly, the child's life may be jeopardized. Under such circumstances, your ability to provide quick, effective first aid may mean the difference between life and death.

This section presents the most up-to-date procedures for all the most common emergencies and mishaps. To help you act quickly and correctly, each procedure combines clear, simple instructions printed in large type with easy to follow step-by-step illustrations. As a further help, the back cover of this book is thumb-indexed to give you immediate access to the procedures for the most serious emergencies. Each procedure is also listed in the Contents in the front of the book. Follow the given instructions carefully, and be sure to pay attention to all the information contained under the IMPORTANT headings.

There are a number of crucial points to keep in mind whenever you have to come to someone's aid:

● It is, of course, terribly distressing to see a loved one suffering from an illness or injury, but if you are to alleviate the emergency, you must do your best to remain calm and clearheaded so you can follow the appropriate procedures correctly.

● You should also do your best to calm and reassure a child who is sick or injured. Anxiety and fear only make things worse.

● In any serious emergency, especially if the child is unconscious, always check the ABCs (Airway, Breathing and Circulation); see **CHECKING THE ABCs,** pages 224-232.

● As a protection against blood-transmitted diseases, wash your hands thoroughly if the child is bleeding and, if possible, put on sterile latex gloves before starting first aid.

● Never give an unconscious child anything to drink.

● If you are unsure about the nature or extent of an emergency, see **ASSESSING THE EMERGENCY,** pages 127-128, before attempting any first aid. There are times when doing the incorrect thing can be more injurious than not doing anything at all.

● Also check for medical alert tags and other instruc-

tions about special medical needs. If your child is allergic to certain medications or subject to a particular illness, make sure he always carries that information with him. He should also always have in his possession some form of personal ID so you can be immediately notified if an emergency arises.

● In all but the most minor cases, contact your doctor after administering first aid, even if the child seems to have recovered completely. Some sort of follow-up treatment may be necessary. You can't be too careful.

To reiterate Dr. Solomon's advice in the Introduction, we suggest that you read through this section as soon as possible to familiarize yourself with the recommended procedures before you ever need to use them. Don't forget that the basic purpose of first aid is to preserve the victim's life and prevent further physical and psychological harm until help arrives. We also suggest that you keep this book in an accessible place known to your baby-sitters and to other members of your family.

It is always better for someone giving first aid to be professionally trained. To obtain the best possible preparation for medical emergencies, sign up for the first-aid courses offered by the local chapter of the American Red Cross. The basic and advanced programs provide training and supervised practice in virtually every aspect of emergency care. **Special training for cardio-pulmonary resuscitation (CPR), the first-aid technique for heart failure, is especially important.** The procedure can cause serious harm if used unnecessarily or incorrectly.

Make sure that all the first-aid supplies you might need in an emergency are always on hand and readily available. For a list of the necessary items, see **STOCKING UP,** on page 106 of **PART TWO: BE PREPARED.** Also make sure to fill out and keep up to date the list of **EMERGENCY TELEPHONE NUMBERS** on page 384, the **EMERGENCY MEDICAL INFORMATION** chart on page 107 and the **IMMUNIZATION RECORD** on page 109. Use the **IMMUNIZATION SCHEDULE** on page 108 as a guide to keeping your children's tetanus and other immunizations current. With the proper foresight, many medical emergencies can be averted altogether. For this same reason, we also strongly urge you to study **PART ONE** of this book, **PREVENTIONS: REDUCING THE ODDS.**

IMPORTANT

- **If the injury seems at all serious, immediately send someone for professional medical assistance while you administer first aid.** Have him call 911 or Operator; see **EMS,** page 272.

- Remain calm and offer reassurance and comfort.

- Look for emergency medical information tags or cards.

- Treat the most serious injuries first.

- **Do not** move the child **unless** you absolutely must. You may cause further injury. If it does become necessary, see **TRANSPORTING THE INJURED,** pages 374-380.

1 **Survey the scene:** Is it safe for you to intervene, or are there immediate dangers that may jeopardize your own safety? What happened? (Ask the child or any witnesses.) How many are injured? Is there anyone else around who can help?

2 **Determine if the child is responsive** by calling him loudly, tapping him on the shoulder or shaking him gently. If he is unresponsive, yell for help and have someone call 911 or Operator; see **EMS,** page 272. **If the child is under 8** and no one answers your repeated shouts for help, administer first aid for 1 minute, then call EMS yourself. Return immediately and continue first aid. **If the child is over 8** and no one responds, call EMS yourself without waiting any longer, then return immediately and begin first aid.

3 **Check the ABCs (AIRWAY, BREATHING and CIRCULATION); see CHECKING THE ABCs,** pages 224-232.

CONTINUED ON NEXT PAGE

4 **Check for bleeding.** Quickly and gently examine the child's head and body for injuries. Make sure to look carefully for wounds that may not be obvious. Control the most serious bleeding first. See **BLEEDING: CUTS & WOUNDS,** pages 156-177.

5 If there are burns or stains on the child's mouth or other signs of poisoning (pills, chemicals, poisonous plants, etc.), see **POISONING,** pages 344-352.

6 If the child is injured, observe for **SHOCK;** see pages 354-356.

7 For broken bones, see **BREAKS: FRACTURES & DISLOCATIONS,** pages 183-200.

8 In cool or cold weather, particularly if it is windy and the child is wet, see **HYPOTHERMIA (COLD EXPO-SURE),** pages 332-335.

9 **Recheck the ABCs (AIRWAY, BREATHING and CIR-CULATION),** and reexamine the child from head to toe.

10 If necessary, place him in the **RECOVERY POSI-TION;** see page 353.

ABRASIONS

IMPORTANT

- **Seek medical aid immediately if an eye or a large area of the body is affected, if dirt or foreign substances have been ground into the wound or if there are signs of infection. Do not** treat these abrasions yourself.

- Wash your hands thoroughly and, if possible, put on sterile latex gloves before starting first aid.

- Do not apply medication unless your doctor so advises.

- Check with your doctor to make sure the child's tetanus immunization is still current.

SIGNS & SYMPTOMS

Surface of the skin is scraped, scratched or rubbed away. Reddening of the affected area. May or may not bleed, depending on severity.

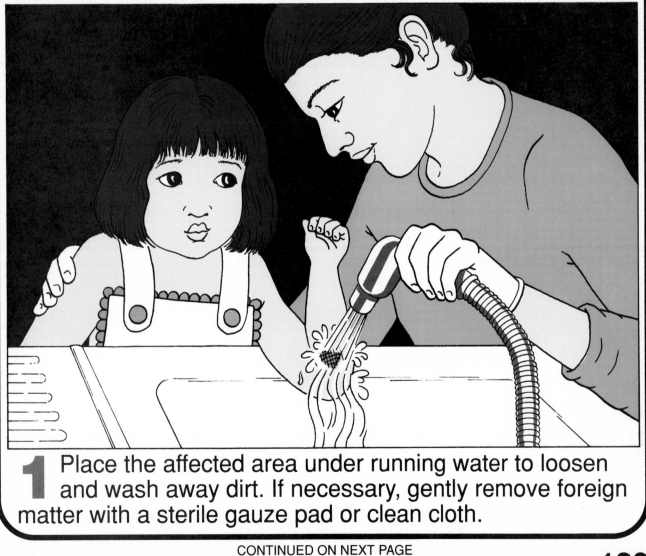

1 Place the affected area under running water to loosen and wash away dirt. If necessary, gently remove foreign matter with a sterile gauze pad or clean cloth.

CONTINUED ON NEXT PAGE

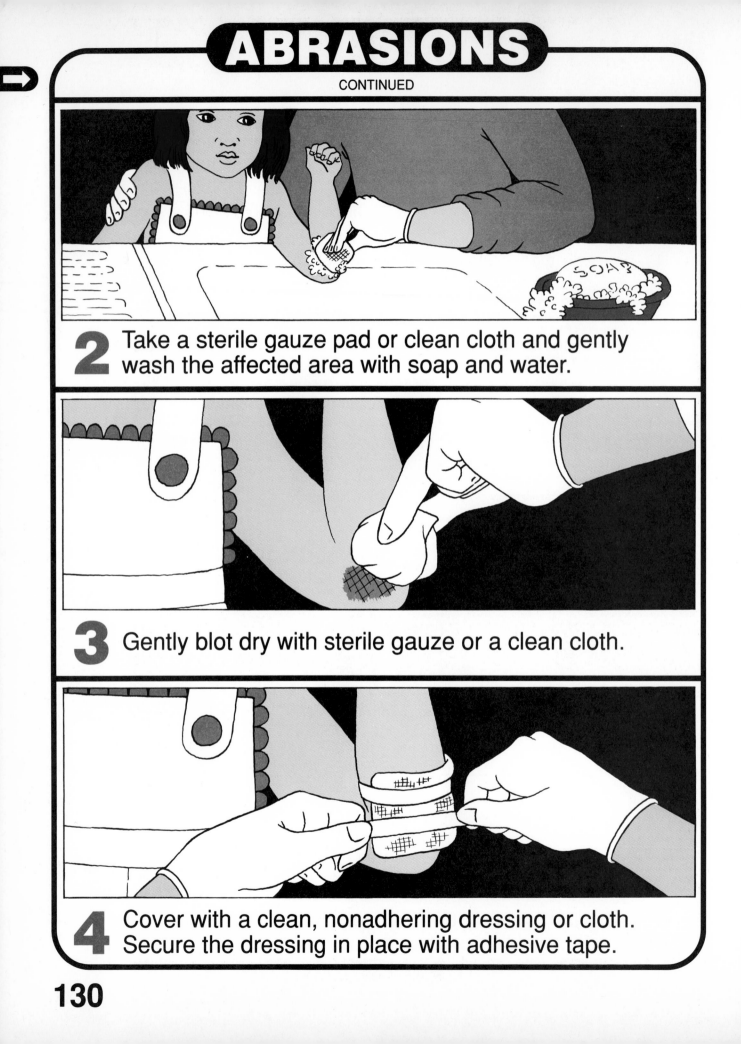

2 Take a sterile gauze pad or clean cloth and gently wash the affected area with soap and water.

3 Gently blot dry with sterile gauze or a clean cloth.

4 Cover with a clean, nonadhering dressing or cloth. Secure the dressing in place with adhesive tape.

ANAPHYLACTIC SHOCK

IMPORTANT

- **Anaphylactic shock is a life-threatening emergency caused by a sudden severe allergic reaction to an insect bite or, less commonly, certain foods or medications.**

- **Seek medical aid immediately.** Call 911 or Operator; see **EMS,** page 272.

- Check the child's ABCs (Airway, Breathing and Circulation); see **CHECKING THE ABCs,** pages 224-232.

- Observe for **SHOCK,** pages 354-356.

- **If she has emergency allergy medication, help her take it.**

- If she has been stung by an insect, see **BITES & STINGS: INSECTS,** pages 139-144.

- **Do not** place a pillow under her head or give her anything by mouth if she has difficulty breathing.

- If she has problems with allergies, ask your doctor if you should keep epinephrine on hand for use in an emergency.

SIGNS & SYMPTOMS

Extreme weakness. Pale or bluish skin. Coughing. Wheezing. Dizziness. Difficulty breathing. Hives. Intense itching. Severe swelling at the site of an insect bite or elsewhere. Stomach cramps. Nausea. Vomiting. Anxiety. Convulsions. Collapse. Unconsciousness.

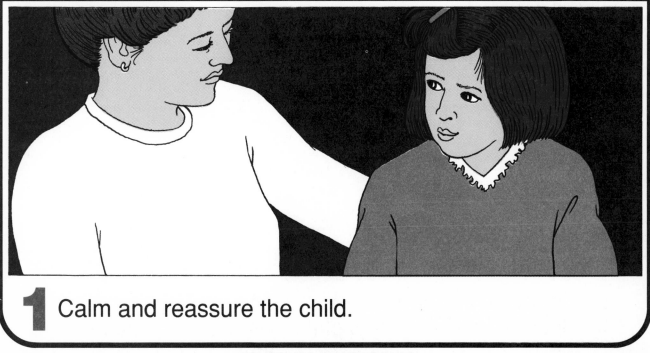

1 Calm and reassure the child.

CONTINUED ON NEXT PAGE

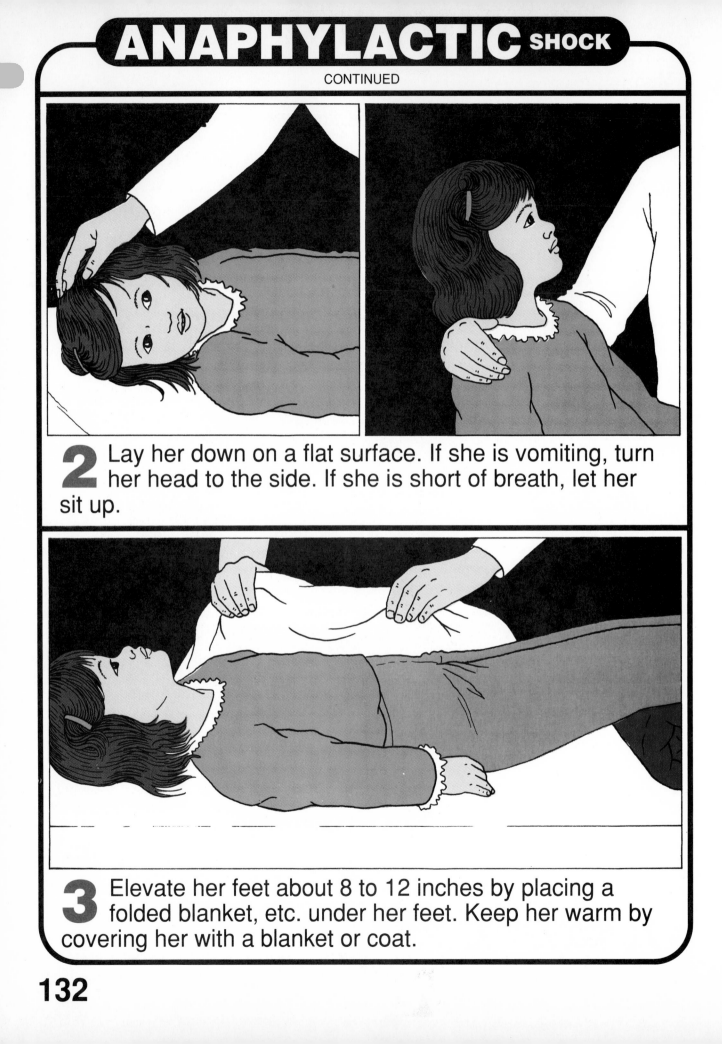

2 Lay her down on a flat surface. If she is vomiting, turn her head to the side. If she is short of breath, let her sit up.

3 Elevate her feet about 8 to 12 inches by placing a folded blanket, etc. under her feet. Keep her warm by covering her with a blanket or coat.

ASTHMA ATTACK

IMPORTANT

- **Seek medical aid if the attack is severe or occurring for the first time.** Call 911 or Operator; see **EMS,** page 272.

- Watch breathing closely. If necessary, see **BREATHING: ARTIFICIAL RESPIRATION,** pages 201-215.

- Someone with a history of asthma should avoid known or suspected causes of attacks.

SIGNS & SYMPTOMS

In early stages: Respiratory discomfort resembling a cold. Coughing. Nasal congestion. **May progress to:** Labored breathing with whistling or wheezing sounds. Anxiety. **In advanced cases:** Feeling of suffocation. Pale or bluish lips, gums, skin and fingernails. **May progress to:** Respiratory failure.

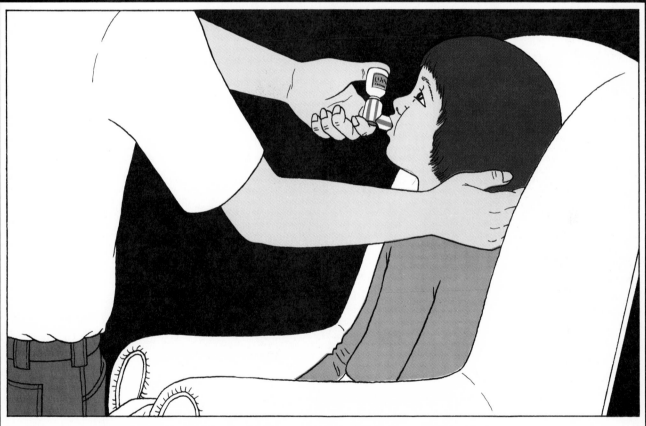

1 As soon as symptoms are noticed, take the child to a quiet area and place her in the most comfortable position possible, preferably seated with her shoulders relaxed. Provide good ventilation. If medicine has been prescribed, help her take it.

CONTINUED ON NEXT PAGE

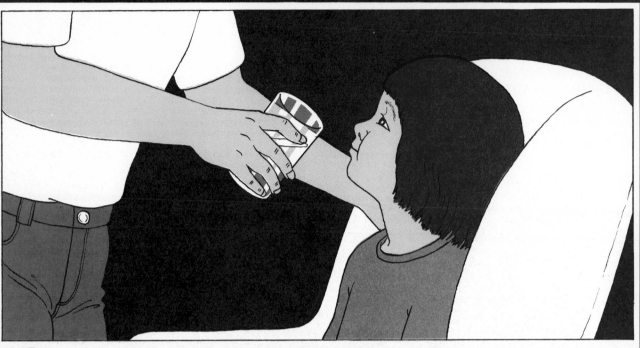

2 Have the child rest. Comfort and reassure her; anxiety may worsen the attack. Encourage her to drink plenty of liquids (preferably at room temperature) — water, fruit juices, etc., but **not** milk.

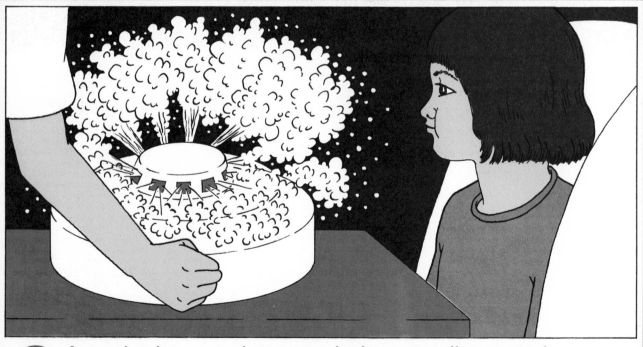

3 A cool-mist vaporizer may help ease distressed breathing.

IMPORTANT

- **Seek medical aid immediately. For a serious injury,** call 911 or Operator; see **EMS,** page 272.

- **Do not** bend or twist the neck or body.

- **Do not** move the child unless you absolutely must. If it does become necessary, see **TRANSPORTING THE INJURED,** pages 374-376.

- Check the child's ABCs (Airway, Breathing and Circulation); see **CHECKING THE ABCs,** pages 224-232.

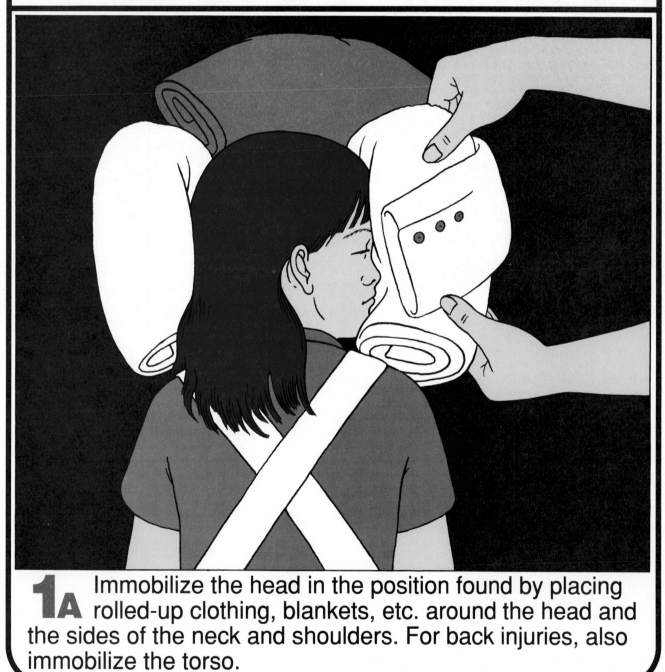

1A Immobilize the head in the position found by placing rolled-up clothing, blankets, etc. around the head and the sides of the neck and shoulders. For back injuries, also immobilize the torso.

CONTINUED ON NEXT PAGE

135

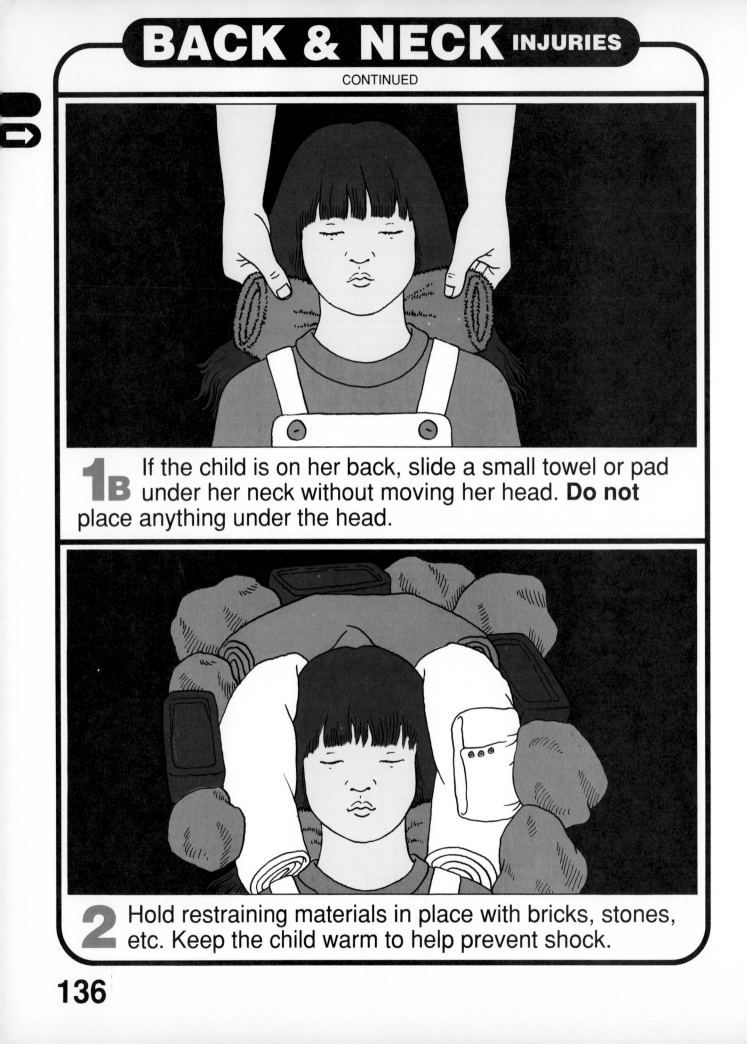

1B If the child is on her back, slide a small towel or pad under her neck without moving her head. **Do not** place anything under the head.

2 Hold restraining materials in place with bricks, stones, etc. Keep the child warm to help prevent shock.

BITES & STINGS

ANIMAL & HUMAN BITES

IMPORTANT

- **If the skin is penetrated, seek medical aid immediately.** Bites can be extremely dangerous.

- **If there is severe bleeding,** call 911 or Operator; see **EMS,** page 272.

- **If possible,** confine the animal. Be careful not to get bitten yourself. **Do not** try to capture the animal. Call the police or Animal Control (if available) to capture and examine it for rabies.

- Wash your hands thoroughly and, if possible, put on sterile latex gloves before starting first aid.

- Observe for **SHOCK,** pages 354-356.

- **Seek medical aid immediately** if any signs of infection develop, such as increased tenderness or pain after 24 hours, redness, swelling, throbbing, pus, red streaks leading from the wound, fever or swollen glands.

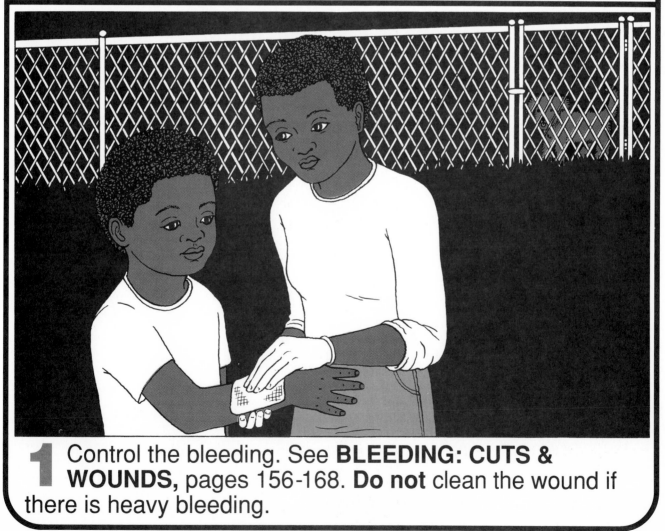

1 Control the bleeding. See **BLEEDING: CUTS & WOUNDS,** pages 156-168. **Do not** clean the wound if there is heavy bleeding.

CONTINUED ON NEXT PAGE

ANIMAL & HUMAN BITES
CONTINUED

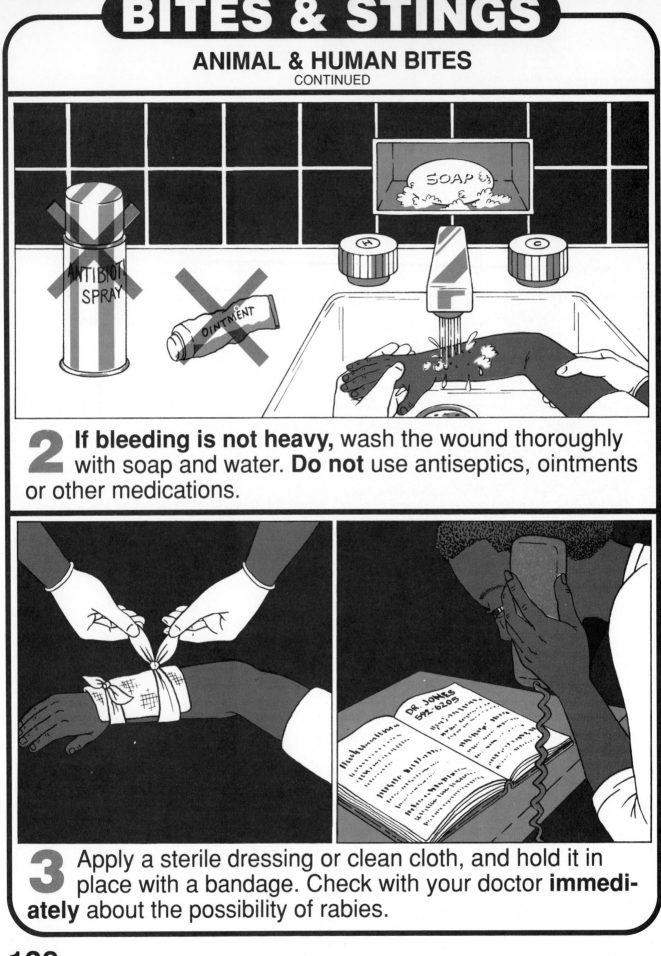

2 **If bleeding is not heavy,** wash the wound thoroughly with soap and water. **Do not** use antiseptics, ointments or other medications.

3 Apply a sterile dressing or clean cloth, and hold it in place with a bandage. Check with your doctor **immediately** about the possibility of rabies.

138

BITES & STINGS

INSECTS

IMPORTANT

- **Seek medical aid immediately for bites and stings from BLACK WIDOW and BROWN RECLUSE SPIDERS and SCORPIONS.** Call your local Poison Control Center or take the child to the nearest hospital emergency room. If necessary, call 911 or Operator; see **EMS,** page 272.

- **Seek medical aid immediately if the child is subject to hay fever, asthma or allergic reactions or if there is severe swelling anywhere on his body.** Call 911 or Operator; see **EMS,** page 272. Observe for **ANAPHYLACTIC SHOCK,** pages 131-132, and **SHOCK,** pages 354-356.

- A severely allergic child should always carry some form of medical identification. Ask your doctor if he recommends an emergency self-treatment kit.

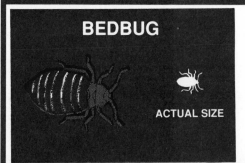

BEDBUG

ACTUAL SIZE

SIGNS & SYMPTOMS

Welts. Swelling. Irritation.

WHAT TO DO

Wash thoroughly with soap and water.

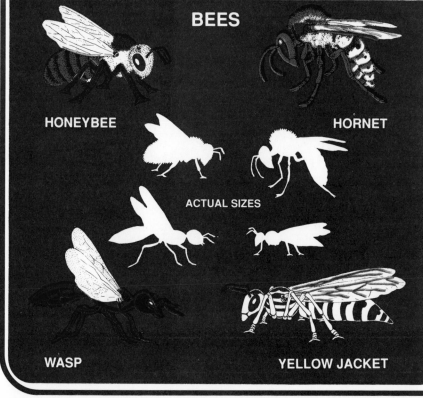

BEES

HONEYBEE

HORNET

ACTUAL SIZES

WASP

YELLOW JACKET

SIGNS & SYMPTOMS

Pain. Local swelling. Burning and itching. Allergic reaction may also cause nausea, shock, unconsciousness and severe swelling.

WHAT TO DO

Seek medical aid immediately if the child is subject to

CONTINUED ON NEXT PAGE

INSECTS
CONTINUED

allergic reactions or there is severe swelling; see **IMPORTANT** on previous page. For a bee sting, remove the venom sac by scraping gently with the edge of your fingernail or the blunt edge of a knife, not by squeezing. (Wasps, hornets and yellow jackets do not leave venom sacs.) Wash with soap and water. Apply ice wrapped in a cloth to reduce swelling and pain. Watch breathing closely. If necessary, see **BREATHING: ARTIFICIAL RESPIRATION,** pages 201-215. For a severe reaction, follow first aid for **BLACK WIDOW** below.

SIGNS & SYMPTOMS

Slight redness and swelling. Severe pain. Profuse sweating. Muscle cramps. Stomach cramps. Difficulty breathing. Nausea.

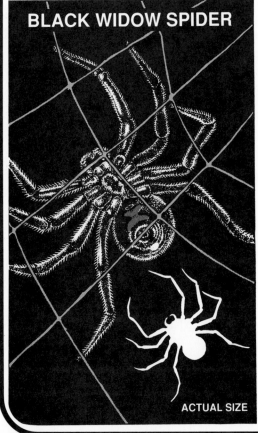

BLACK WIDOW SPIDER

ACTUAL SIZE

WHAT TO DO

Seek medical aid immediately; see **IMPORTANT** on previous page. Check the child's ABCs (Airway, Breathing and Circulation); see **CHECKING THE ABCs,** pages 224-232. Keep the child quiet, offer reassurance and avoid unnecessary movement. Remove any items that may restrict circulation. Try to keep the affected parts below heart level. Wash the wound with soap and water, then apply cold compresses. **Do not** give the child food, liquids or any unprescribed medication.

CONTINUED ON NEXT PAGE

BITES & STINGS

INSECTS
CONTINUED

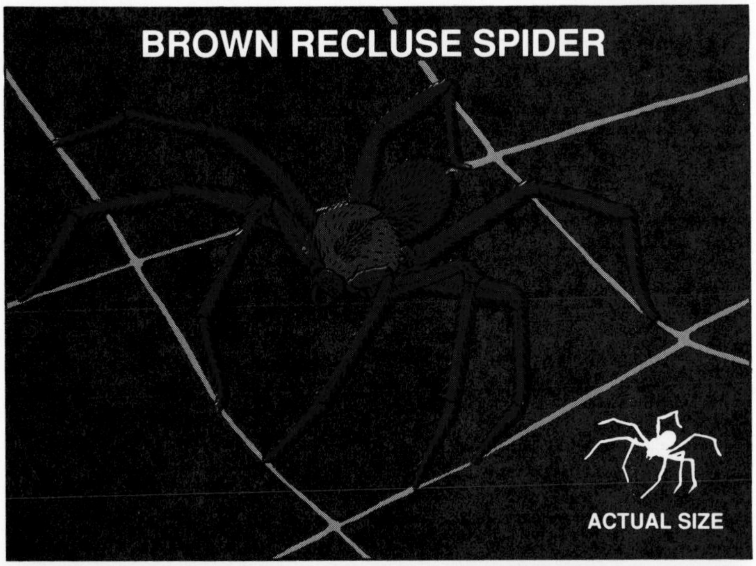

BROWN RECLUSE SPIDER

ACTUAL SIZE

SIGNS & SYMPTOMS

The bite may be hardly noticed, but hours later severe pain, swelling and blisters occur.

WHAT TO DO

Follow first aid for **BLACK WIDOW, page 140.**

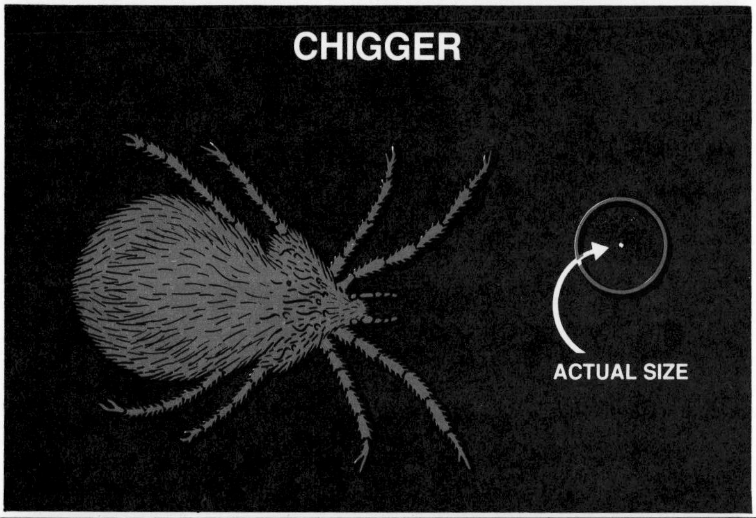

CHIGGER

ACTUAL SIZE

SIGNS & SYMPTOMS

Itching. Irritation. Local pain. Small red welts.

WHAT TO DO

Wash with soap and water. Soothe irritation with cold compresses or calamine lotion.

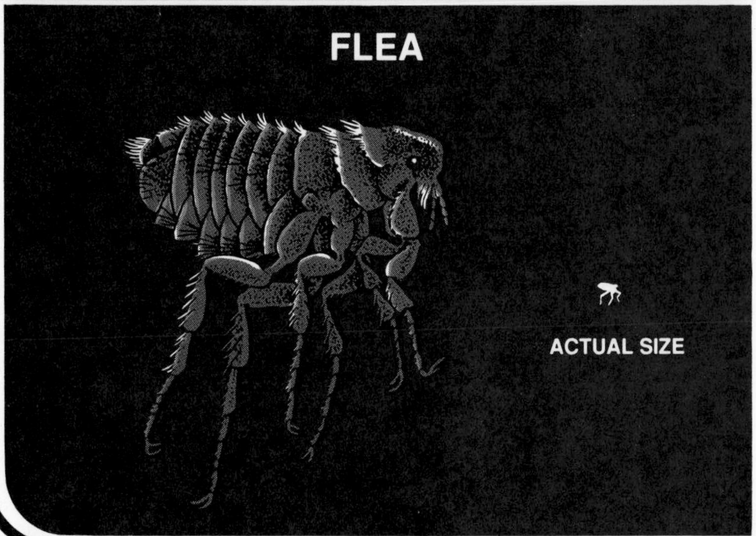

FLEA

ACTUAL SIZE

SIGNS & SYMPTOMS

Itching. Irritation. Local pain. Small red welts.

WHAT TO DO

Wash with soap and water. Soothe irritation with cold compresses or calamine lotion.

CONTINUED ON NEXT PAGE

INSECTS
CONTINUED

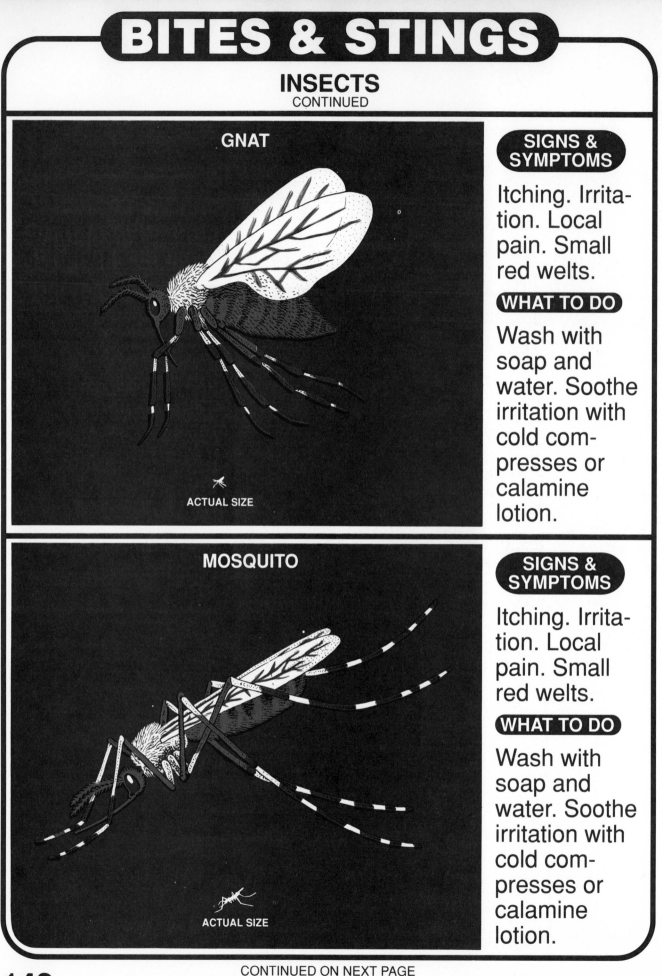

GNAT

ACTUAL SIZE

SIGNS & SYMPTOMS

Itching. Irritation. Local pain. Small red welts.

WHAT TO DO

Wash with soap and water. Soothe irritation with cold compresses or calamine lotion.

MOSQUITO

ACTUAL SIZE

SIGNS & SYMPTOMS

Itching. Irritation. Local pain. Small red welts.

WHAT TO DO

Wash with soap and water. Soothe irritation with cold compresses or calamine lotion.

CONTINUED ON NEXT PAGE

INSECTS
CONTINUED

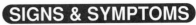

SCORPION

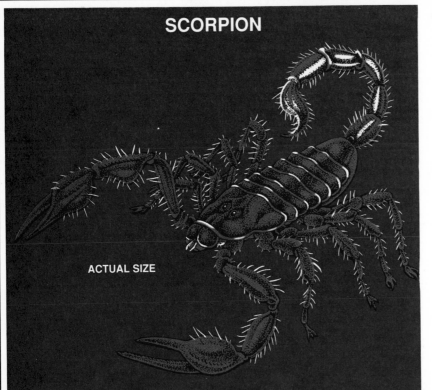

ACTUAL SIZE

SIGNS & SYMPTOMS

Excruciating pain at the sting. Swelling. Fever. Nausea. Stomach pains. Difficulty speaking. Worsening convulsions. Coma.

WHAT TO DO

Follow first aid for **BLACK WIDOW,** page 140.

TARANTULA

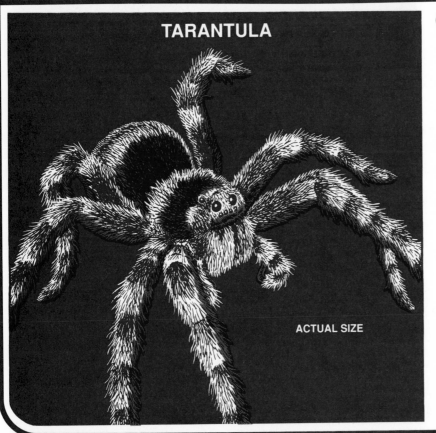

ACTUAL SIZE

SIGNS & SYMPTOMS

May vary from pinprick to severe wound.

WHAT TO DO

Wash with soap and water. Cover lightly with a sterile dressing or clean cloth. For severe reactions, follow first aid for **BLACK WIDOW,** page 140.

CONTINUED ON NEXT PAGE

INSECTS
CONTINUED

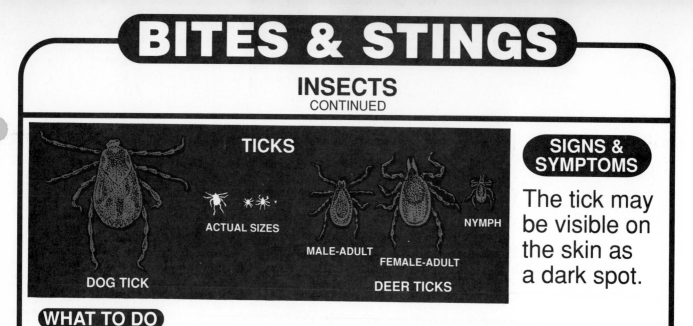

TICKS

ACTUAL SIZES

NYMPH

MALE-ADULT

FEMALE-ADULT

DOG TICK

DEER TICKS

SIGNS & SYMPTOMS

The tick may be visible on the skin as a dark spot.

WHAT TO DO

Do not try to burn the tick off. Grab the tick by the head with tweezers and slowly pull it straight out, taking care not to leave any of the mouth parts behind. Tape the tick to a card and write down the current date in case it has to be examined later. Clean the bite with an antiseptic, rubbing alcohol or soap and water. Get medical help if parts of the tick remain embedded. Ticks can transmit Lyme disease, Rocky Mountain spotted fever and other serious diseases. **Seek medical aid immediately** if over the next days or months the child develops any of the following signs and symptoms: rash, fever, chills, headache, swollen glands, stiff neck, fatigue, restlessness, muscle and joint pains, dizziness, loss of appetite, swelling around the eyes or on the inner eyelids, measles-like spots on the palms and soles, swollen hands and feet. The best way for your child to protect himself against tick bites is by wearing protective clothing (long sleeve shirts, long pants tucked into thick socks) and insect repellent when walking in the woods during the summer tick season. Light-colored clothing and white socks will make it easier to find any ticks he might have brought back with him. Always check your child for ticks when he returns from the woods. Brush him off with a broom or towel, and comb and brush his hair thoroughly. Teach him not to leave his clothes on the ground when he is camping.

BITES & STINGS

MARINE LIFE

IMPORTANT

- **Seek medical aid immediately. For a serious injury,** call 911 or Operator; see **EMS,** page 272.

- Check the child's ABCs (Airway, Breathing and Circulation); see **CHECKING THE ABCs,** pages 224-232.

- Check for bleeding. If necessary, see **BLEEDING: CUTS & WOUNDS,** pages 156-168. If bleeding is not severe, gently clean the wound and rinse it in salt water.

- Try to determine the cause of the bite and kill the creature if possible so it can be identified later. Be careful not to get bitten or stung yourself.

- Keep the child quiet, offer reassurance and avoid unnecessary movement.

- Remove any items that may restrict circulation.

- Try to keep the affected part below heart level.

- **Do not** give the child any stimulants or unprescribed medication.

- Observe for **SHOCK,** pages 354-356.

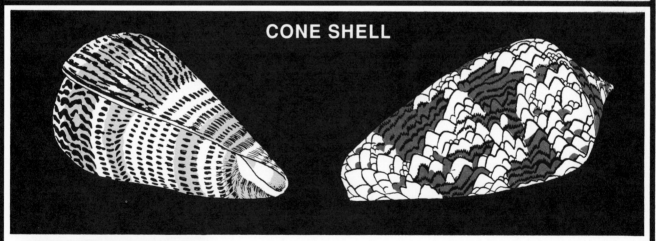

CONE SHELL

SIGNS & SYMPTOMS

Vary from a slight sting to severe pain. Numbness. Tingling. Difficulty swallowing. Tightness in the chest. Partial paralysis. Impaired vision. Collapse.

WHAT TO DO

Soak the wound in hot water or apply hot compresses until pain is relieved.

CONTINUED ON NEXT PAGE

BITES & STINGS

MARINE LIFE
CONTINUED

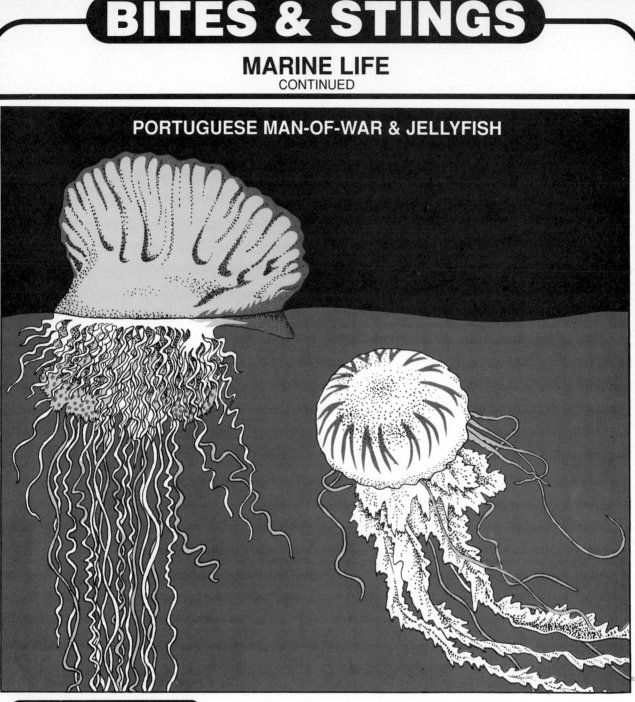

PORTUGUESE MAN-OF-WAR & JELLYFISH

SIGNS & SYMPTOMS

Burning pain. Rash. Swelling. Difficulty breathing. Cramps. Nausea. Vomiting. Collapse.

WHAT TO DO

Wearing gloves, if possible, gently wipe off the tentacles with a towel or cloth. Rinse the affected area with water or seawater, or apply rubbing alcohol or diluted ammonia until pain subsides.

CONTINUED ON NEXT PAGE

MARINE LIFE
CONTINUED

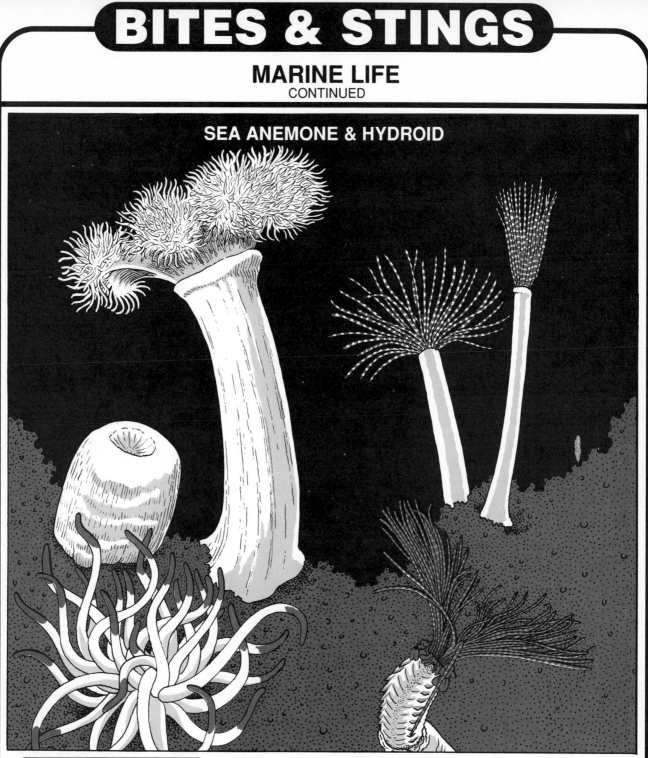

SEA ANEMONE & HYDROID

SIGNS & SYMPTOMS

Burning or stinging pain. Stomach cramps. Chills. Diarrhea.

WHAT TO DO

Gently try to remove the stinger. Wash the affected area with soap and warm water, then soak in hot water or apply hot compresses until pain is relieved.

CONTINUED ON NEXT PAGE

MARINE LIFE
CONTINUED

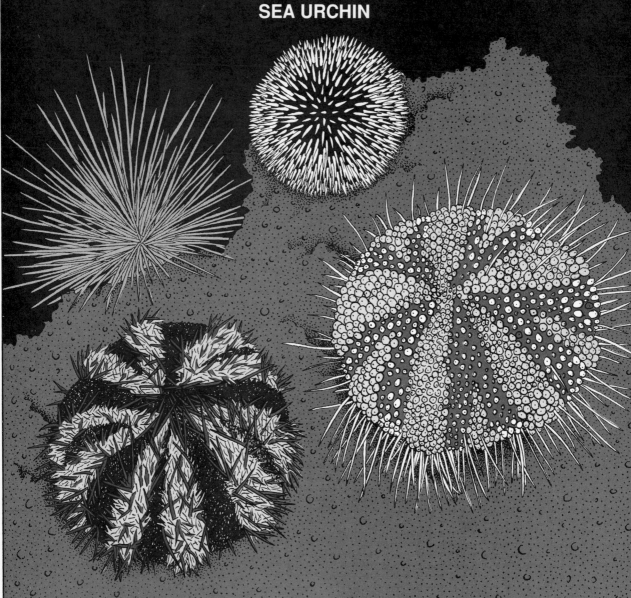

SEA URCHIN

SIGNS & SYMPTOMS

Pain. Dizziness. Muscle tremors. Paralysis.

WHAT TO DO

Gently remove any spines that are not deeply embedded or located near a joint. Wash the affected area with soap and warm water, then soak in hot water or apply hot compresses until pain is relieved.

CONTINUED ON NEXT PAGE

MARINE LIFE
CONTINUED

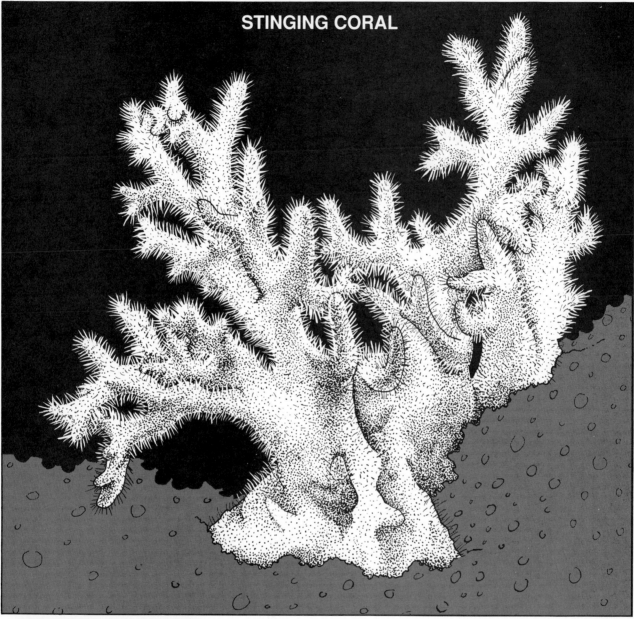

STINGING CORAL

SIGNS & SYMPTOMS

Burning or stinging pain. Sharp cuts.

WHAT TO DO

Wash the affected area with soap and warm water, then soak in hot water or apply hot compresses until pain is relieved. If necessary, treat the cuts; see **BLEEDING: CUTS & WOUNDS,** pages 156-168.

CONTINUED ON NEXT PAGE

MARINE LIFE
CONTINUED

STINGRAY

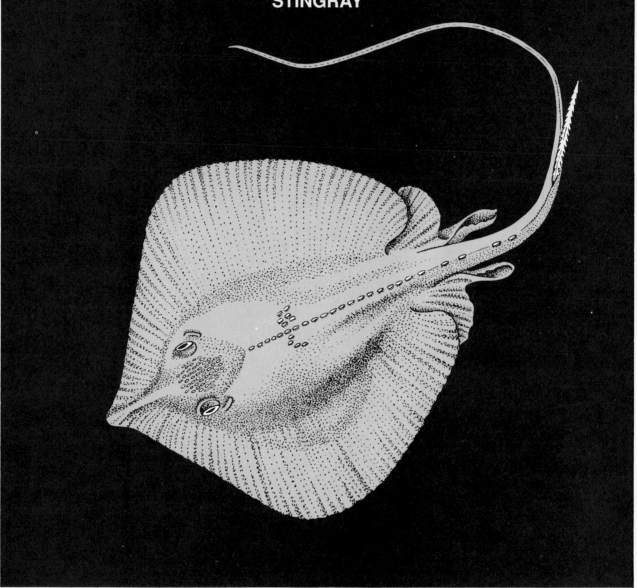

SIGNS & SYMPTOMS

Painful cut or puncture. Swelling. Discoloration. Nausea. Vomiting. Muscle spasms. Convulsions. Difficulty breathing.

WHAT TO DO

Carefully remove the stinger if possible. Rinse the wound in seawater, then soak it in very hot water until pain subsides. Apply a dry dressing.

BITES & STINGS

SNAKEBITE: POISONOUS SNAKE IDENTIFICATION

The main types of poisonous snakes found in the United States are **pit vipers** (**rattlesnakes, copperheads,** and **cottonmouths,** which are also known as **water moccasins**) and **coral snakes.**

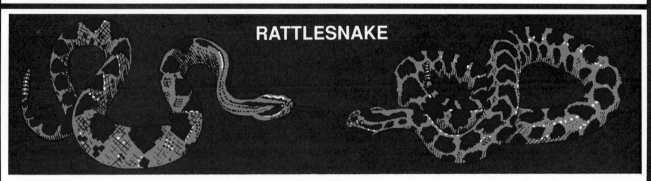

RATTLESNAKE

Habitat: Found throughout the United States.

Appearance: Like other pit vipers, has a triangular head, deep poison pits between its nostrils and slitlike eyes, and 2 long fangs. Easily identified by the distinctive rattles at the end of its tail, which produce a sound like escaping steam before the snake strikes.

Length: Up to 8 feet.

Behavior: May strike without provocation. Able to bite deeply. May leave visible puncture wounds and teeth marks.

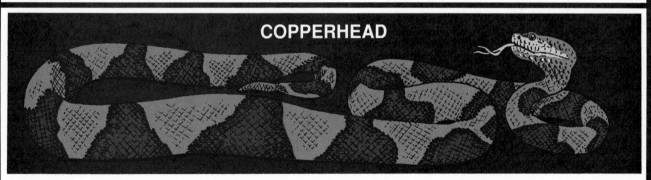

COPPERHEAD

Habitat: Mainly found in the southeast and south-central parts of the United States.

Appearance: Like other pit vipers, has a triangular head, deep poison pits between its nostrils and slitlike eyes, and 2 long fangs. Its color ranges from pink to copper red to brown, with darker bands. Has diamond-shaped markings down its back.

Length: Up to 4 feet.

Behavior: May strike without provocation. Able to bite deeply. May leave visible puncture wounds and teeth marks.

CONTINUED ON NEXT PAGE

SNAKEBITE: POISONOUS SNAKE IDENTIFICATION
CONTINUED

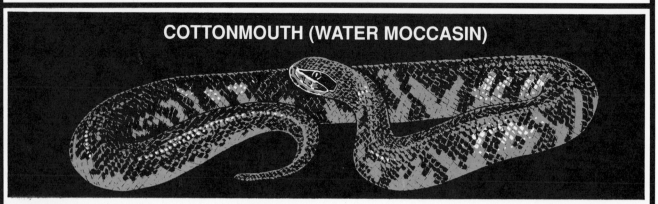

COTTONMOUTH (WATER MOCCASIN)

Habitat: Mainly found in the southeast and south-central parts of the United States.

Appearance: Like other pit vipers, has a triangular head, deep poison pits between its nostrils and slitlike eyes, and 2 long fangs. Its color ranges from olive to brown to black, with a lighter underside. Its mouth is bordered with dark bands and lined with white.

Length: Up to 4 feet.

Behavior: May strike without provocation. Able to bite deeply. May leave visible puncture wounds and teeth marks.

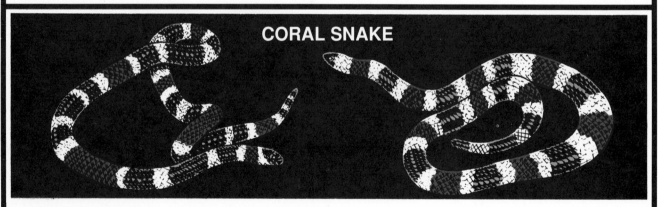

CORAL SNAKE

Habitat: Mainly found in the southeast.

Appearance: Has rounded eyes and a black nose. Colored with bright red, yellow (or white) and black bands. The yellow (or white) bands are narrow and always come between the red and the black.

Length: Up to 3 feet.

Behavior: Usually only strikes when provoked. Because of its short fangs and small mouth it only bites at small targets such as fingers and toes. Leaves teeth marks that look like small, bloody scratches, sometimes without visible fang punctures.

BITES & STINGS

SNAKEBITE: FIRST AID

IMPORTANT

- **Seek medical aid for any suspected snakebite.**
- Calm and reassure the child.
- Remove any constricting items around the affected area; snakebites swell.
- **Do not** cut through a snakebite and draw out the venom unless you are trained in the procedure and are more than several hours away from medical aid.
- **Do not** apply a constricting band around the bite unless you are trained in the procedure.
- **Before administering first aid, try to identify the snake and determine whether it is poisonous or non-poisonous;** see pages 151-152. Most snakes found in the United States are non-poisonous.

SIGNS & SYMPTOMS OF POISONOUS SNAKEBITE

Mild to moderate: Pain. Swelling. Discolored skin. Dizziness. Nausea. Drowsiness. Sweating. Headache. Drooling. Thirst. Weakness. **Severe:** Slurred speech. Blurred vision. Severe nausea. Vomiting. Difficulty breathing. Shock. Delirium. Paralysis. Convulsions. **May progress to:** Unconsciousness. No breathing or circulation.

SIGNS & SYMPTOMS OF NON-POISONOUS SNAKEBITE

Swelling. Itching.

IF THE SNAKE IS POISONOUS OR YOU ARE NOT ABSOLUTELY CERTAIN THAT IT ISN'T

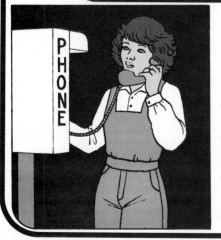

1 **Seek medical aid immediately.** If possible, call 911 or Operator; see **EMS,** page 272. If that isn't possible, transport the child to a hospital emergency room yourself; see **TRANSPORTING THE INJURED,** pages 377-380. Try to call ahead so the appropriate antivenin will be waiting.

CONTINUED ON NEXT PAGE

CONTINUED ON NEXT PAGE

153

SNAKEBITE: FIRST AID
CONTINUED

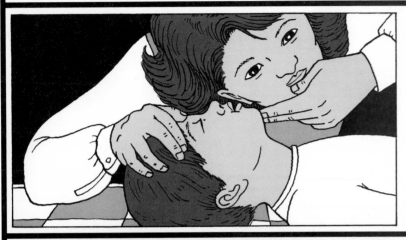

2 Keep a close watch over the child's ABCs (Airway, Breathing and Circulation); see **CHECKING THE ABCs,** pages 224-232.

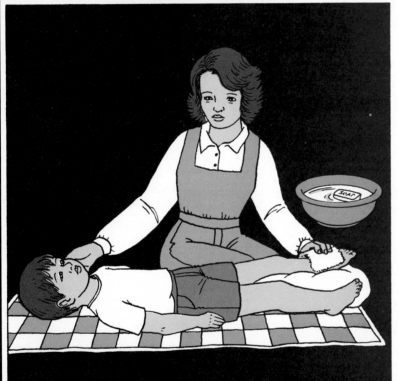

3 Keep the affected part at heart level until medical aid is obtained. Wash the wound with soap and water, but **do not** apply cold compresses or pack in ice. **Do not** let the child walk or move the affected part unless absolutely necessary. Try to keep him warm. **Do not** give him any food, drink or medication.

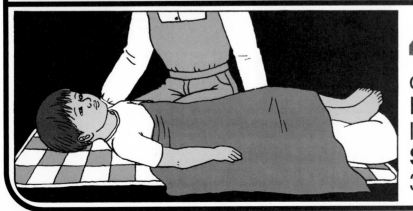

4 Continue to monitor the child's ABCs (Airway, Breathing and Circulation). Observe for **SHOCK;** see pages 354-356.

CONTINUED ON NEXT PAGE

SNAKEBITE: FIRST AID
CONTINUED

IF THE SNAKE IS NON-POISONOUS

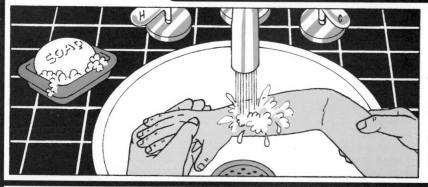

1 Wash the wound thoroughly with soap and water, and bandage if necessary.

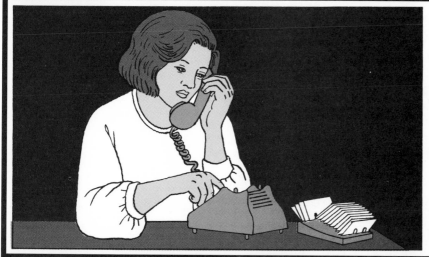

2 Consult your doctor as soon as possible to determine if further treatment is required and to make sure the child's tetanus immunization is still current.

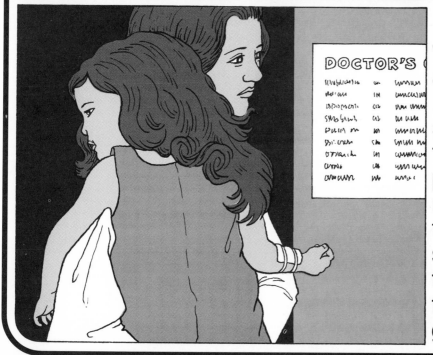

3 **Seek medical aid immediately** if any signs of infection develop, such as increased tenderness and pain after 24 hours, redness, swelling, throbbing, pus, red streaks leading from the wound, fever or swollen glands.

155

DIRECT PRESSURE

IMPORTANT

- **Seek medical aid for any serious bleeding. For a serious injury,** call 911 or Operator; see **EMS,** page 272.

- Wash your hands thoroughly both before and after administering first aid. If possible, put on sterile latex gloves, especially if **you** have any open sores, cuts or wounds. If gloves aren't available, place several layers of dressing between you and the wound.

- **Do not** apply direct pressure on breaks, injuries to the eye or head, or wounds that contain embedded objects.

- **Do not** probe or try to pull an embedded object from a wound.

- **Do not** try to clean a large wound, even after bleeding has been controlled.

- **Do not** try to remove a dressing that has become soaked with blood. Place a fresh dressing on top of it.

- Calm and reassure the child while administering first aid.

- Observe for **SHOCK,** pages 354-356.

- **Seek medical aid immediately** if any signs of infection develop, such as increased tenderness or pain after 24 hours, redness, swelling, throbbing, pus, red streaks leading from the wound, fever or swollen glands.

- Check with your doctor to make sure the child's tetanus immunization is still current.

- **FIRST TRY TO CONTROL THE BLEEDING BY DIRECT PRESSURE; SEE NEXT PAGE.**

- **IF THE BLEEDING DOESN'T STOP, USE PRESSURE POINTS WHILE CONTINUING DIRECT PRESSURE; SEE BLEEDING: CUTS & WOUNDS (PRESSURE POINTS), PAGES 159-160.**

- **ONLY IF SERIOUS BLOOD LOSS CONTINUES AND BECOMES CRITICAL, APPLY A TOURNIQUET AS A LAST RESORT; SEE BLEEDING: CUTS & WOUNDS (TOURNIQUET), PAGES 161-164.**

CONTINUED ON NEXT PAGE

DIRECT PRESSURE
CONTINUED

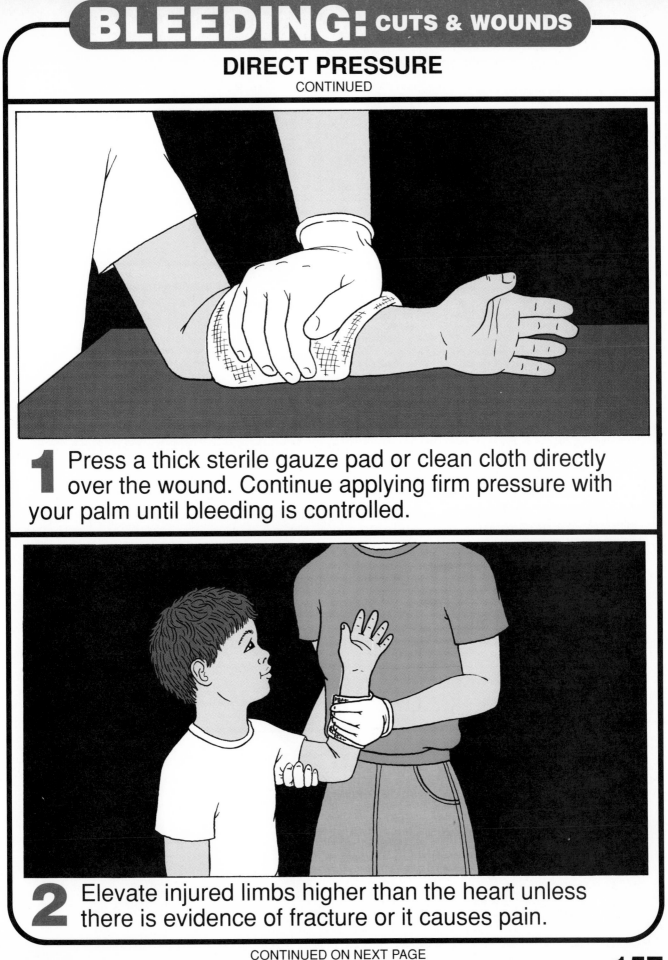

1 Press a thick sterile gauze pad or clean cloth directly over the wound. Continue applying firm pressure with your palm until bleeding is controlled.

2 Elevate injured limbs higher than the heart unless there is evidence of fracture or it causes pain.

CONTINUED ON NEXT PAGE

DIRECT PRESSURE
CONTINUED

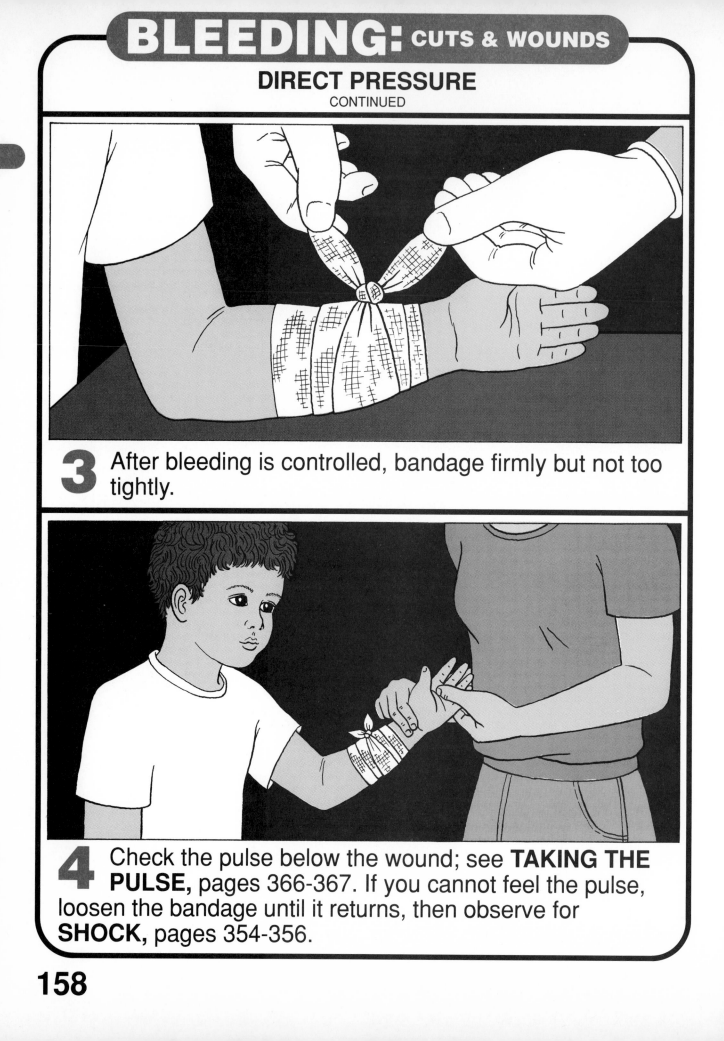

3 After bleeding is controlled, bandage firmly but not too tightly.

4 Check the pulse below the wound; see **TAKING THE PULSE,** pages 366-367. If you cannot feel the pulse, loosen the bandage until it returns, then observe for **SHOCK,** pages 354-356.

PRESSURE POINTS

IMPORTANT

- **Seek medical aid for any serious bleeding. For a serious injury,** call 911 or Operator; see **EMS,** page 272.

- Observe for **SHOCK,** pages 354-356.

- **IF BLEEDING DOESN'T STOP WITH DIRECT PRESSURE, PAGES 156-158, TRY TO CONTROL IT WITH PRESSURE POINTS WHILE CONTINUING DIRECT PRESSURE.**

- **ONLY IF SERIOUS BLOOD LOSS CONTINUES AND BECOMES CRITICAL, APPLY A TOURNIQUET AS A LAST RESORT; SEE PAGES 161-164.**

ARM

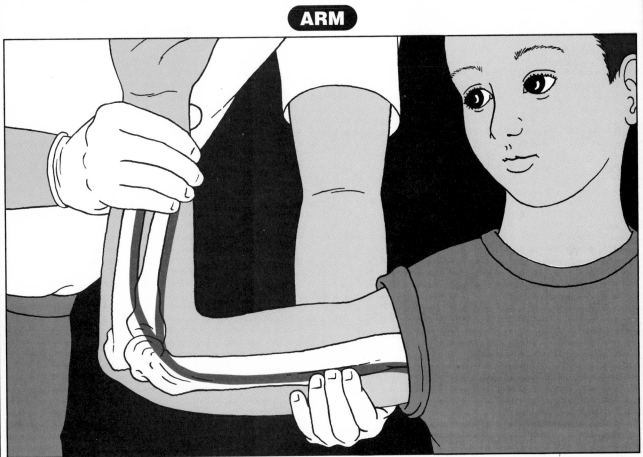

Elevate the injured arm higher than the heart unless there is evidence of fracture. Place your fingers on the inner side of the arm, pressing in the groove between the muscles. Keeping your thumb on the outside of the arm, compress toward the bone until bleeding stops.

CONTINUED ON NEXT PAGE

PRESSURE POINTS
CONTINUED

LEG

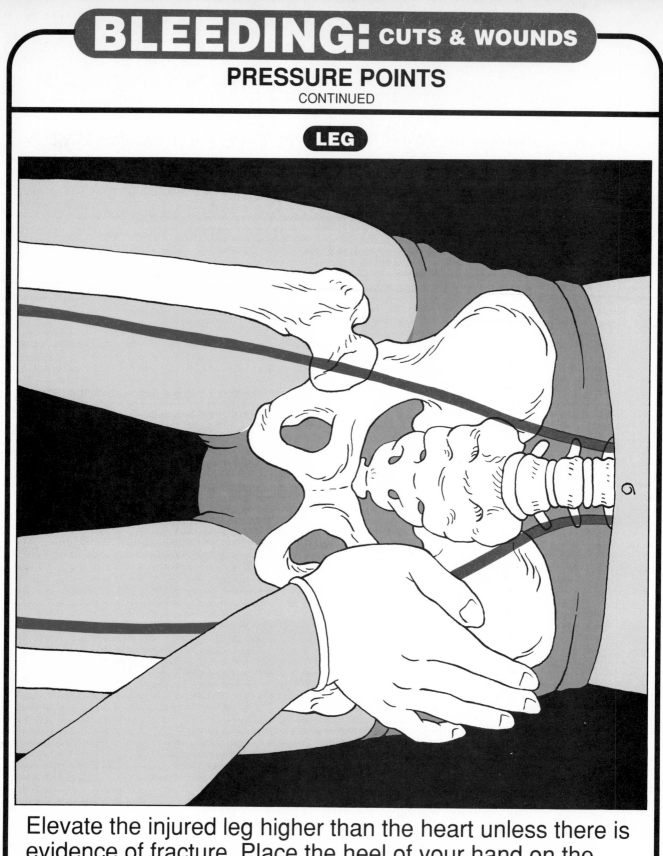

Elevate the injured leg higher than the heart unless there is evidence of fracture. Place the heel of your hand on the inner thigh at the midpoint of the crease of the groin. With your arm straight and your elbow locked, press down against the bone until bleeding stops.

TOURNIQUET

IMPORTANT

- **Seek medical aid immediately.** Call 911 or Operator; see **EMS,** page 272.

- **Use of a tourniquet may lead to later amputation of the limb. Do not use except in a critical emergency where all other methods fail to control serious bleeding and it is a matter of life and death. First try direct pressure and pressure points; see BLEEDING: CUTS & WOUNDS (DIRECT PRESSURE), pages 156-158, and BLEEDING: CUTS & WOUNDS (PRESSURE POINTS), pages 159-160.**

- **The tourniquet band should be at least 2 inches wide.**

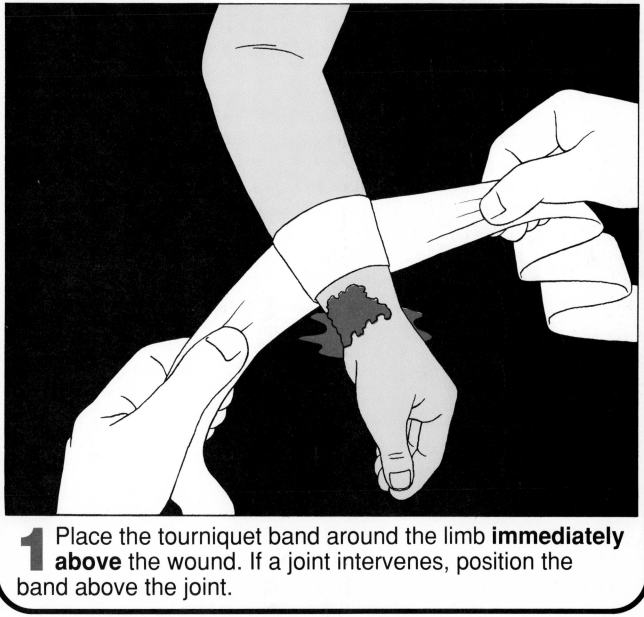

1 Place the tourniquet band around the limb **immediately above** the wound. If a joint intervenes, position the band above the joint.

CONTINUED ON NEXT PAGE

TOURNIQUET
CONTINUED

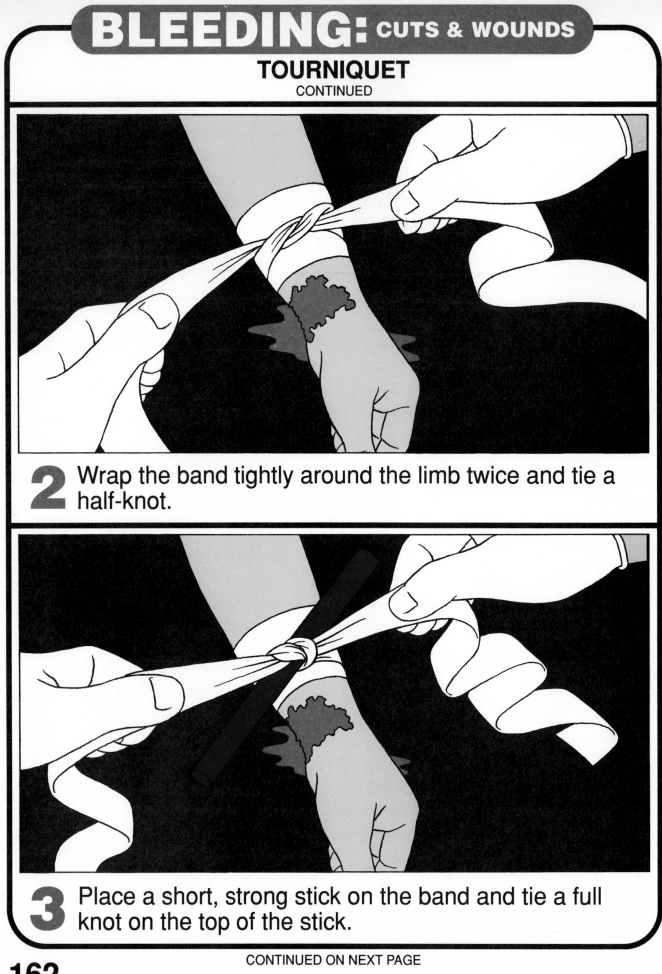

2 Wrap the band tightly around the limb twice and tie a half-knot.

3 Place a short, strong stick on the band and tie a full knot on the top of the stick.

CONTINUED ON NEXT PAGE

TOURNIQUET
CONTINUED

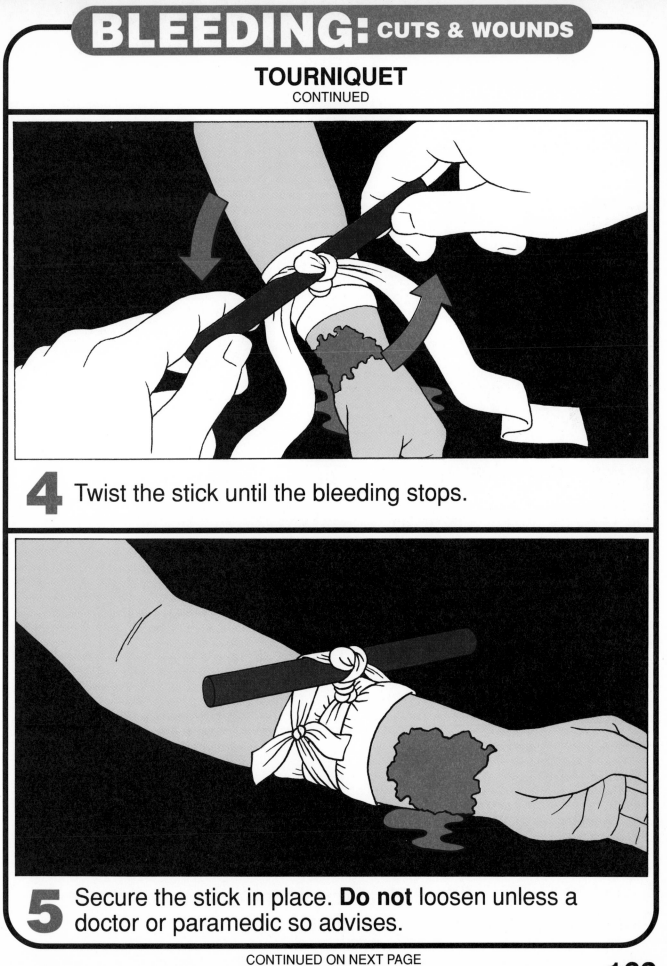

4 Twist the stick until the bleeding stops.

5 Secure the stick in place. **Do not** loosen unless a doctor or paramedic so advises.

CONTINUED ON NEXT PAGE

TOURNIQUET
CONTINUED

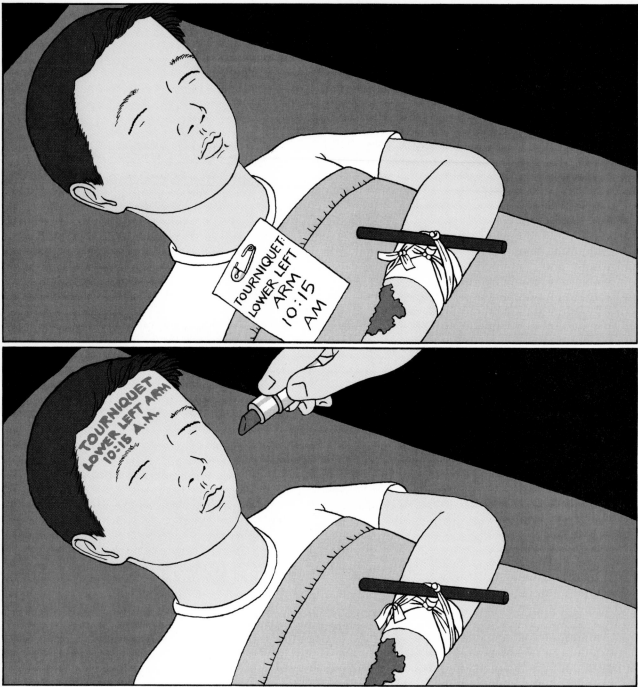

6 Write down the location of the tourniquet and the exact time it was applied. Attach it as a note to the child's clothing or write it on his forehead with lipstick, etc. Treat for **SHOCK,** pages 354-356, and **get to the hospital immediately. Do not** cover the tourniquet.

LACERATIONS

IMPORTANT

- **Seek medical aid for any serious bleeding. For a serious injury,** call 911 or Operator; see **EMS,** page 272.

- **Seek medical aid** for lacerations on the neck or the palms of the hand, or if caused by a dirty object.

- **Seek medical aid** if any foreign material is embedded in the wound. **Do not** try to remove it yourself.

- **Wash your hands thoroughly** both before and after administering first aid. If possible, put on sterile latex gloves, especially if **you** have any open sores, cuts or wounds. If gloves aren't available, place several layers of dressing between you and the wound.

- **Do not** try to clean a severe wound, even after bleeding has been controlled.

- **Do not** probe or breathe on the wound.

- **Do not** try to push back exposed or protruding body parts. Cover them with sterile material and call EMS.

- **Do not** apply ointments or other medications unless your doctor so advises.

- **Do not** try to remove a dressing that has become soaked with blood. Place a fresh dressing on top of it.

- Observe for **SHOCK,** pages 354-356.

- **Seek medical aid immediately** if any signs of infection develop, such as increased tenderness and pain after 24 hours, redness, swelling, throbbing, pus, red streaks leading from the wound, fever or swollen glands.

- Check with your doctor to make sure the child's tetanus immunization is still current.

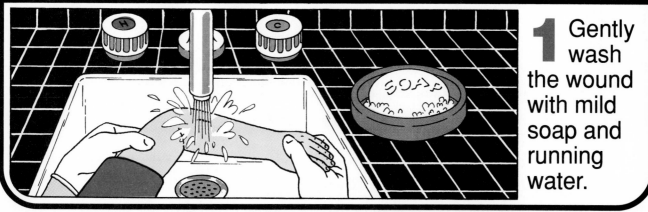

1 Gently wash the wound with mild soap and running water.

CONTINUED ON NEXT PAGE

LACERATIONS
CONTINUED

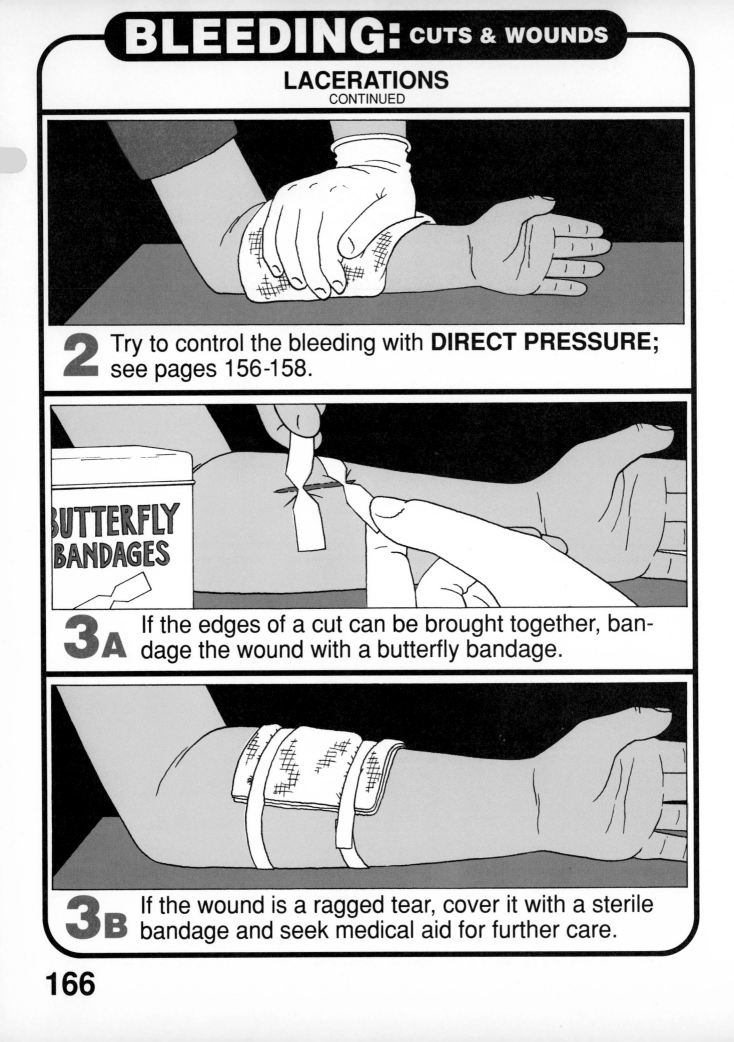

2 Try to control the bleeding with **DIRECT PRESSURE**; see pages 156-158.

3A If the edges of a cut can be brought together, bandage the wound with a butterfly bandage.

3B If the wound is a ragged tear, cover it with a sterile bandage and seek medical aid for further care.

BLEEDING: CUTS & WOUNDS

PUNCTURE WOUNDS

IMPORTANT

- **Seek medical aid for any serious bleeding. For a serious injury,** call 911 or Operator; see **EMS,** page 272.

- **Seek medical aid immediately** if a puncture caused by a sharp object penetrates a vitally important area, such as the eye, skull, chest, abdomen or a joint.

- **Seek medical aid immediately** if the puncture is caused by an impaled object; see **IMPALED OBJECTS,** pages 171-172.

- **Seek medical aid immediately** if it seems likely that dirt, bacteria or any other potentially harmful material is lodged in the wound, or metal or glass is embedded under the skin.

- **Wash your hands thoroughly** both before and after administering first aid. If possible, put on sterile latex gloves, especially if **you** have any open sores, cuts or wounds. If gloves aren't available, place several layers of dressing between you and the wound.

- **Do not** try to clean a severe puncture wound.

- **Do not** probe or breathe on the wound.

- **Do not** try to push back exposed body parts.

- **Do not** try to remove foreign material from the wound.

- **Do not** apply antibiotic ointments unless a doctor so advises.

- Observe for **SHOCK,** pages 354-356.

- **Seek medical aid immediately** if any signs of infection develop, such as increased tenderness or pain after 24 hours, redness, swelling, throbbing, pus, red streaks leading from the wound, fever or swollen glands.

- Check with your doctor to make sure the child's tetanus immunization is still current.

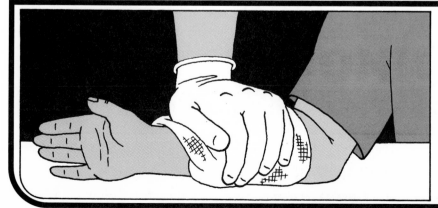

1A **If the wound is bleeding severely,** try to control the bleeding with **DIRECT PRESSURE;** see pages 156-158.

CONTINUED ON NEXT PAGE

BLEEDING: CUTS & WOUNDS

PUNCTURE WOUNDS
CONTINUED

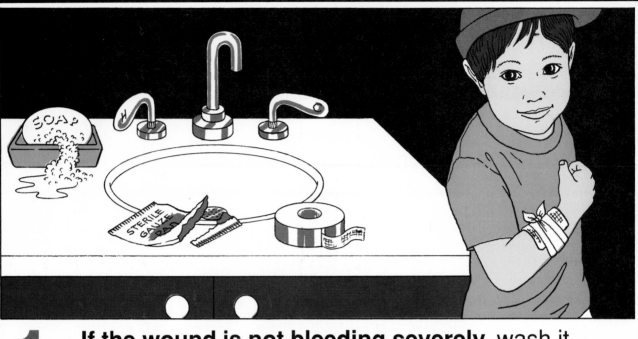

1B **If the wound is not bleeding severely,** wash it thoroughly with soap and water, then bandage with a sterile gauze pad. **Do not** tape the puncture closed.

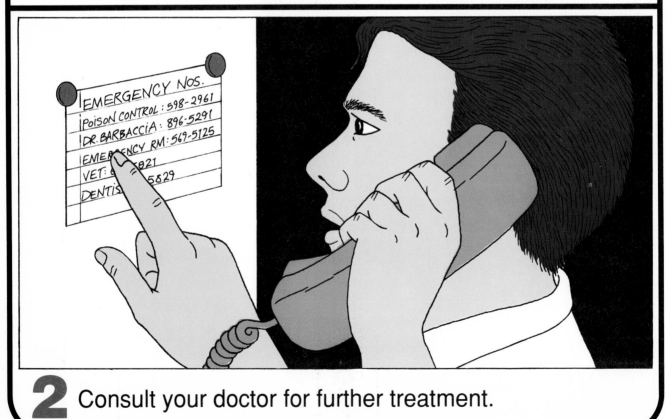

2 Consult your doctor for further treatment.

FISHHOOKS

IMPORTANT

- **Do not** attempt to remove a fishhook from the face or near an artery. **Seek medical aid immediately.**

- Wash your hands thoroughly and, if possible, put on sterile latex gloves before starting first aid.

- **Seek medical aid immediately** if any signs of infection develop, such as increased tenderness or pain after 24 hours, redness, swelling, throbbing, pus, red streaks leading from the wound, fever or swollen glands.

- Check with your doctor to make sure the child's tetanus immunization is still current.

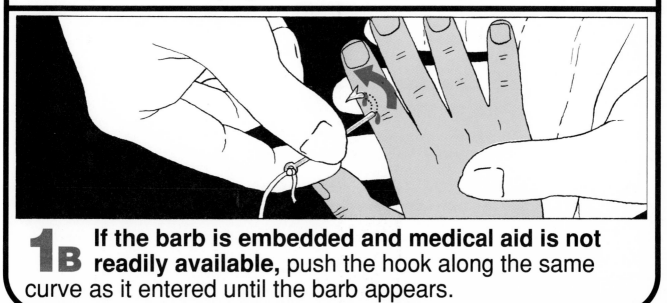

1A **If only the point is in the skin,** gently remove it by backing it out at the same angle it entered. Then go to **Step 4 on next page.**

1B **If the barb is embedded and medical aid is not readily available,** push the hook along the same curve as it entered until the barb appears.

CONTINUED ON NEXT PAGE

FISHHOOKS
CONTINUED

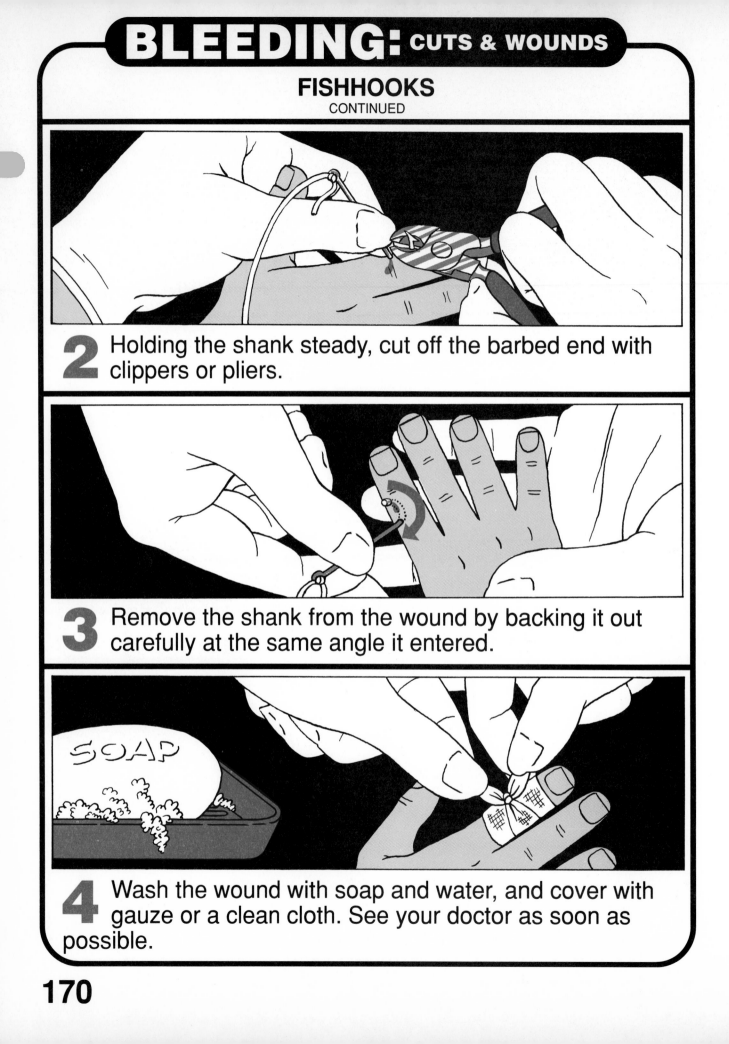

2 Holding the shank steady, cut off the barbed end with clippers or pliers.

3 Remove the shank from the wound by backing it out carefully at the same angle it entered.

4 Wash the wound with soap and water, and cover with gauze or a clean cloth. See your doctor as soon as possible.

IMPALED OBJECTS

IMPORTANT

- **Call for an ambulance** (dial 911 or Operator; see **EMS,** page 272) **or get to a hospital immediately.** If necessary, see **TRANSPORTING THE INJURED: PULLS, CARRIES & STRETCHERS,** pages 377-380.

- **Do not** move or remove the impaled object.

- **Do not** try to cut it off unless it is absolutely necessary in order to transport the child to the hospital.

- **Do not** move a child off an impaling object unless her life is in imminent danger. If you must, remove her as gently as possible, then tend to her wounds immediately and treat for **SHOCK,** pages 354-356.

- **Do not** try to clean the wound.

- **Seek medical aid immediately** if any signs of infection develop, such as increased tenderness or pain after 24 hours, redness, swelling, throbbing, pus, red streaks leading from the wound, fever or swollen glands.

- Check with your doctor to make sure the child's tetanus immunization is still current.

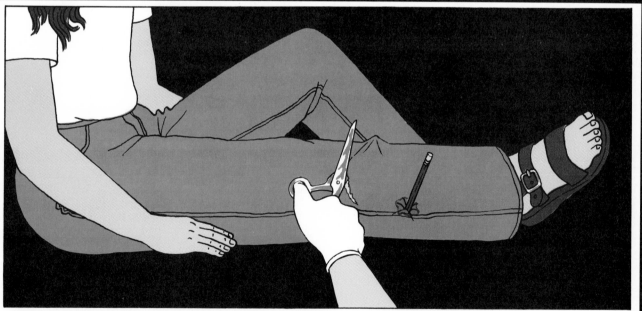

1 Carefully cut away the clothing from around the wound. Wash your hands thoroughly and, if possible, put on sterile latex gloves, then control any serious bleeding with indirect pressure. See **BLEEDING: CUTS & WOUNDS (PRESSURE POINTS),** pages 159-160.

CONTINUED ON NEXT PAGE

IMPALED OBJECTS
CONTINUED

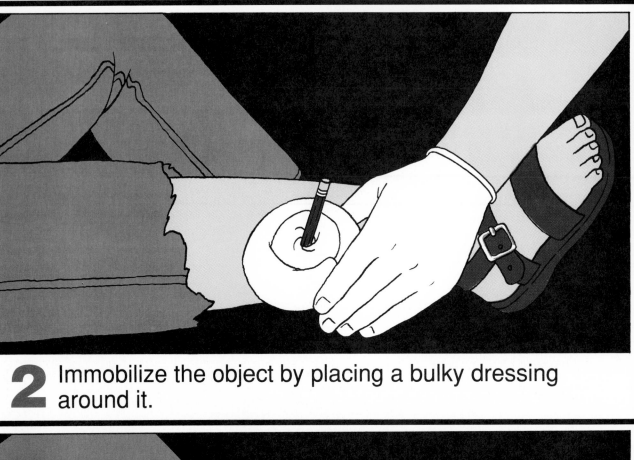

2 Immobilize the object by placing a bulky dressing around it.

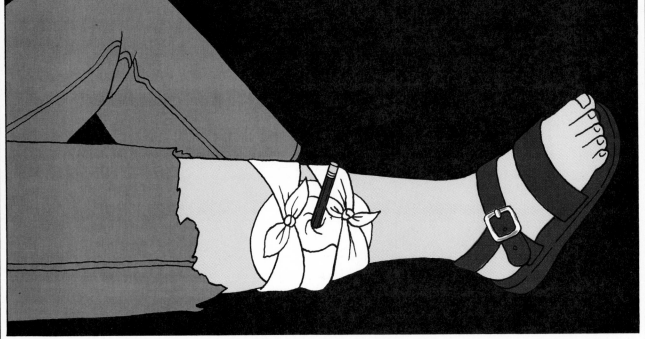

3 Secure the dressing in place with bandages. Treat for **SHOCK,** pages 354-356.

AMPUTATIONS

IMPORTANT

- **Stay calm and act quickly. Bleeding must be stopped as soon as possible.**

- **Seek medical aid immediately.** Call 911 or Operator; see **EMS**, page 272.

- Check the child's ABCs (Airway, Breathing and Circulation); see **CHECKING THE ABCs,** pages 224-232.

- Calm and reassure the child.

- Wash your hands thoroughly and, if possible, put on sterile latex gloves before starting first aid.

- **Do not** put severed parts in water, alcohol or any other liquid. Avoid freezing.

- Check with your doctor to make sure the child's tetanus immunization is still current.

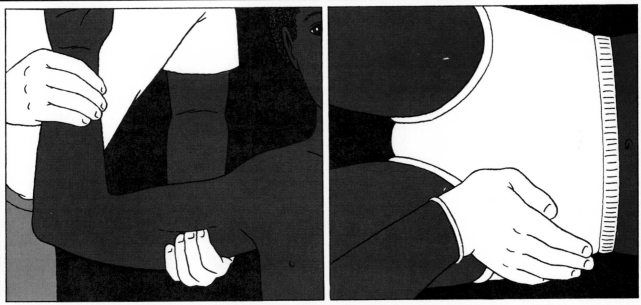

1 Control the bleeding through direct pressure and pressure points; see **BLEEDING: CUTS & WOUNDS (DIRECT PRESSURE),** pages 156-158, and **BLEEDING: CUTS & WOUNDS (PRESSURE POINTS),** pages 159-160. As a last resort, a tourniquet may be necessary; see **BLEEDING: CUTS & WOUNDS (TOURNIQUET),** pages 161-164.

CONTINUED ON NEXT PAGE

AMPUTATIONS
CONTINUED

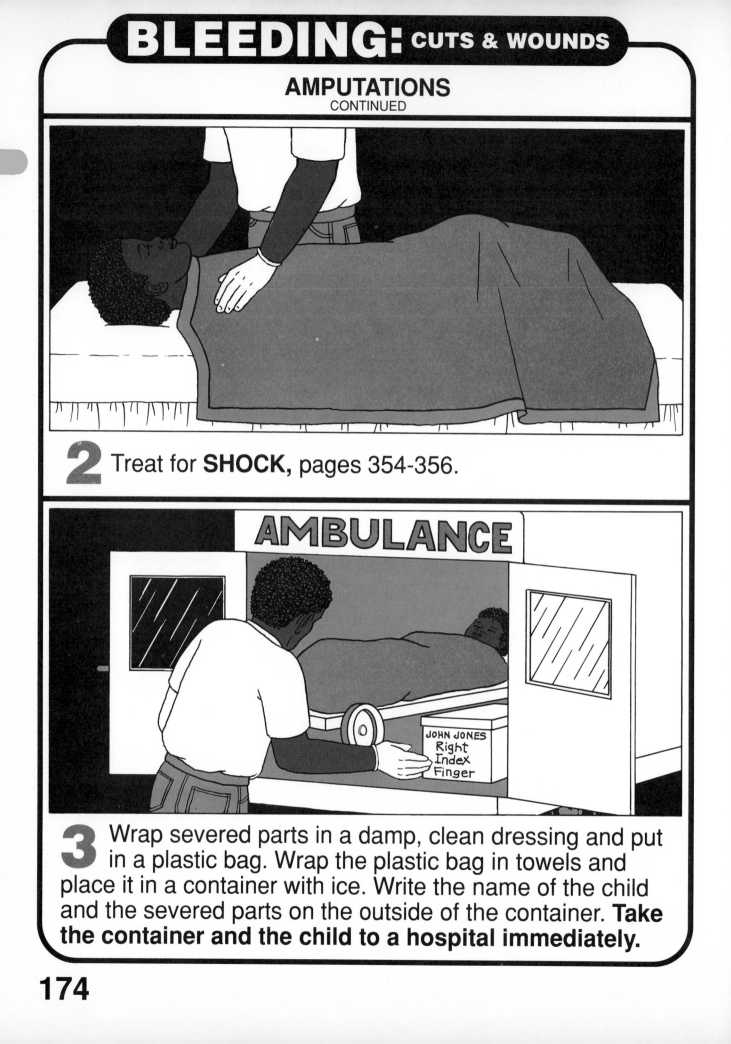

2 Treat for **SHOCK,** pages 354-356.

3 Wrap severed parts in a damp, clean dressing and put in a plastic bag. Wrap the plastic bag in towels and place it in a container with ice. Write the name of the child and the severed parts on the outside of the container. **Take the container and the child to a hospital immediately.**

INTERNAL BLEEDING

IMPORTANT

- To be suspected if the child has had a sharp blow or crushing injury to the abdomen, chest or torso. Symptoms may not appear until days or weeks later.

- **Seek medical aid immediately.** Call 911 or Operator; see **EMS,** page 272.

- Check the child's ABCs (Airway, Breathing and Circulation); see **CHECKING THE ABCs,** pages 224-232.

- **Do not** give the child anything to eat or drink.

- Check for other injuries.

SIGNS & SYMPTOMS

Stomach: Vomit is bright red, dark red or the color and size of large coffee grounds. (Save a sample for later examination.)
Intestines: Excrement contains dark tar-like material or bright red blood.
Chest and Lungs: Bright red foamy blood is coughed up.
May also include: Paleness. Cold, clammy skin. Rapid but weak pulse. Swollen abdomen. Thirst. Lightheadedness. Restlessness. Anxiety. Disorientation.

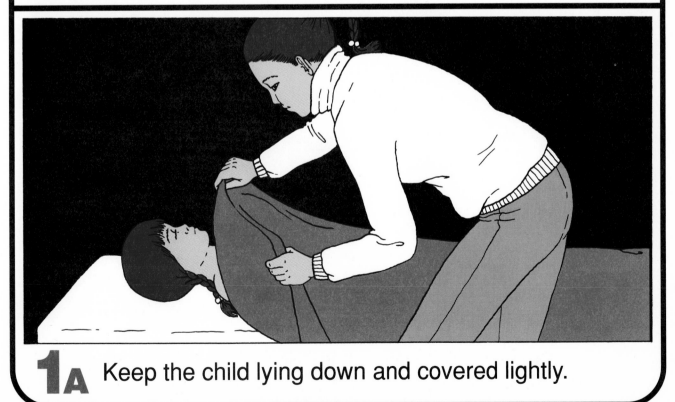

1A Keep the child lying down and covered lightly.

CONTINUED ON NEXT PAGE

INTERNAL BLEEDING
CONTINUED

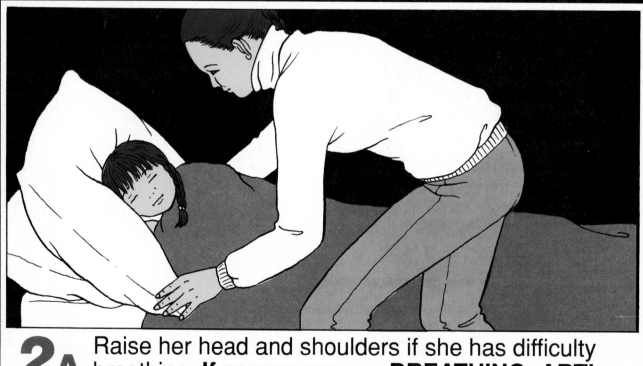

1B **If she is nauseous or likely to vomit,** turn her to one side to keep the airway clear. **If a chest injury is suspected,** place the injured side down.

2A Raise her head and shoulders if she has difficulty breathing. **If necessary,** see **BREATHING: ARTIFICIAL RESPIRATION,** pages 201-215.

CONTINUED ON NEXT PAGE

INTERNAL BLEEDING
CONTINUED

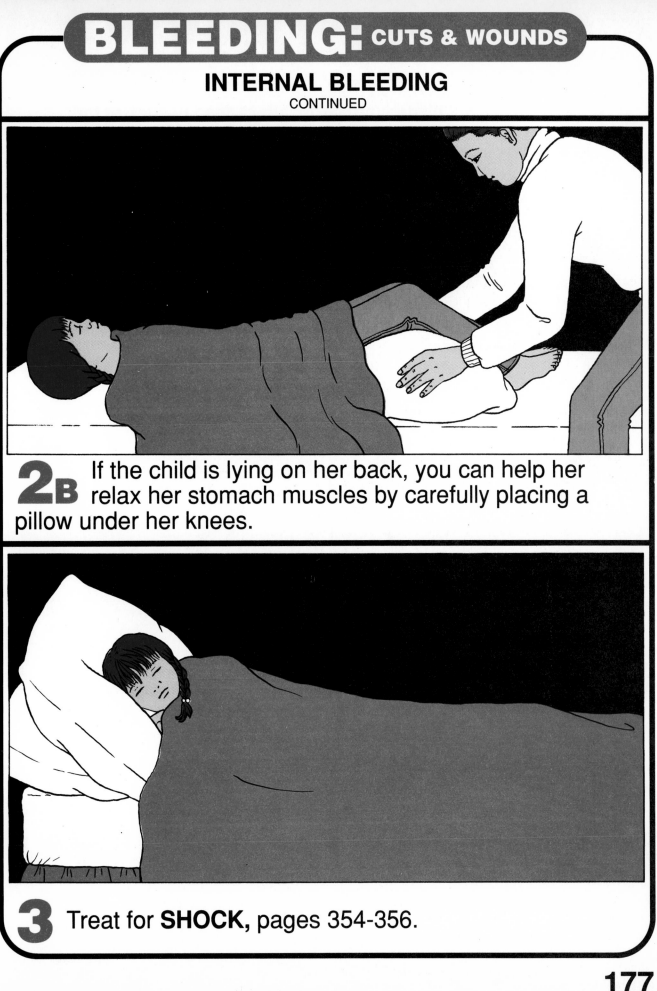

2B If the child is lying on her back, you can help her relax her stomach muscles by carefully placing a pillow under her knees.

3 Treat for **SHOCK,** pages 354-356.

BLISTERS

- **Seek medical aid if blisters are large, affect deep tissues of the hands or soles of the feet, cover a large portion of the body or become infected.**

- **Do not** break or open blisters caused by burns, frostbite or irritation from insect bites, poison ivy or heat rash.

- **Do not** break any blister unless absolutely necessary, as in the case of hiking or walking long distances.

- Wash your hands thoroughly and, if possible, put on sterile latex gloves before beginning first aid.

SIGNS & SYMPTOMS

A well-defined cushion-like raised area filled with clear fluid. May be uncomfortable or painful, particularly if broken.

IF THE BLISTER IS UNBROKEN

Try to keep the blister from breaking by improvising a protective shield: Cut a hole in the center of several gauze pads slightly larger than the affected area. Place the hole in each pad over the blister, taking care not to touch the blister. Add sufficient layers to protect the blister from contact, then cover the opening with a pad fastened loosely in place with adhesive tape. If possible, try to keep the child from using the affected area.

CONTINUED ON NEXT PAGE

IF YOU MUST BREAK THE BLISTER

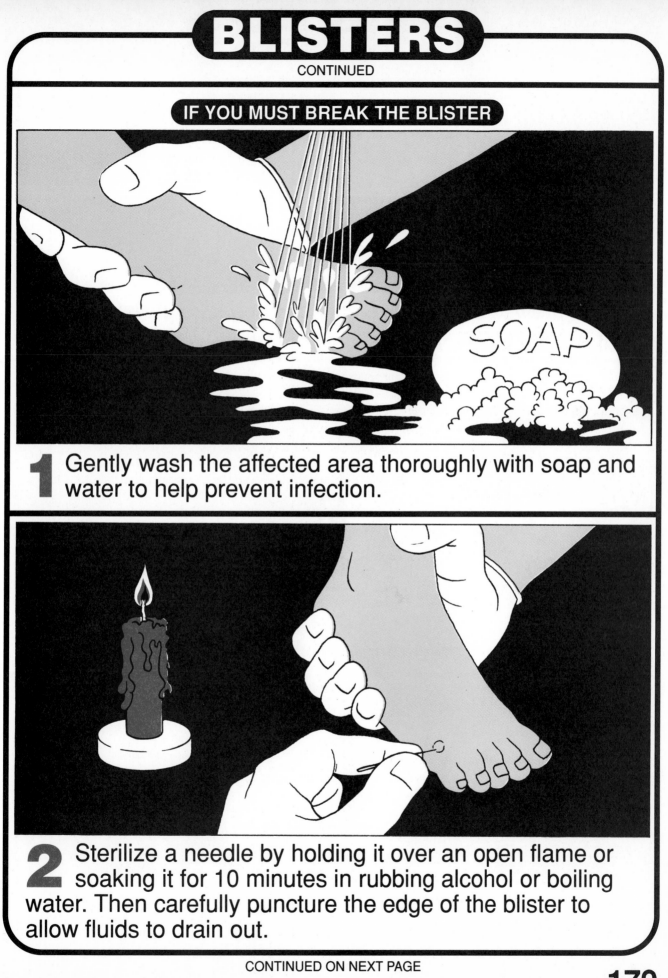

1 Gently wash the affected area thoroughly with soap and water to help prevent infection.

2 Sterilize a needle by holding it over an open flame or soaking it for 10 minutes in rubbing alcohol or boiling water. Then carefully puncture the edge of the blister to allow fluids to drain out.

CONTINUED ON NEXT PAGE

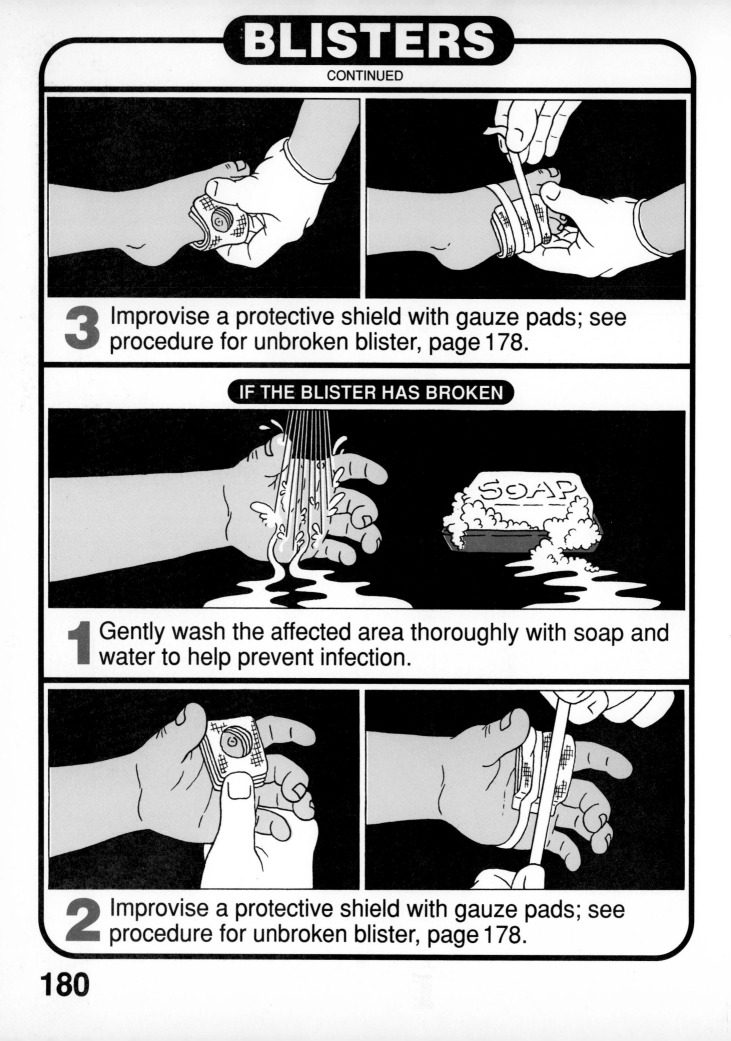

3 Improvise a protective shield with gauze pads; see procedure for unbroken blister, page 178.

IF THE BLISTER HAS BROKEN

1 Gently wash the affected area thoroughly with soap and water to help prevent infection.

2 Improvise a protective shield with gauze pads; see procedure for unbroken blister, page 178.

IMPORTANT

- **Seek medical aid, particularly if the central area of the face, underarm or groin is affected, or if the boils spread, form clusters (carbuncles) or keep recurring.**

- **Do not** puncture or squeeze boils.

- Wash your hands thoroughly and, if possible, put on sterile latex gloves before starting first aid.

SIGNS & SYMPTOMS

An abscess caused by inflamed and infected hair follicles. Usually take 3 to 5 days to develop. Commonly occur on the face, neck, chest or buttocks. Itching. Redness. Tenderness or acute pain. Possible throbbing. May come to a head, open and drain a mixture of pus and blood. **In severe cases:** May spread and form clusters. Chills. Fever.

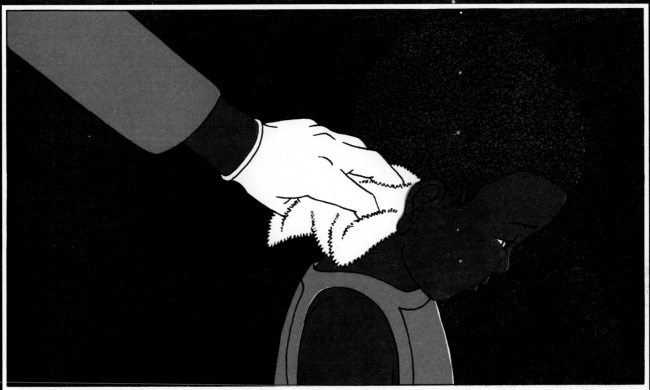

1 Apply hot wet compresses to affected area for 10 minutes, 3 to 4 times a day. Between compresses, prevent pressure or friction by covering the affected area with a gauze pad or clean cloth loosely fastened in place with adhesive tape. Continue until the boil comes to a head, opens by itself and begins to drain.

CONTINUED ON NEXT PAGE

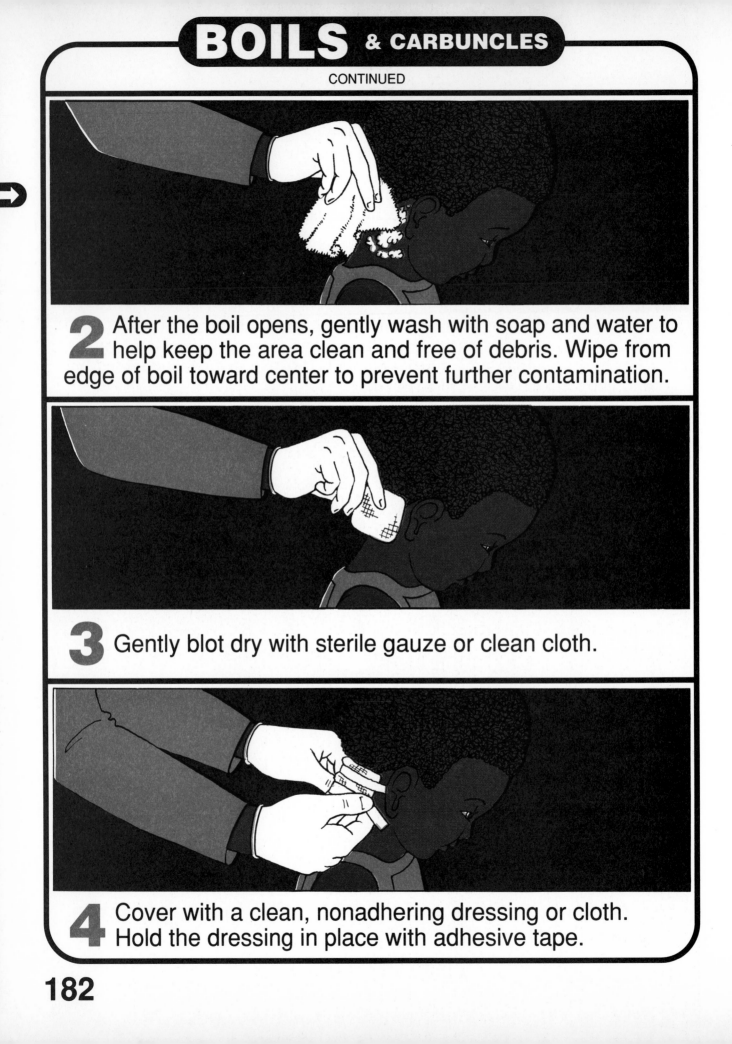

2 After the boil opens, gently wash with soap and water to help keep the area clean and free of debris. Wipe from edge of boil toward center to prevent further contamination.

3 Gently blot dry with sterile gauze or clean cloth.

4 Cover with a clean, nonadhering dressing or cloth. Hold the dressing in place with adhesive tape.

COLLARBONE & SHOULDER

IMPORTANT

- **Seek medical aid.** Call 911 or Operator; see **EMS,** page 272.

- **Keep the child as still as possible until medical aid arrives.** If medical aid cannot be obtained within 1 hour or you must transport her to an emergency room or doctor, **do not** move her until the injured part has been immobilized; see below.

- **Do not** try to reset dislocations yourself. Treat the same as fractures.

- If the child is bleeding, wash your hands thoroughly and, if possible, put on sterile latex gloves before starting first aid.

- If any bones protrude, control the bleeding, then cover the bone and the wound with a large clean dressing or cloth. **Do not** clean the wound. See **BLEEDING: CUTS & WOUNDS (PRESSURE POINTS),** pages 159-160.

- Observe for **SHOCK,** pages 354-356.

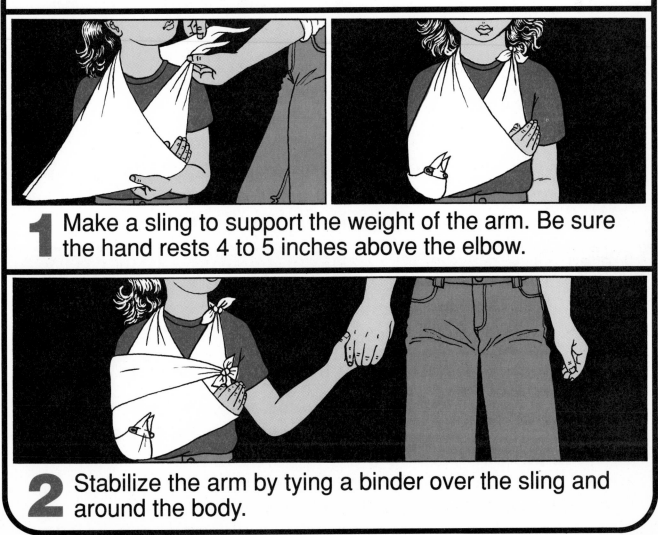

1 Make a sling to support the weight of the arm. Be sure the hand rests 4 to 5 inches above the elbow.

2 Stabilize the arm by tying a binder over the sling and around the body.

BENT ELBOW

IMPORTANT

- **Seek medical aid.** Call 911 or Operator; see **EMS,** page 272.

- **Keep the child as still as possible until medical aid arrives.** If medical aid cannot be obtained within 1 hour or you must transport him to an emergency room or doctor, **do not** move him until the injured part has been immobilized; see below.

- **Do not** try to reset dislocations yourself. Treat the same as fractures.

- If the child is bleeding, wash your hands thoroughly and, if possible, put on sterile latex gloves before starting first aid.

- If any bones protrude, control the bleeding, then cover the bone and the wound with a large clean dressing or cloth. **Do not** clean the wound. See **BLEEDING: CUTS & WOUNDS (PRESSURE POINTS),** pages 159-160.

- Observe for **SHOCK,** pages 354-356.

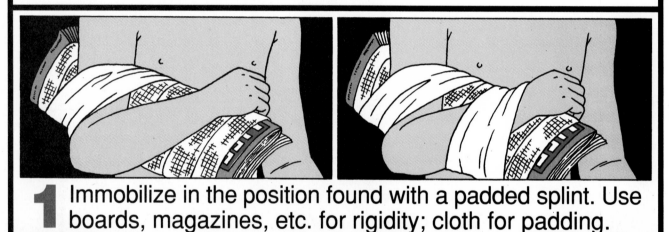

1 Immobilize in the position found with a padded splint. Use boards, magazines, etc. for rigidity; cloth for padding.

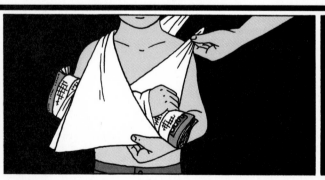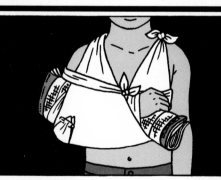

2 Make a sling to support the weight of the arm and bind it to the body. Be sure the fingers are above elbow level. Check the fingertips for circulation. If they become blue or swollen, loosen the binding.

STRAIGHT ELBOW

IMPORTANT

- **Seek medical aid.** Call 911 or Operator; see **EMS,** page 272.

- **Keep the child as still as possible until medical aid arrives.** If medical aid cannot be obtained within 1 hour or you must transport her to an emergency room or doctor, **do not** move her until the injured part has been immobilized; see below.

- **Do not** try to reset dislocations yourself. Treat the same as fractures.

- If the child is bleeding, wash your hands thoroughly and, if possible, put on sterile latex gloves before starting first aid.

- If any bones protrude, control the bleeding, then cover the bone and the wound with a large clean dressing or cloth. **Do not** clean the wound. See **BLEEDING: CUTS & WOUNDS (PRESSURE POINTS),** pages 159-160.

- Observe for **SHOCK,** pages 354-356.

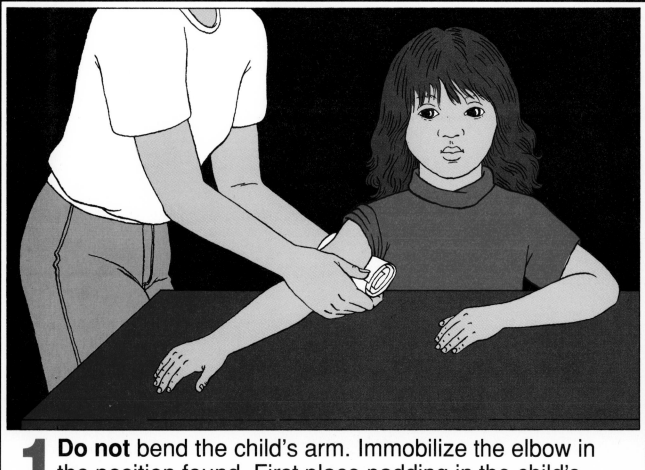

1 **Do not** bend the child's arm. Immobilize the elbow in the position found. First place padding in the child's armpit.

CONTINUED ON NEXT PAGE

STRAIGHT ELBOW
CONTINUED

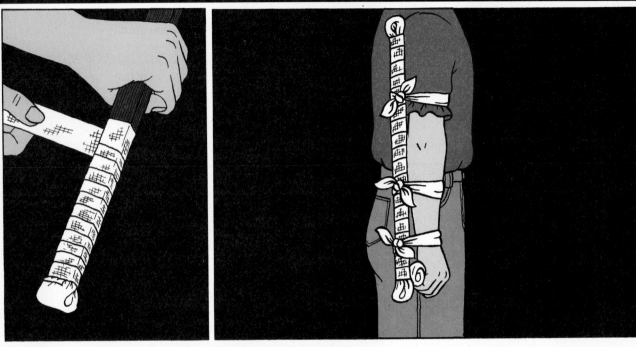

2A Then place padded splints along one or two sides of the arm from the shoulder to the hand. Use boards, magazines, etc. for rigidity; cloth for padding. Bind in place.

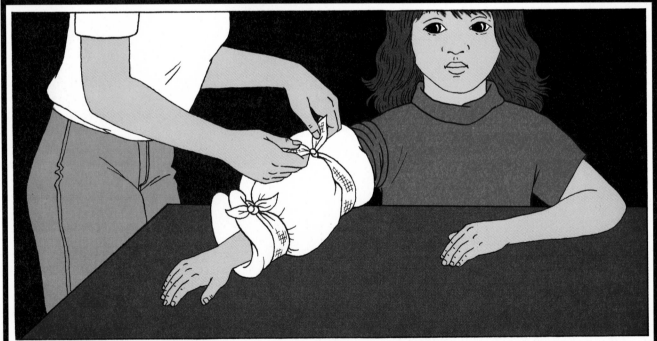

2B **If no splints are readily available,** use a pillow, centered at the elbow. Bind in place.

ARM, WRIST & HAND

IMPORTANT

- **Seek medical aid.** Call 911 or Operator; see **EMS,** page 272.

- **Keep the child as still as possible until medical aid arrives.** If medical aid cannot be obtained within 1 hour or you must transport her to an emergency room or doctor, **do not** move her until the injured part has been immobilized; see below.

- **Do not** try to reset dislocations yourself. Treat the same as fractures.

- If the child is bleeding, wash your hands thoroughly and, if possible, put on sterile latex gloves before starting first aid.

- Observe for **SHOCK,** pages 354-356.

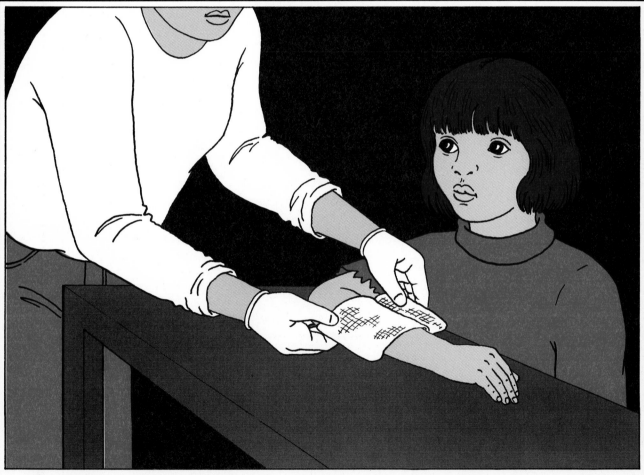

1 If any bones protrude, control the bleeding, then cover the bone and the wound with a large clean dressing or cloth. **Do not** clean the wound. See **BLEEDING: CUTS & WOUNDS (PRESSURE POINTS),** pages 159-160.

CONTINUED ON NEXT PAGE

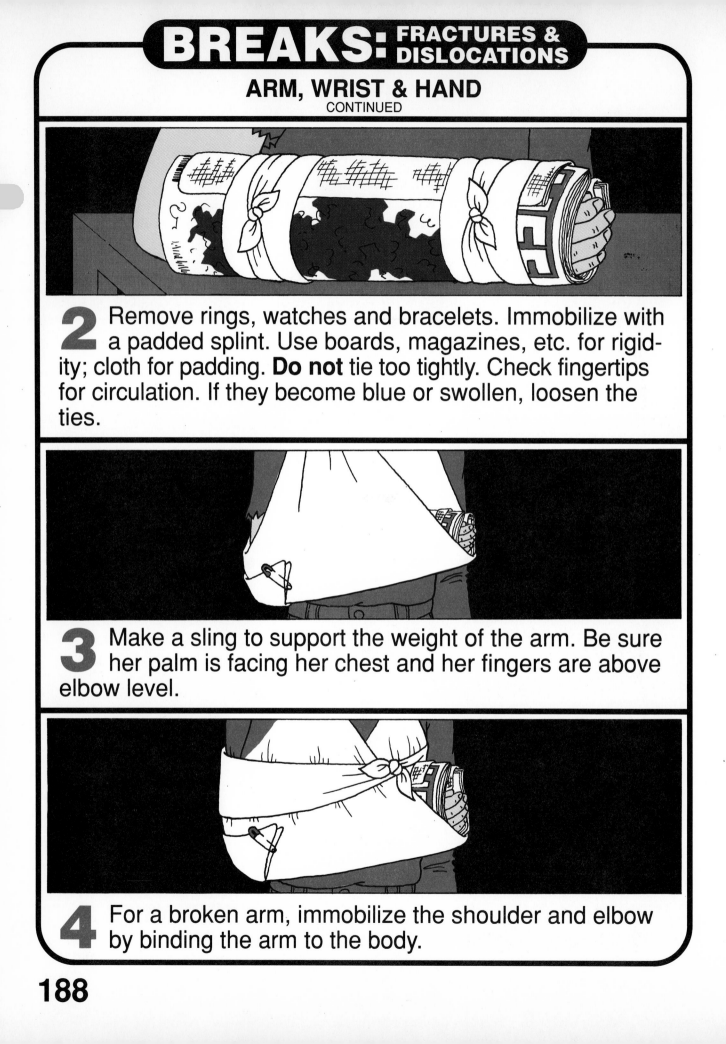

2 Remove rings, watches and bracelets. Immobilize with a padded splint. Use boards, magazines, etc. for rigidity; cloth for padding. **Do not** tie too tightly. Check fingertips for circulation. If they become blue or swollen, loosen the ties.

3 Make a sling to support the weight of the arm. Be sure her palm is facing her chest and her fingers are above elbow level.

4 For a broken arm, immobilize the shoulder and elbow by binding the arm to the body.

FINGER

IMPORTANT

- **Seek medical aid.**

- **Do not** try to straighten the finger.

- **Do not** try to reset dislocations yourself. Treat the same as fractures.

- If the child is bleeding, wash your hands thoroughly and, if possible, put on sterile latex gloves before starting first aid.

- If any bones protrude, control the bleeding, then cover the bone and the wound with a large clean dressing or cloth. **Do not** clean the wound. See **BLEEDING: CUTS & WOUNDS (PRESSURE POINTS),** pages 159-160.

- Observe for **SHOCK,** pages 354-356.

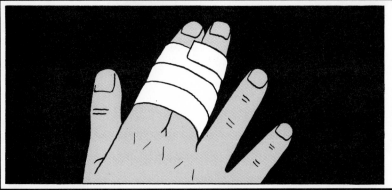

1 Apply cold compresses to the finger and elevate the hand until pain subsides. Repeat if necessary.

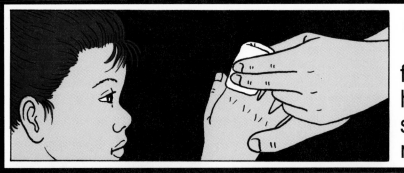

2A Before transporting the child to medical aid, splint the injured finger by gently taping it to the next uninjured finger for support.

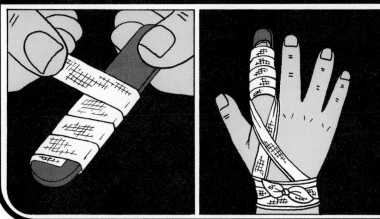

2B Or immobilize it in the position found with a padded splint made from a tongue depressor, etc. Bind the splint to the finger with cloth or tape.

189

PELVIS

IMPORTANT

- **Seek medical aid immediately.** Call 911 or Operator; see **EMS,** page 272.

- **Keep the child as still as possible until medical aid arrives. Do not move him unless absolutely necessary. If medical aid cannot be obtained within 1 hour or you must transport him to an emergency room or doctor, do not move him until the injured part has been immobilized; see below.**

- **Do not** try to reset dislocations yourself. Treat the same as fractures.

- If the child is bleeding, wash your hands thoroughly and, if possible, put on sterile latex gloves before starting first aid.

- If any bones protrude, cover the bone and the wound with a large clean dressing or cloth. **Do not** clean the wound.

- Observe for **SHOCK,** pages 354-356.

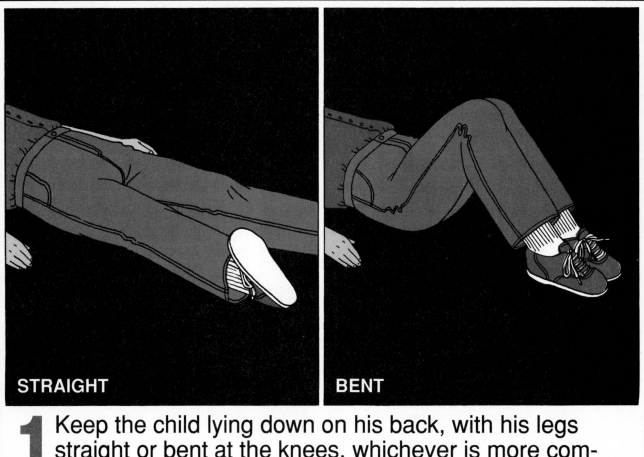

STRAIGHT

BENT

1 Keep the child lying down on his back, with his legs straight or bent at the knees, whichever is more comfortable.

CONTINUED ON NEXT PAGE

PELVIS
CONTINUED

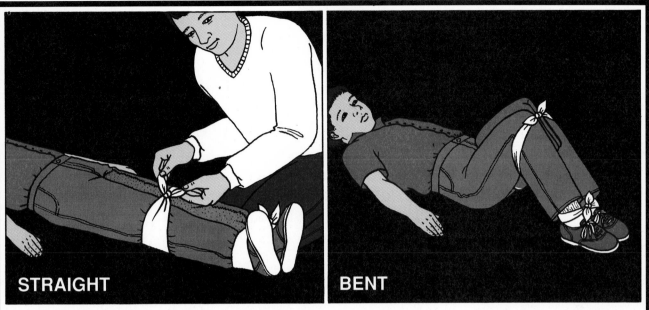

STRAIGHT

BENT

2 Immobilize him by placing a blanket or other thick padding between his thighs, then tying his legs together at the ankles and knees. Make sure the knots do not press against his legs. **Do not** tie too tightly. Loosen if his toes get numb.

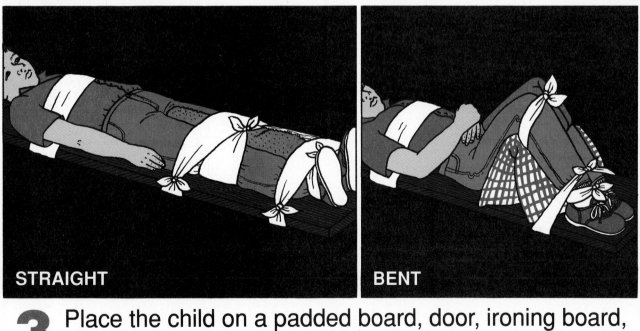

STRAIGHT

BENT

3 Place the child on a padded board, door, ironing board, etc., then secure him in place with bandages, belts, etc. See **TRANSPORTING THE INJURED,** pages 377-380.

HIP & UPPER LEG

IMPORTANT

- For an injured **lower leg,** see pages 198-199.

- **Seek medical aid immediately.** Call 911 or Operator; see **EMS,** page 272. **This is a particularly dangerous fracture and could be life-threatening.**

- **Keep the child as still as possible until medical aid arrives. Do not move him unless absolutely necessary. If medical aid cannot be obtained within 1 hour or you must transport him to an emergency room or doctor, do not move him until the injured part has been immobilized. Carefully follow the instructions below.**

- **Do not** try to straighten the injured bones.

- **Do not** try to reset dislocations yourself. Treat the same as fractures.

- If the child is bleeding, wash your hands thoroughly and, if possible, put on sterile latex gloves before starting first aid.

- If any bones protrude, cover the bone and the wound with a large clean dressing or cloth. **Do not** clean the wound.

- Observe for **SHOCK,** pages 354-356.

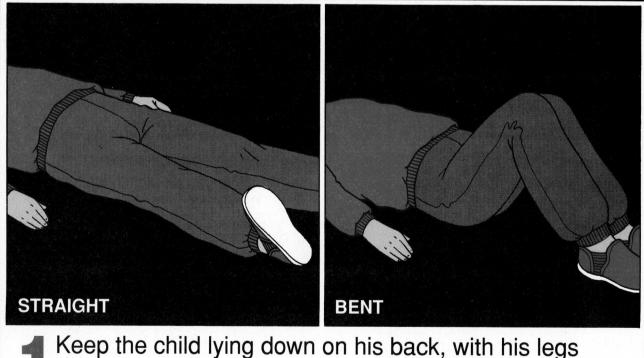

STRAIGHT

BENT

1 Keep the child lying down on his back, with his legs straight or bent at the knees, whichever is more comfortable.

CONTINUED ON NEXT PAGE

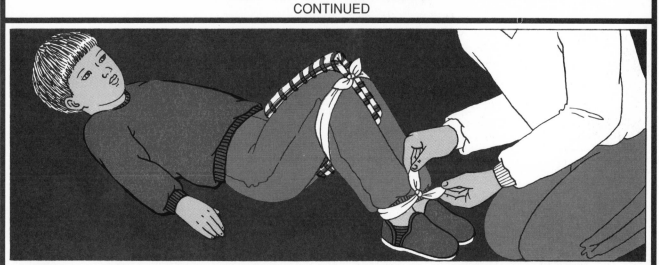

2A **If his legs are bent,** immobilize them by gently placing a blanket or other thick padding between his thighs, then tying his legs together at the ankles and knees. Make sure the knots do not press against the injured part. **Do not** tie too tightly. Loosen if the toes get numb.

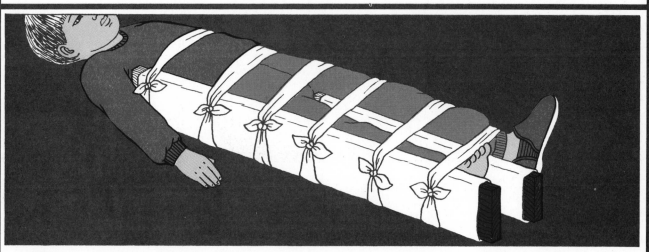

2B **If his legs are straight, immobilize them with a padded splint:** Place a padded board, straight branch, etc. on the outside of the injured leg extending from the armpit to below the foot. Then place another padded board on the inside of the leg extending from the groin to below the foot. Tie them in place in 6 or 7 spots, making sure the knots do not press against the injury. **Do not** tie too tightly. Loosen if the toes get numb.

CONTINUED ON NEXT PAGE

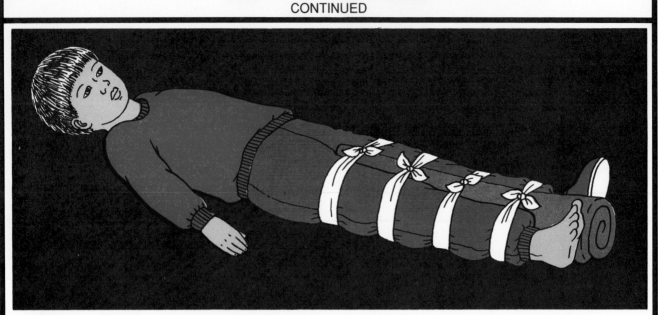

2c **If his legs are straight and you are unable to improvise a padded splint:** Gently place a blanket or other thick padding between the child's legs and tie them together at 4 or 5 spots. **Do not** place binding over the injury or tie too tightly. Loosen if the toes get numb.

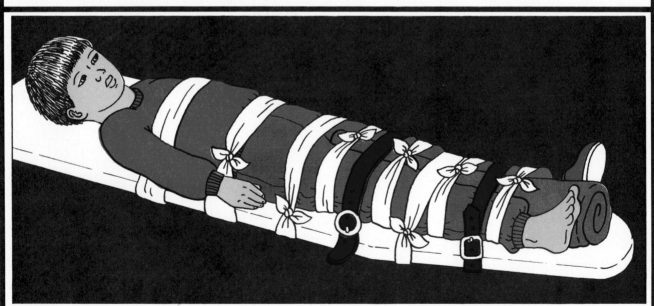

3 To transport the child, place him on a padded board, door, ironing board, etc., then secure him in place with bandages, belts, etc. See **TRANSPORTING THE INJURED,** pages 377-380.

KNEE

IMPORTANT

- **Seek medical aid.** Call 911 or Operator; see **EMS,** page 272.

- **Keep the child as still as possible until medical aid arrives.** If medical aid cannot be obtained within 1 hour or you must transport him to an emergency room or doctor, **do not** move him until the injured part has been immobilized; see below.

- **Do not** try to reset dislocations yourself. Treat the same as fractures.

- If the child is bleeding, wash your hands thoroughly and, if possible, put on sterile latex gloves before starting first aid.

- If any bones protrude, control the bleeding, then cover the bone and the wound with a large clean dressing or cloth. **Do not** clean the wound. See **BLEEDING: CUTS & WOUNDS (PRESSURE POINTS),** pages 159-160.

- Observe for **SHOCK,** pages 354-356.

BENT KNEE

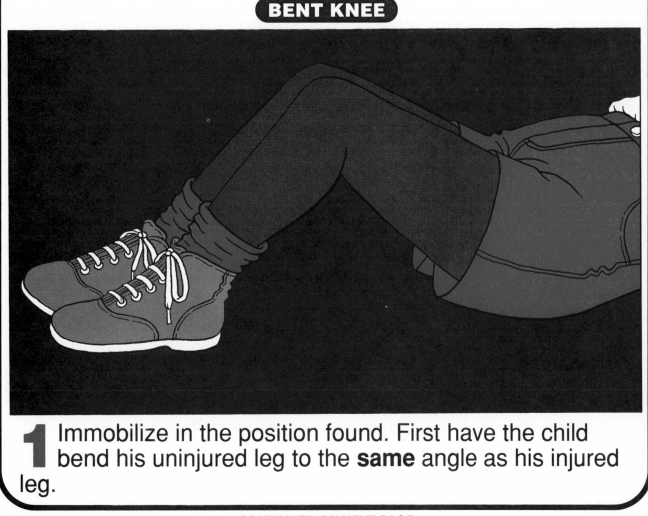

1 Immobilize in the position found. First have the child bend his uninjured leg to the **same** angle as his injured leg.

CONTINUED ON NEXT PAGE

KNEE
CONTINUED

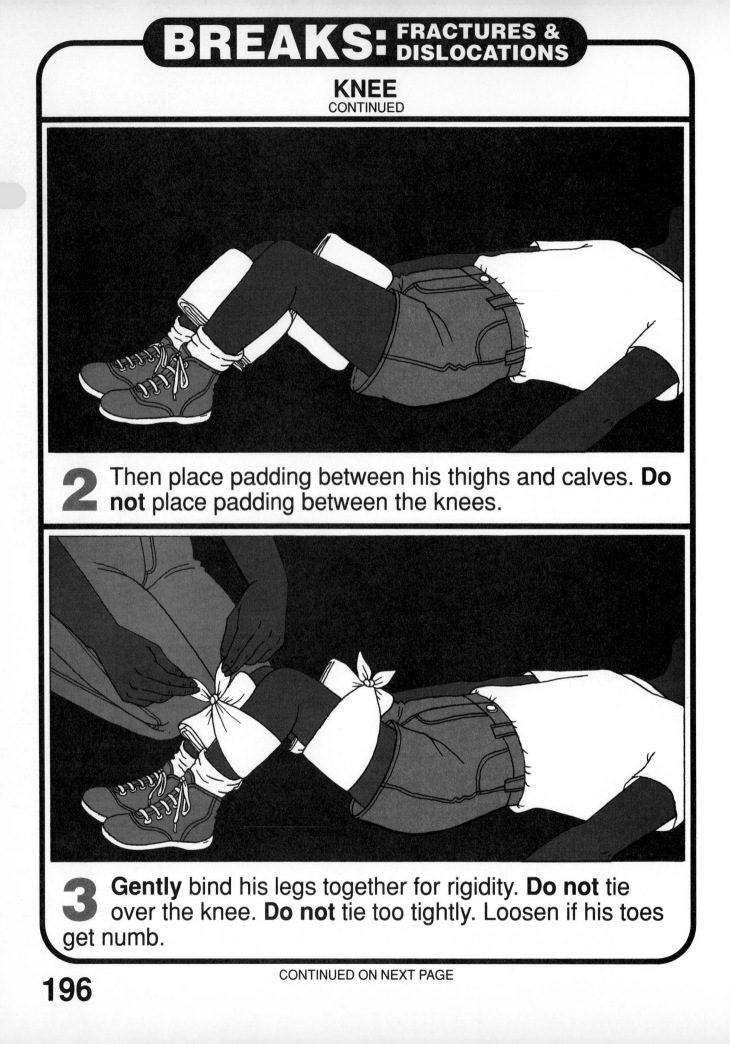

2 Then place padding between his thighs and calves. **Do not** place padding between the knees.

3 **Gently** bind his legs together for rigidity. **Do not** tie over the knee. **Do not** tie too tightly. Loosen if his toes get numb.

CONTINUED ON NEXT PAGE

KNEE
CONTINUED

STRAIGHT KNEE

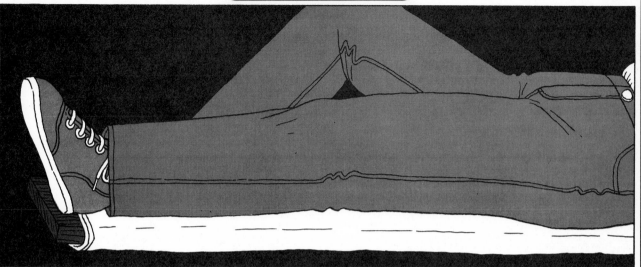

1 Immobilize in the position found with a padded splint at least 4 inches wide. Use boards, magazines, etc. for rigidity; cloth for padding. Extend the splint from the buttock to beyond the heel.

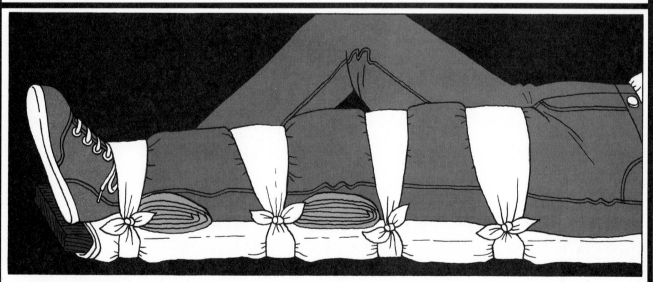

2 **Gently** place additional padding under the ankle and knee. Then tie the leg in place at the 4 spots shown — around the ankle, below and above the knee, and around the thigh. **Do not** tie over the knee. **Do not** tie too tightly. Loosen if the toes get numb.

LOWER LEG

IMPORTANT

- For an injured **upper leg,** see **HIP & UPPER LEG,** pages 192-194.

- **Seek medical aid immediately.** Call 911 or Operator; see **EMS,** page 272.

- **Keep the child as still as possible until medical aid arrives.** If medical aid cannot be obtained within 1 hour or you must transport him to an emergency room or doctor, **do not** move him until the injured leg has been immobilized; see below.

- **Do not** try to reset dislocations yourself. Treat the same as fractures.

- If the child is bleeding, wash your hands thoroughly and, if possible, put on sterile latex gloves before starting first aid.

- If any bones protrude, control the bleeding, then cover the bone and the wound with a large clean dressing or cloth. **Do not** clean the wound. See **BLEEDING: CUTS & WOUNDS (PRESSURE POINTS),** pages 159-160.

- Observe for **SHOCK,** pages 354-356.

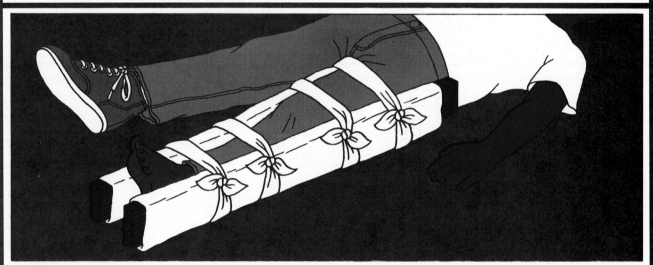

1A Immobilize the injured leg with a padded splint: **Do not** try to straighten the injured bones. Place a padded board, straight branch, etc. on the outside of the injured leg extending from the hip to below the foot. Then place another padded board on the inside of the leg extending from the groin to below the foot. Tie them in place in 4 or 5 spots, making sure the knots do not press against the injury. **Do not** tie too tightly. Loosen if the toes get numb.

CONTINUED ON NEXT PAGE

LOWER LEG
CONTINUED

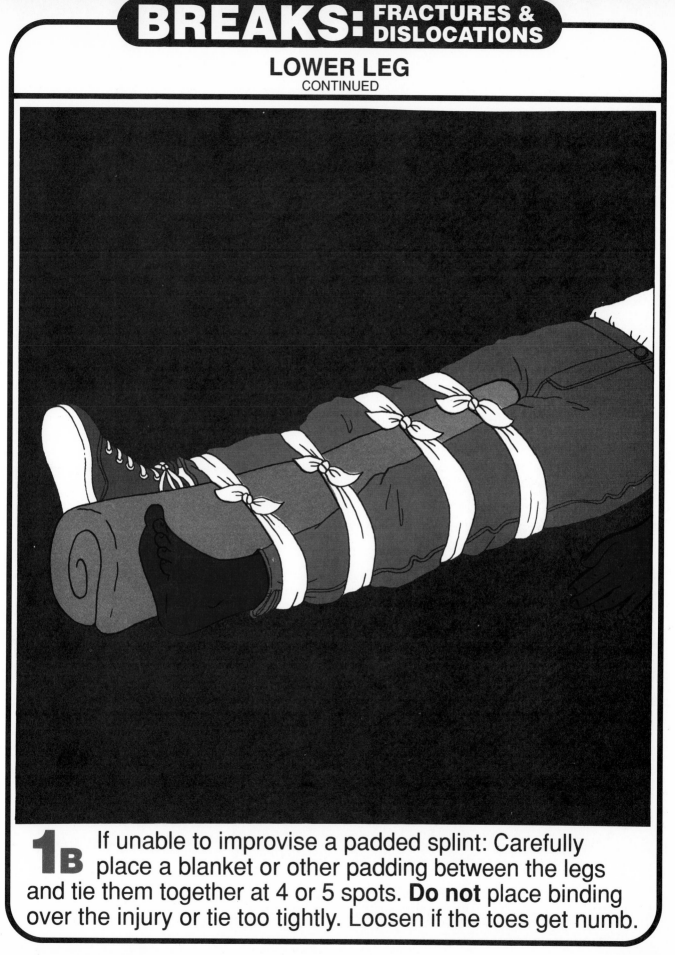

1B If unable to improvise a padded splint: Carefully place a blanket or other padding between the legs and tie them together at 4 or 5 spots. **Do not** place binding over the injury or tie too tightly. Loosen if the toes get numb.

ANKLE, FOOT & TOE

IMPORTANT

- **Seek medical aid.** Call 911 or Operator; see **EMS,** page 272.

- **Keep the child as still as possible until medical aid arrives.** If medical aid cannot be obtained within 1 hour or you must transport him to an emergency room or doctor, **do not** move him until the injured part has been immobilized; see below.

- **Do not** try to reset dislocations yourself. Treat the same as fractures.

- If the child is bleeding, wash your hands thoroughly and, if possible, put on sterile latex gloves before starting first aid.

- If any bones protrude, control the bleeding, then cover the bone and the wound with a large clean dressing or cloth. **Do not** clean the wound. See **BLEEDING: CUTS & WOUNDS (PRESSURE POINTS),** pages 159-160.

- **For an injured toe:** Apply cold compresses or ice wrapped in a cloth and elevate the foot to avoid swelling.

- Observe for **SHOCK,** pages 354-356.

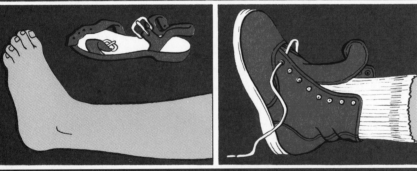

1 Remove or cut away the shoe or boot if possible. (If not possible, then loosen it.)

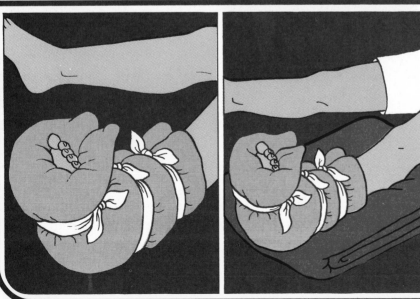

2 Immobilize with a padded splint made from a blanket, pillow, etc. Tie it snugly but not too tightly. Leave the toes exposed. Elevate the foot to minimize swelling.

INFANT (TO 1 YEAR OLD)

IMPORTANT

- Determine if the infant is responsive by calling him loudly, tapping him on the shoulder or shaking him gently.

- **If he is unresponsive,** yell for help and have someone call 911 or Operator; see **EMS,** page 272. **If no one answers your repeated shouts for help, administer first aid for 1 minute, then call EMS yourself.** Return immediately and continue first aid.

- Even if the child is responsive, seek medical aid as soon as possible. Call 911 or Operator; see **EMS,** page 272.

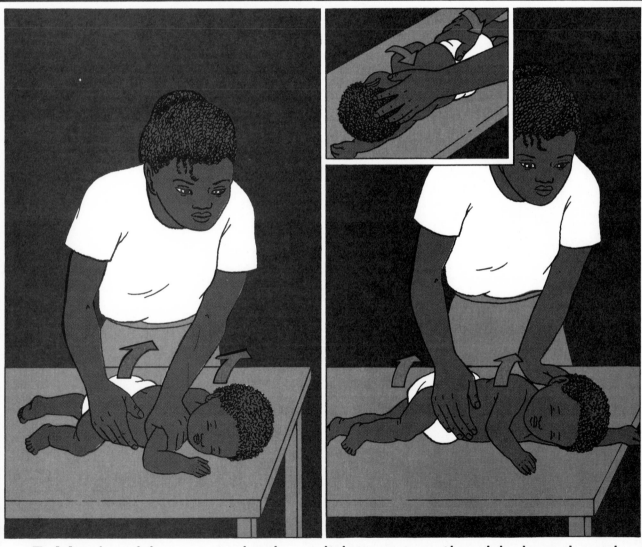

1 Moving him as a single unit by supporting his head and neck, roll the infant onto his back on a firm surface. Stand or kneel facing him from the side.

CONTINUED ON NEXT PAGE

INFANT (TO 1 YEAR OLD)
CONTINUED

HEAD-TILT/CHIN-LIFT

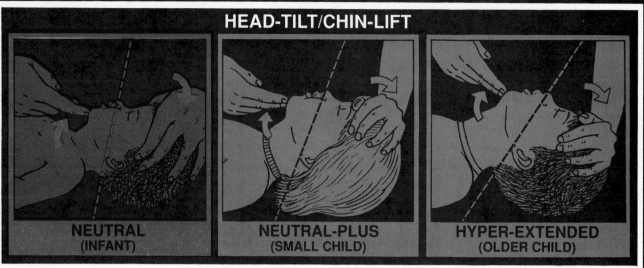

NEUTRAL (INFANT) **NEUTRAL-PLUS (SMALL CHILD)** **HYPER-EXTENDED (OLDER CHILD)**

2A **If there is no neck or back injury, open the airway** by using the **head-tilt/chin-lift:** Place your hand — the one closest to his head — on his forehead. Place 1 or 2 fingers (but **not** the thumb) of your other hand under the bony part of his jaw at the chin. Gently tilt his head back to the **neutral** position (as shown) by applying gentle backward pressure on his forehead and lifting his chin. **Do not** close his mouth completely.

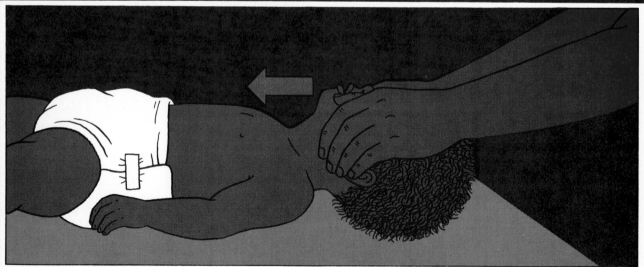

2B **If there is a neck or back injury, open the airway** by gently moving his jaw forward **without** tilting or moving his head.

CONTINUED ON NEXT PAGE

INFANT (TO 1 YEAR OLD)
CONTINUED

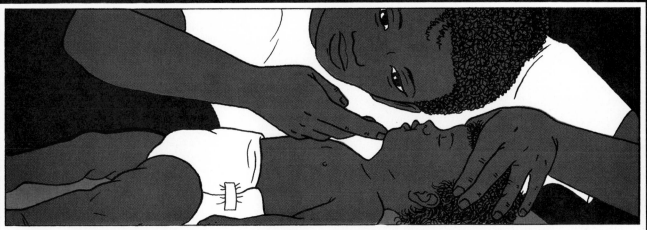

3 Taking 3 to 5 seconds, check for breathing by looking, listening and feeling for air leaving his lungs. (**Look** at his chest for movement. **Listen** for sounds of breathing. And **feel** for his breath on your cheek.)

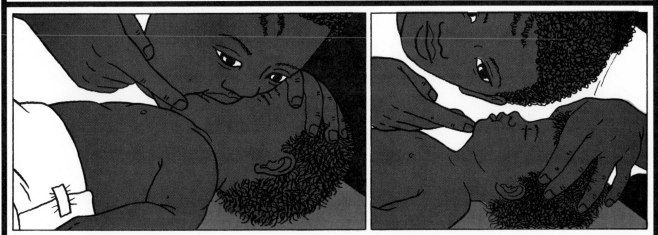

4 **If the infant is not breathing:** Place your open mouth over his nose and mouth, forming an airtight seal, and give 2 slow, gentle breaths (1 to 1½ seconds each), allowing the lungs to deflate fully between each breath. Remove your mouth between breaths, and look and listen for air leaving his lungs. **If the entry or return of air seems blocked, or his chest does not rise, try again to open his airway** (see Step 2A or 2B) and give 2 slow, gentle breaths. **If the airway still seems blocked,** see CHOKING, pages 239-245.

CONTINUED ON NEXT PAGE

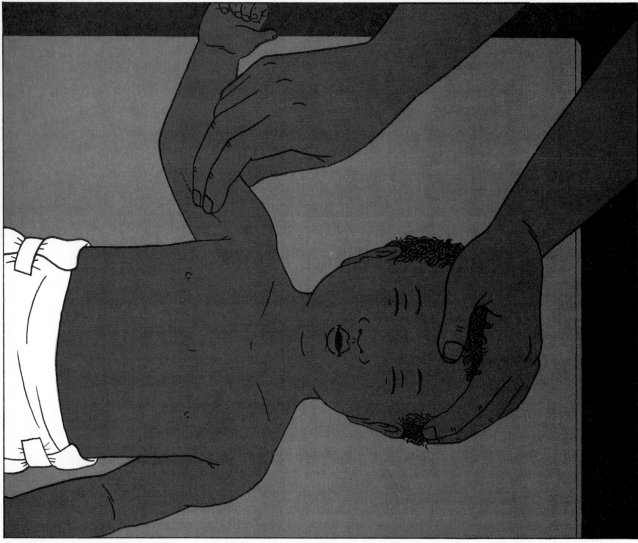

5 Continue to hold the infant's head in the **neutral** position with your hand on his forehead. **Check his pulse slowly and carefully** by placing the fingertips of your other hand (but **not** your thumb) on the inside of his upper arm between the elbow and shoulder. **It is extremely important to find the pulse if one is present. Take between 5 and 10 seconds to find it. Do not rush.** It is easily missed under emergency conditions.

6A **If you cannot feel the pulse,** see **HEART FAILURE,** pages 303-308.

CONTINUED ON NEXT PAGE

INFANT (TO 1 YEAR OLD)
CONTINUED

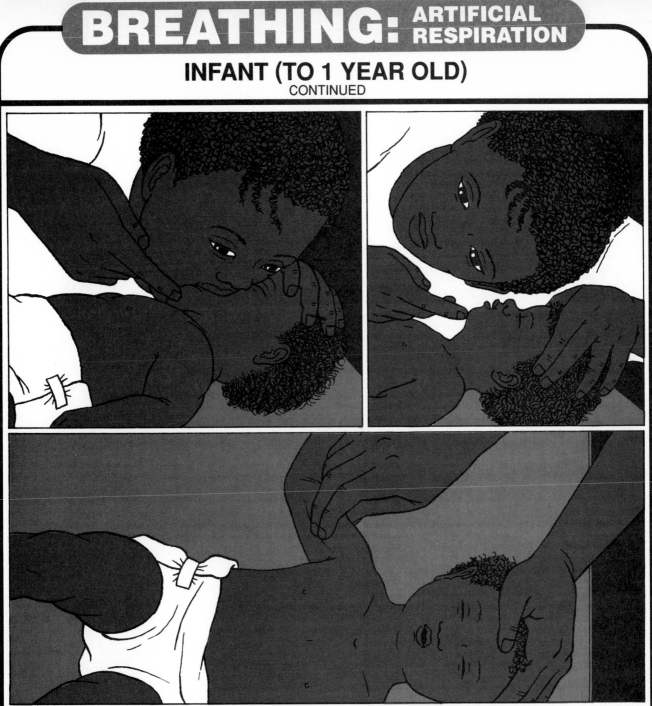

6B **If a pulse is present,** then give the infant a new breath every 3 seconds (20 per minute), using slow, gentle breaths lasting 1 to 1½ seconds each. **Remove your mouth between breaths, and look and listen for air leaving his lungs.** Recheck the pulse and breathing after the first minute of artificial respiration, then recheck every few minutes thereafter. Continue rescue breathing until the infant breathes on his own or professional help arrives. Treat for **SHOCK;** see pages 354-356.

SMALL CHILD (1 TO 8 YEARS OLD)

IMPORTANT

- Determine if the child is responsive by calling her loudly, tapping her on the shoulder or shaking her gently.

- **If she is unresponsive,** yell for help and have someone call 911 or Operator; see **EMS,** page 272. **If no one answers your repeated shouts for help, administer first aid for 1 minute, then call EMS yourself.** Return immediately and continue first aid.

- Even if the child is responsive, seek medical aid as soon as possible. Call 911 or Operator; see **EMS,** page 272.

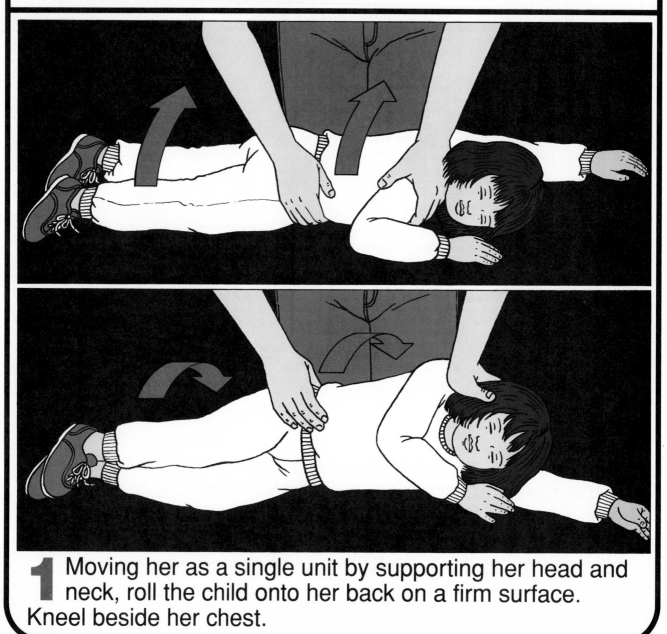

1 Moving her as a single unit by supporting her head and neck, roll the child onto her back on a firm surface. Kneel beside her chest.

CONTINUED ON NEXT PAGE

SMALL CHILD (1 TO 8 YEARS OLD)
CONTINUED

HEAD-TILT/CHIN-LIFT

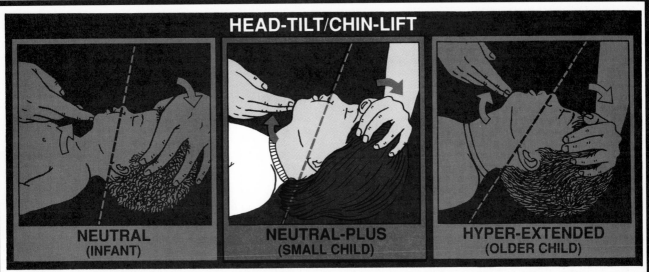

NEUTRAL
(INFANT)

NEUTRAL-PLUS
(SMALL CHILD)

HYPER-EXTENDED
(OLDER CHILD)

2A **If there is no neck or back injury, open the airway** by using the **head-tilt/chin-lift:** Place your hand — the one closest to her head — on her forehead. Place 2 or 3 fingers (but **not** the thumb) of your other hand under the bony part of her jaw at the chin. Gently tilt her head back to the **neutral-plus** position (as shown) by applying gentle backward pressure on her forehead and lifting her chin. **Do not** close her mouth completely.

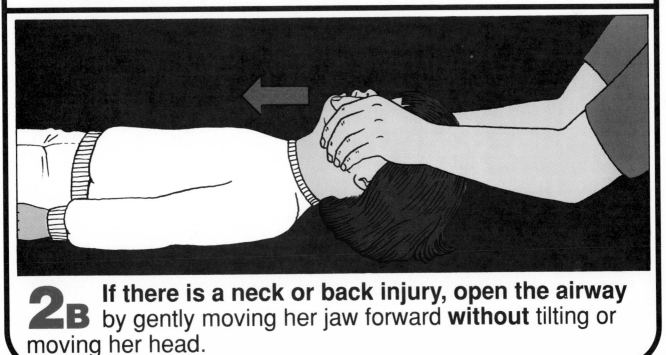

2B **If there is a neck or back injury, open the airway** by gently moving her jaw forward **without** tilting or moving her head.

CONTINUED ON NEXT PAGE

SMALL CHILD (1 TO 8 YEARS OLD)
CONTINUED

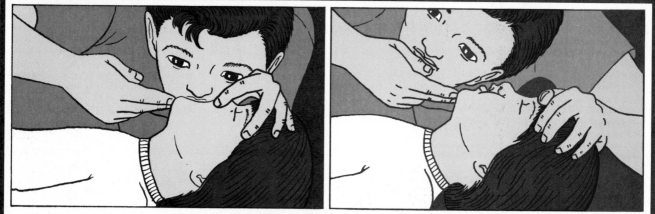

3 Taking 3 to 5 seconds, check for breathing by looking, listening and feeling for air leaving her lungs. (**Look** at her chest for movement. **Listen** for sounds of breathing. And **feel** for her breath on your cheek.)

4 **If the child is not breathing:** Pinch her nose closed with the thumb and index finger of the hand that is on her forehead. Place your open mouth over her open mouth, forming an airtight seal. Give 2 slow, gentle breaths (1 to 1½ seconds each), allowing the lungs to deflate fully between each breath. Remove your mouth between breaths, and look and listen for air leaving her lungs. **If the entry or return of air seems blocked, or her chest does not rise, try again to open her airway** (see Step 2A or 2B) and give 2 slow, gentle breaths. **If the airway still seems blocked,** see **CHOKING,** pages 246-252.

CONTINUED ON NEXT PAGE

SMALL CHILD (1 TO 8 YEARS OLD)
CONTINUED

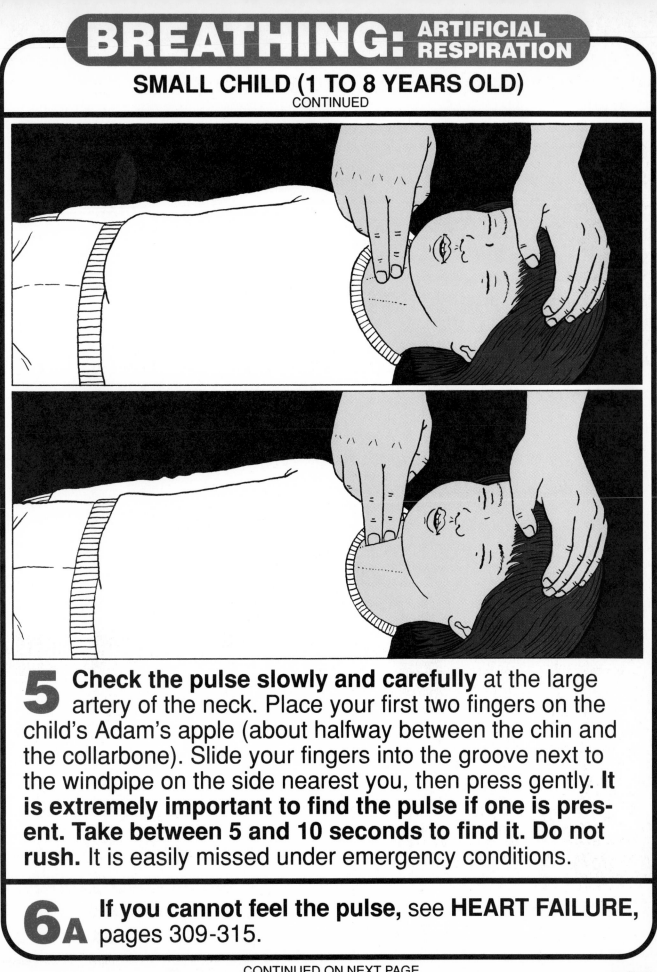

5 **Check the pulse slowly and carefully** at the large artery of the neck. Place your first two fingers on the child's Adam's apple (about halfway between the chin and the collarbone). Slide your fingers into the groove next to the windpipe on the side nearest you, then press gently. **It is extremely important to find the pulse if one is present. Take between 5 and 10 seconds to find it. Do not rush.** It is easily missed under emergency conditions.

6A **If you cannot feel the pulse,** see **HEART FAILURE,** pages 309-315.

CONTINUED ON NEXT PAGE

SMALL CHILD (1 TO 8 YEARS OLD)

CONTINUED

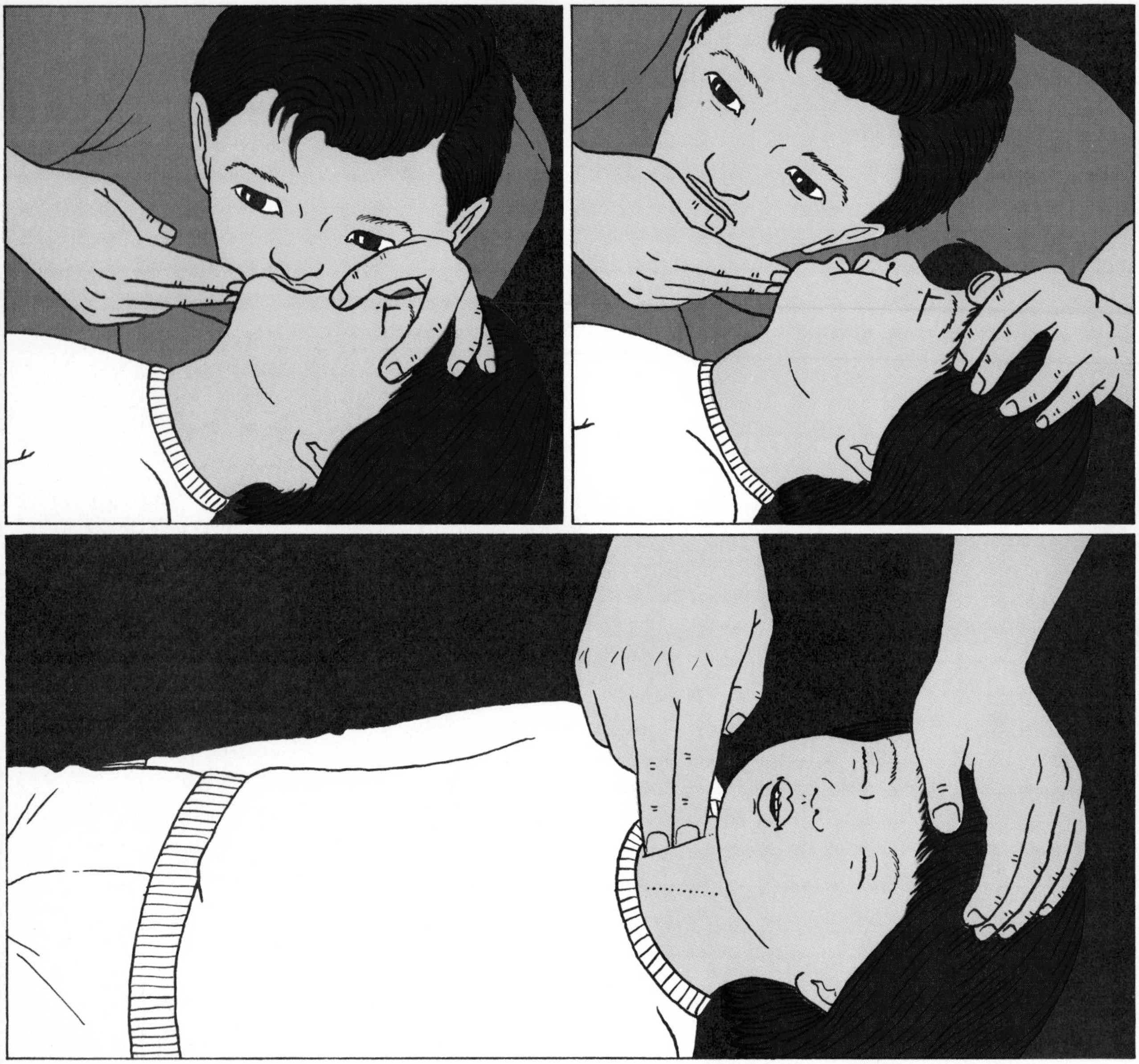

6B **If a pulse is present,** then give the child a new breath every 4 seconds (15 per minute), using slow, gentle breaths lasting 1 to 1½ seconds each. **Remove your mouth between breaths, and look and listen for air leaving her lungs.** Recheck the pulse and breathing after the first minute of artificial respiration, then recheck every few minutes thereafter. Continue rescue breathing until the child breathes on her own or professional help arrives. Treat for **SHOCK;** see pages 354-356.

OLDER CHILD (8 YEARS & OLDER)

IMPORTANT

- Determine if the child is responsive by calling him loudly, tapping him on the shoulder or shaking him gently.

- **If he is unresponsive,** have someone call 911 or Operator immediately; see **EMS,** page 272. **If no one is available, call EMS yourself, then return immediately and begin first aid.**

- Even if the child is responsive, seek medical aid as soon as possible. Call 911 or Operator; see **EMS,** page 272.

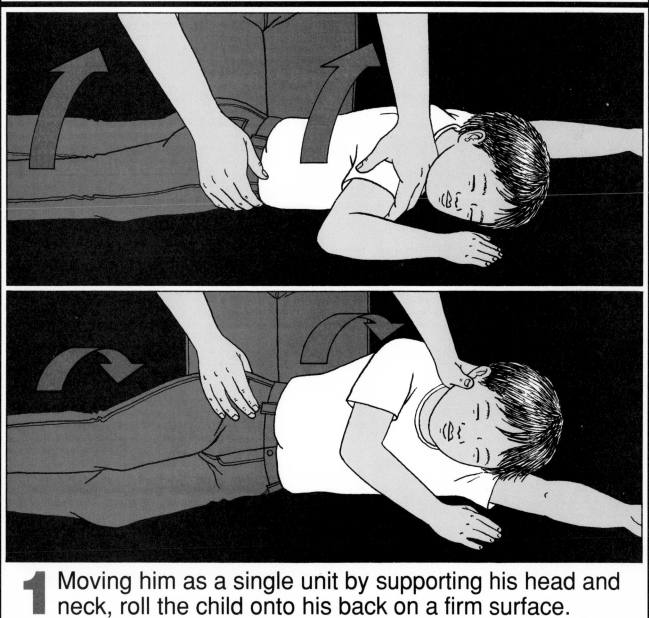

1 Moving him as a single unit by supporting his head and neck, roll the child onto his back on a firm surface. Kneel beside his chest.

CONTINUED ON NEXT PAGE

HEAD-TILT/CHIN-LIFT

NEUTRAL
(INFANT)

NEUTRAL-PLUS
(SMALL CHILD)

HYPER-EXTENDED
(OLDER CHILD)

2A **If there is no neck or back injury, open the airway** by using the **head-tilt/chin-lift:** Place your hand — the one closest to his head — on his forehead. Place 2 or 3 fingers (but **not** the thumb) of your other hand under the bony part of his jaw at the chin. Gently tilt his head back to the **hyper-extended** position (with his chin pointing straight up, as shown) by applying gentle backward pressure on his forehead and lifting his chin. **Do not** close his mouth completely.

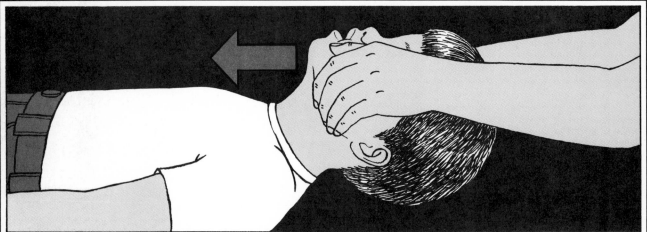

2B **If there is a neck or back injury, open the airway** by gently moving his jaw forward **without** tilting or moving his head.

CONTINUED ON NEXT PAGE

212

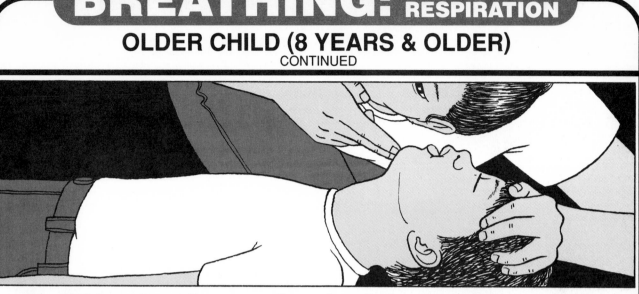

3 Taking 3 to 5 seconds, check for breathing by look-ing, listening and feeling for air leaving his lungs. (**Look** at his chest for movement. **Listen** for sounds of breathing. And **feel** for his breath on your cheek.)

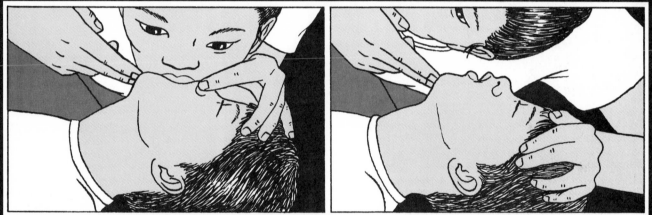

4 **If the child is not breathing:** Pinch his nose closed with the thumb and index finger of the hand that is on his forehead. Place your open mouth over his open mouth, forming an airtight seal. Give 2 slow, full breaths (1½ to 2 seconds each), allowing the lungs to deflate fully between each breath. Remove your mouth between breaths, and look and listen for air leaving his lungs. **If the entry or return of air seems blocked, or his chest does not rise, try again to open his airway** (see Step 2A or 2B) and give 2 slow, full breaths. **If the airway still seems blocked,** see **CHOKING,** pages 246-252.

CONTINUED ON NEXT PAGE

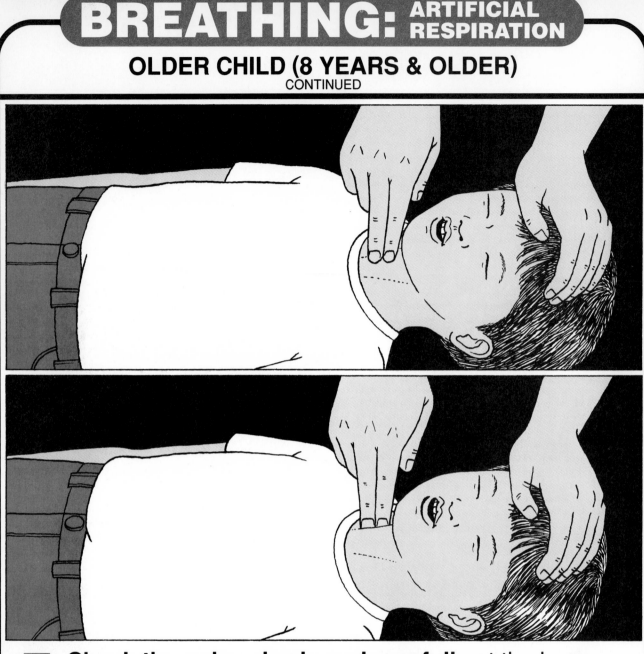

5 **Check the pulse slowly and carefully** at the large artery of the neck. Place your first two fingers on the child's Adam's apple (about halfway between the chin and the collarbone). Slide your fingers into the groove next to the windpipe on the side nearest you, then press gently. **It is extremely important to find the pulse if one is present. Take between 5 and 10 seconds to find it. Do not rush.** It is easily missed under emergency conditions.

6A **If you cannot feel the pulse,** see HEART FAILURE, pages 316-323.

CONTINUED ON NEXT PAGE

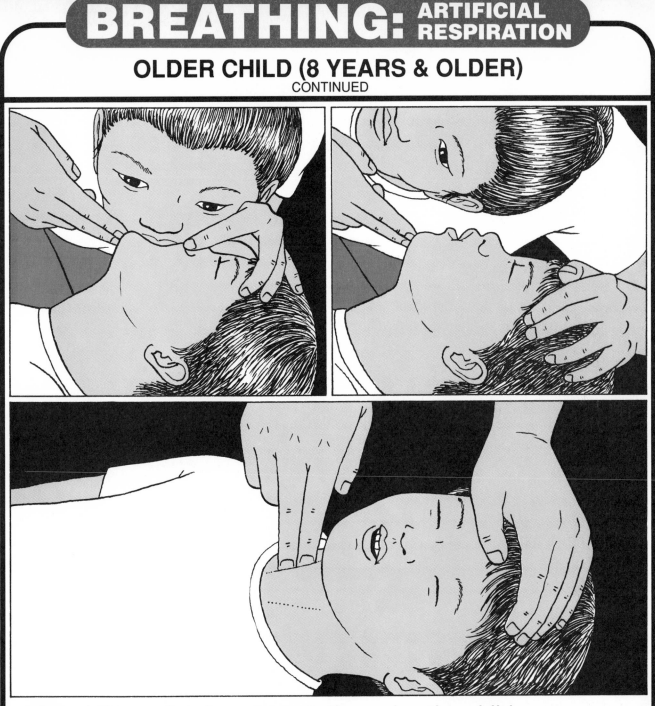

6B **If a pulse is present,** then give the child a new breath every 5 seconds (12 per minute), using slow, full breaths lasting 1½ to 2 seconds each. **Remove your mouth between breaths, and look and listen for air leaving his lungs.** Recheck the pulse and breathing after the first minute of artificial respiration, then recheck every few minutes thereafter. Continue rescue breathing until the child breathes on his own or professional help arrives. Treat for **SHOCK;** see pages 354-356.

BRUISES

IMPORTANT

- **Seek medical aid immediately** if you suspect internal bleeding. If necessary, call 911 or Operator; see **EMS,** page 272.

- Consult your doctor if you think a bone may be broken, there is loss of use or feeling, or if the bruises are very painful, appear for no apparent reason or do not heal in 10 to 14 days.

- If the bruises are around the eyes, see **EYE INJURIES: BLACK EYE,** page 278.

SIGNS & SYMPTOMS

Reddish or purple discoloration under the skin that first turns black and blue, then greenish-yellow. Swelling. Pain. May not appear until several days after an injury occurs. Usually related to an injury but may also be caused by blood-clotting disorders, infections or allergic reactions.

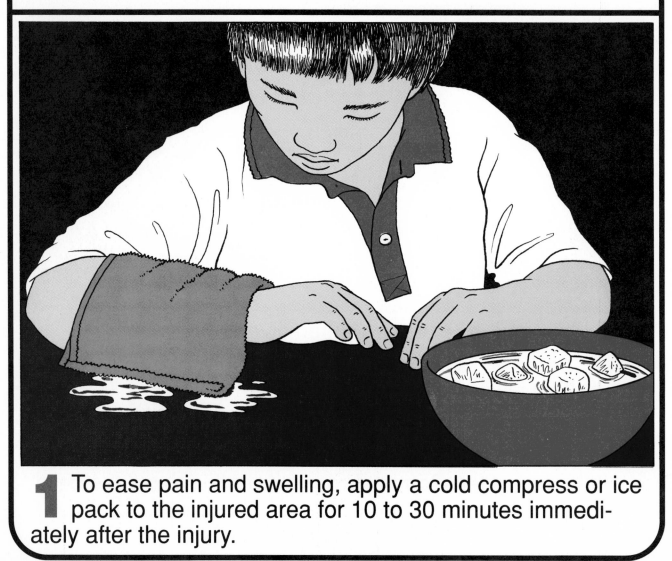

1 To ease pain and swelling, apply a cold compress or ice pack to the injured area for 10 to 30 minutes immediately after the injury.

CONTINUED ON NEXT PAGE

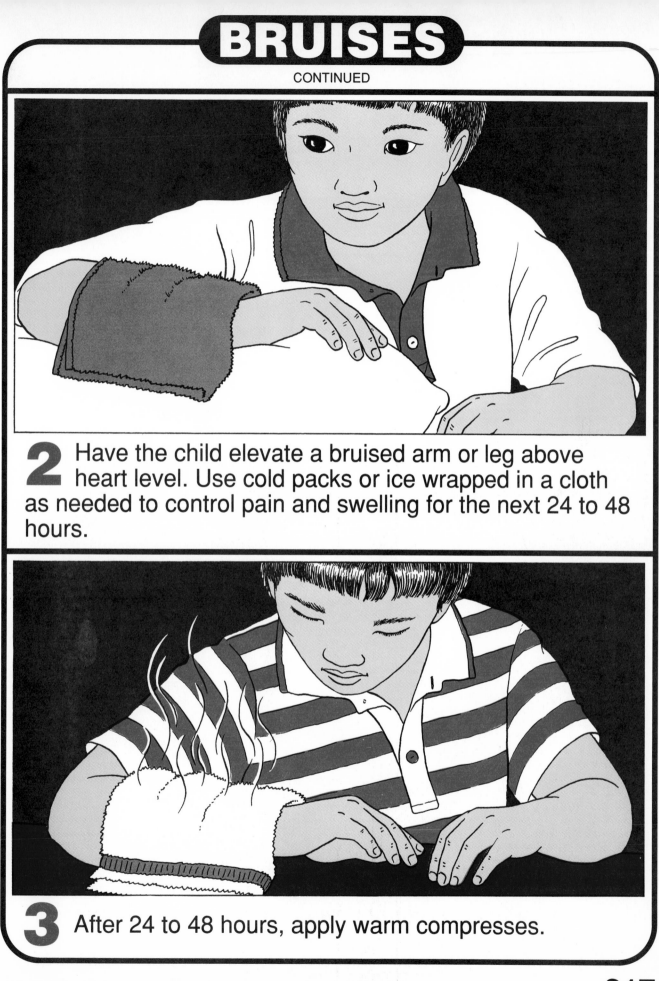

2 Have the child elevate a bruised arm or leg above heart level. Use cold packs or ice wrapped in a cloth as needed to control pain and swelling for the next 24 to 48 hours.

3 After 24 to 48 hours, apply warm compresses.

IMPORTANT

- **Seek medical aid as soon as possible.**
- Try to identify the chemical causing the burn.
- Call your local Poison Control Center for advice.
- **For a serious chemical burn,** call 911 or Operator; see **EMS,** page 272.
- **Do not** apply ointments, salves, etc. unless advised to do so by your Poison Control Center or doctor.
- Be careful not to become contaminated by the chemical.
- If the chemical is dry, brush off as much as possible before beginning first aid.
- **Do not** disturb blisters.
- Observe for signs of toxic reaction that may appear later, such as a rash, bluish or bright red lips and skin, headache, dizziness, difficulty breathing, generalized pains, etc. **If necessary, seek medical aid immediately.**

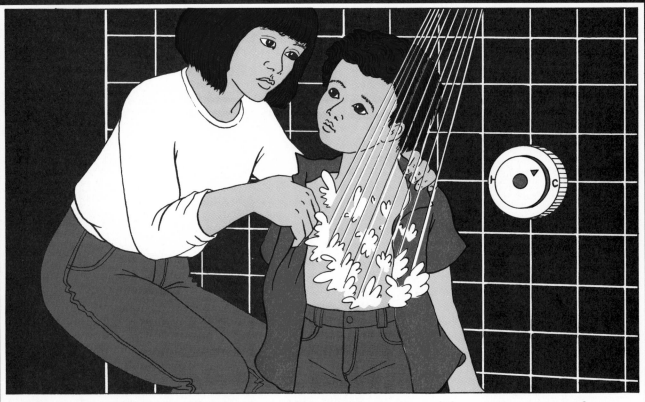

1 Immediately flush the affected area with a stream of cool water. Remove all contaminated clothing. Continue drenching with water for at least 5 minutes, until all traces of the chemical have been washed away.

CONTINUED ON NEXT PAGE

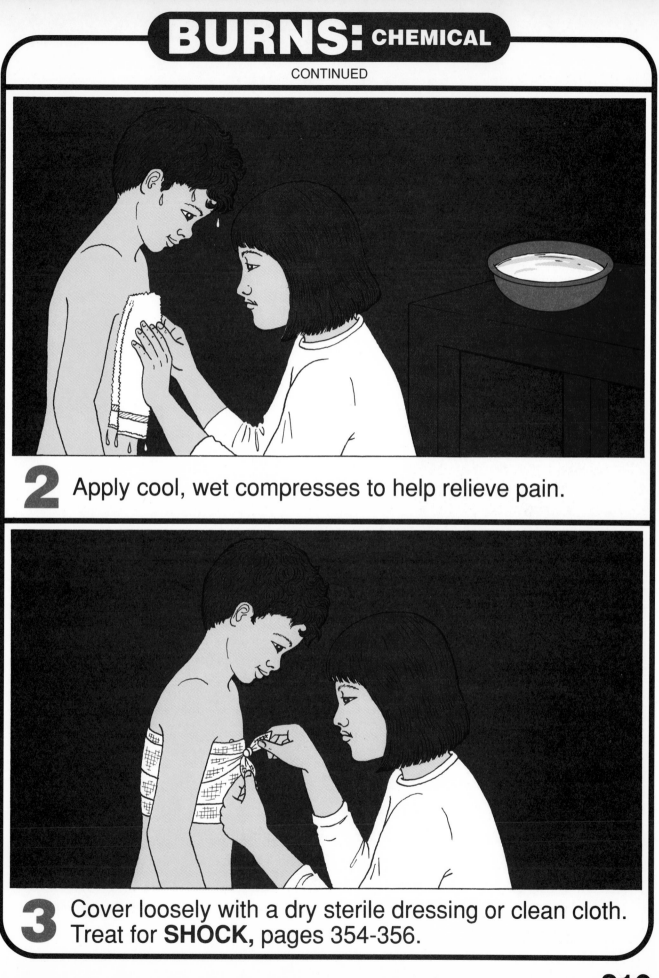

2 Apply cool, wet compresses to help relieve pain.

3 Cover loosely with a dry sterile dressing or clean cloth. Treat for **SHOCK,** pages 354-356.

1st & 2nd DEGREE

IMPORTANT

- Calm and reassure the child.
- **Do not** break blisters.
- **Do not** use antiseptic sprays, ointments or home remedies.
- **Do not** put pressure on burned areas.
- Treat for **SHOCK,** pages 354-356.
- **Seek medical aid, especially for burns involving the eyes, face, hands, genitals or airway.**
- For a minor burn inside the mouth, have the child suck on small chips of ice.
- **Seek medical aid immediately** if any signs of infection develop, such as increased pain, redness and swelling, pus, swollen glands or red streaks leading from the burn.

Determine the degree of the burn and treat accordingly. If the skin is broken or there is any question as to the severity of the burn, treat for Third Degree.
- **First Degree:** Red or discolored skin. **See below.**
- **Second Degree:** Blisters and red or mottled skin. **See below.**
- **Third Degree:** White or charred skin. **See pages 222-223.**

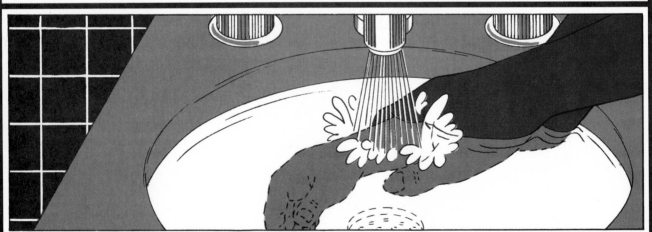

1A **If the skin isn't broken,** immediately immerse in cold (**not ice**) water or place under cold running water until pain subsides. Remove clothing from the burned area if it comes off easily, along with any constricting items such as rings.

CONTINUED ON NEXT PAGE

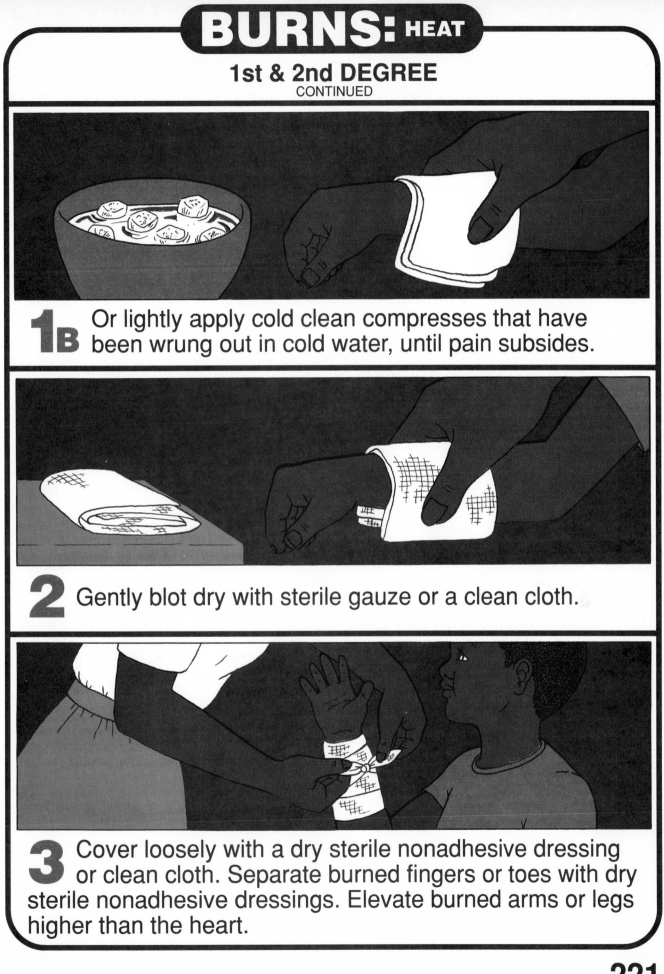

1B Or lightly apply cold clean compresses that have been wrung out in cold water, until pain subsides.

2 Gently blot dry with sterile gauze or a clean cloth.

3 Cover loosely with a dry sterile nonadhesive dressing or clean cloth. Separate burned fingers or toes with dry sterile nonadhesive dressings. Elevate burned arms or legs higher than the heart.

3rd DEGREE

IMPORTANT

- **Seek medical aid immediately.** Call 911 or Operator; see **EMS,** page 272.

- Check the child's ABCs (Airway, Breathing and Circulation); see **CHECKING THE ABCs,** pages 224-232.

- Calm and reassure the child.

- **Do not** apply water, antiseptic sprays, ointments or home remedies.

- **Do not** apply cold compresses or ice, or immerse in cold water.

- **Do not** remove adhered particles of clothing.

- **Do not** remove shreds of tissue or break blisters.

- **Do not** use absorbent cotton.

- **Do not** give the child anything to drink.

- Treat for **SHOCK;** see pages 354-356.

- **Seek medical aid immediately** if any signs of infection develop, such as increased pain, redness and swelling, pus, swollen glands or red streaks leading from the burn.

1A If the **face** has been burned, sit or prop the child up and apply a dry cool compress (an ice bag wrapped in a towel or ice wrapped in a thick towel). Continue to check the child's ABCs (Airway, Breathing and Circulation); see **CHECKING THE ABCs,** pages 224-232.

CONTINUED ON NEXT PAGE

3rd DEGREE
CONTINUED

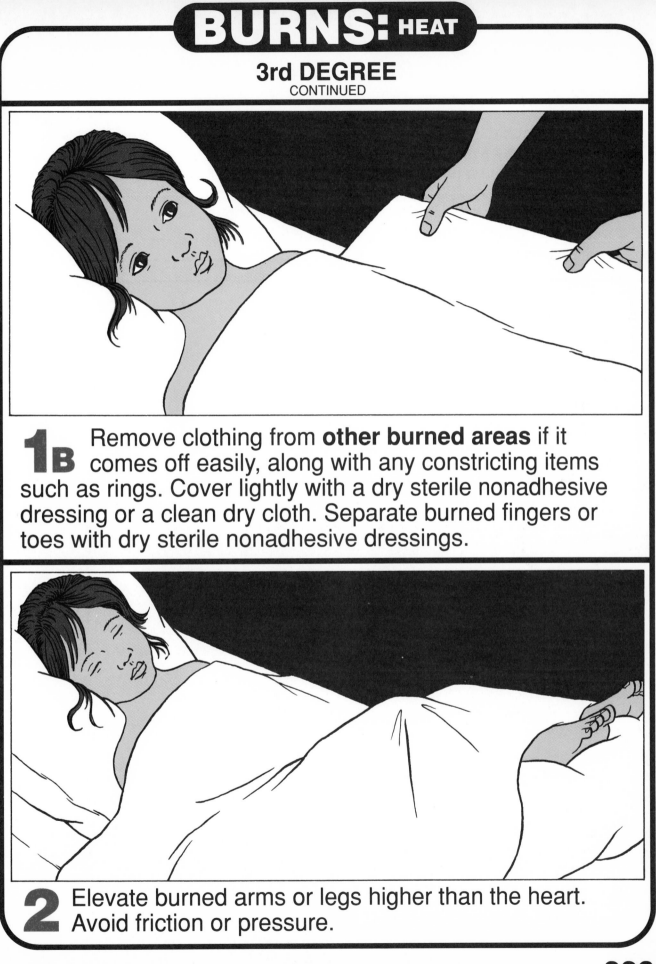

1B Remove clothing from **other burned areas** if it comes off easily, along with any constricting items such as rings. Cover lightly with a dry sterile nonadhesive dressing or a clean dry cloth. Separate burned fingers or toes with dry sterile nonadhesive dressings.

2 Elevate burned arms or legs higher than the heart. Avoid friction or pressure.

CHECKING THE ABCs

(Airway, Breathing & Circulation)

IMPORTANT

- For life to be sustained, the lungs (the respiratory system) and the heart (the circulatory system) must continue to function. To be sure a child's respiratory system is still working, it is necessary to open her **AIRWAY** and check her **BREATHING** to make certain that her lungs are still operating. To be sure her heart is still functioning, it is necessary to check her **CIRCULATION** by checking her pulse.

- **If the child has stopped breathing or her heart has stopped beating, immediate action must be taken. Seek medical aid immediately.** Yell for help and have someone call 911 or Operator; see **EMS,** page 272.

- **If the child is under 8 years old and no one responds to your repeated shouts for help,** administer first aid for 1 minute, then call EMS yourself. Return immediately and continue first aid.

- **If the child is over 8 years old and no one is available,** call EMS yourself, then return immediately and begin first aid.

- Severe bleeding can also interfere with circulation. If necessary, see **BLEEDING: CUTS & WOUNDS,** pages 156-177.

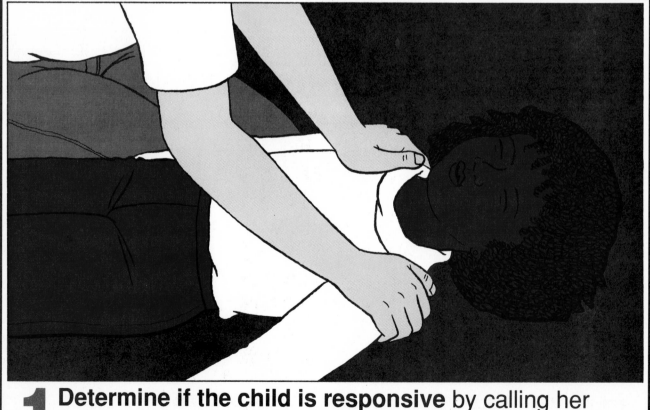

1 **Determine if the child is responsive** by calling her loudly, tapping her on the shoulder or shaking her gently.

CONTINUED ON NEXT PAGE

(Airway, Breathing & Circulation)
CONTINUED

2A **If an infant under 1 year old is unresponsive and there is no neck or back injury, open her AIRWAY** by using the **HEAD-TILT/CHIN-LIFT:** Moving her as a single unit by supporting her head and neck, roll her onto her back on a firm surface. Stand or kneel facing her from the side. Place your hand — the one closest to her head — on her forehead. Place 1 or 2 fingers (but **not** the thumb) of your other hand under the bony part of her jaw at the chin. Gently tilt her head back to the **neutral** position (as shown) by applying gentle backward pressure on her forehead and lifting her chin. **Do not** close her mouth completely. **If there is a neck or back injury, open her AIRWAY** by gently moving her jaw forward **without** tilting or moving her head.

CONTINUED ON NEXT PAGE

(Airway, Breathing & Circulation)
CONTINUED

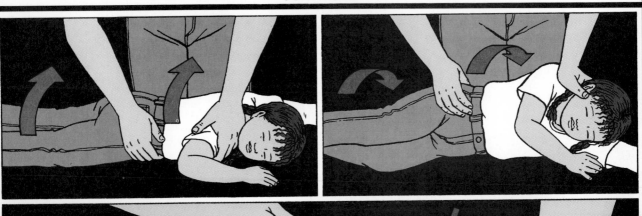

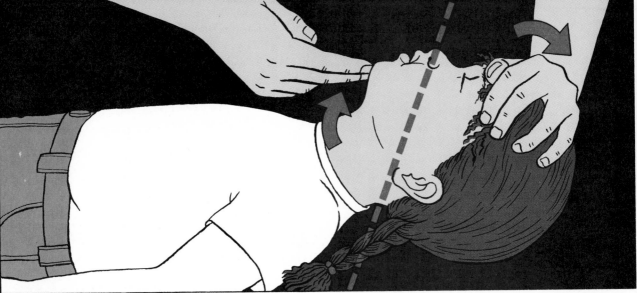

2B If a child between 1 and 8 years old is unresponsive and there is no neck or back injury, open her AIRWAY by using the **HEAD-TILT/CHIN-LIFT**: Moving her as a single unit by supporting her head and neck, roll her onto her back on a firm surface. Kneel beside her chest. Place your hand — the one closest to her head — on her forehead. Place 2 or 3 fingers (but **not** the thumb) of your other hand under the bony part of her jaw at the chin. Gently tilt her head back to the **neutral-plus** position (as shown) by applying gentle backward pressure on her forehead and lifting her chin. **Do not** close her mouth completely. **If there is a neck or back injury, open her AIRWAY** by gently moving her jaw forward **without** tilting or moving her head.

CONTINUED ON NEXT PAGE

(Airway, Breathing & Circulation)
CONTINUED

2c **If a child over 8 years old is unresponsive and there is no neck or back injury, open her AIRWAY** by using the **HEAD-TILT/CHIN-LIFT:** Moving her as a single unit by supporting her head and neck, roll the child onto her back on a firm surface. Kneel beside her chest. Place your hand — the one closest to her head — on her forehead. Place 2 or 3 fingers (but **not** the thumb) of your other hand under the bony part of her jaw at the chin. Gently tilt her head back to the **hyper-extended** position (with her chin pointing straight up, as shown) by applying gentle backward pressure on her forehead and lifting her chin. **Do not** close her mouth completely. **If there is a neck or back injury, open her AIRWAY** by gently moving her jaw forward **without** tilting or moving her head.

CONTINUED ON NEXT PAGE

(Airway, Breathing & Circulation)

CONTINUED

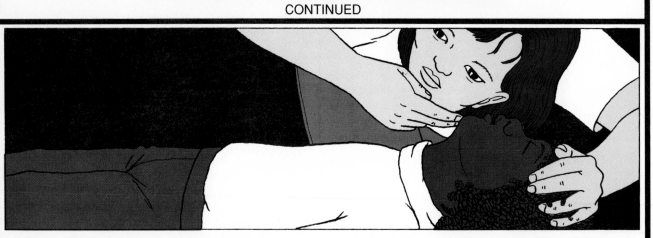

3 Taking 3 to 5 seconds, check the child's BREATH-ING by looking, listening and feeling for air leaving her lungs. (**Look** at her chest for movement. **Listen** for sounds of breathing. And **feel** for her breath on your cheek.)

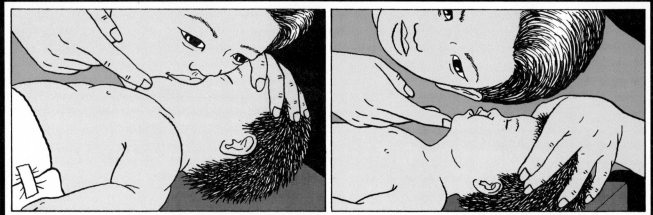

4A **If an infant under 1 year old is not breathing:** Place your open mouth over her nose and mouth, forming an airtight seal. Then give 2 slow, gentle breaths (1 to 1½ seconds each), allowing the lungs to deflate fully between each breath. Remove your mouth between breaths, and look and listen for air leaving her lungs. **If the entry or return of air seems blocked, or her chest does not rise, try again to open her AIRWAY** (see Step 2A) and give 2 slow, gentle breaths. **If the AIRWAY still seems blocked,** see **CHOKING,** pages 239-245. When the obstruction is cleared, continue on to Step 5.

CONTINUED ON NEXT PAGE

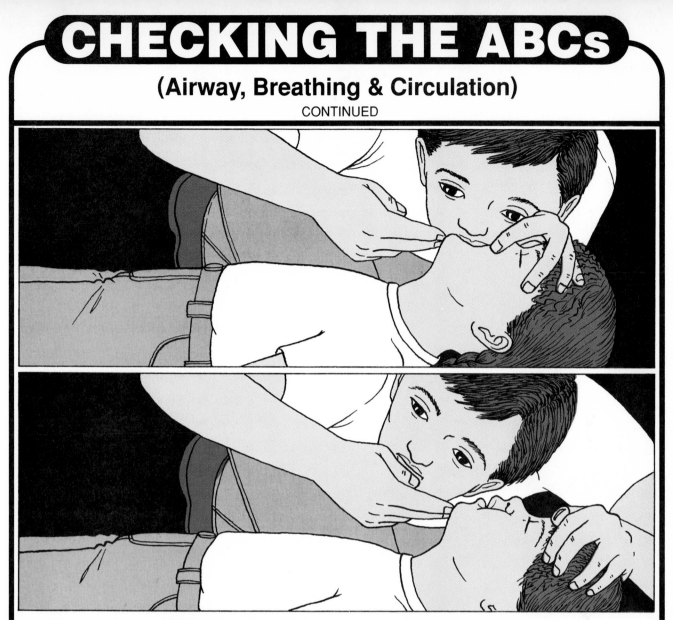

4B **If a child between 1 and 8 years old is not breathing:** Pinch her nose closed with the thumb and index finger of the hand that is on her forehead. Place your open mouth over her open mouth, forming an airtight seal. Then give 2 slow, gentle breaths (1 to 1½ seconds each), allowing the lungs to deflate fully between each breath. Remove your mouth between breaths, and look and listen for air leaving her lungs. **If the entry or return of air seems blocked, or her chest does not rise, try again to open her AIRWAY** (see Step 2B) and give 2 slow, gentle breaths. **If the AIRWAY still seems blocked,** see **CHOK-ING,** pages 246-252. When the obstruction is cleared, continue on to Step 5.

CONTINUED ON NEXT PAGE

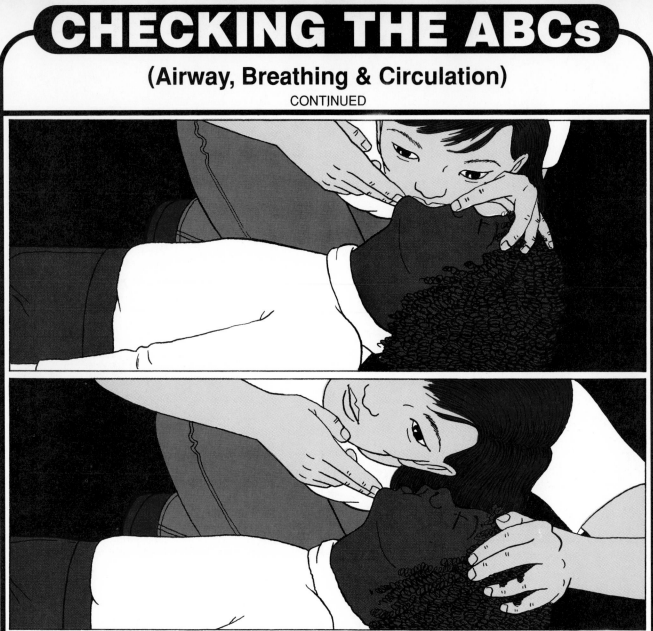

4c **If a child over 8 years old is not breathing:** Pinch her nose closed with the thumb and index finger of the hand that is on her forehead. Place your open mouth over her open mouth, forming an airtight seal. Then give 2 slow, full breaths (1½ to 2 seconds each), allowing the lungs to deflate fully between each breath. Remove your mouth between breaths, and look and listen for air leaving her lungs. **If the entry or return of air seems blocked, or her chest does not rise, try again to open her AIRWAY** (see Step 2C) and give 2 slow, full breaths. **If the AIRWAY still seems blocked,** see **CHOKING,** pages 246-252. When the obstruction is cleared, continue on to Step 5.

CONTINUED ON NEXT PAGE

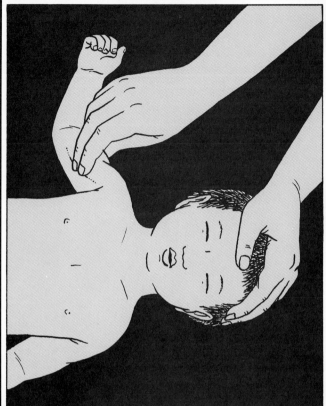

INFANT (UNDER 1 YEAR OLD)

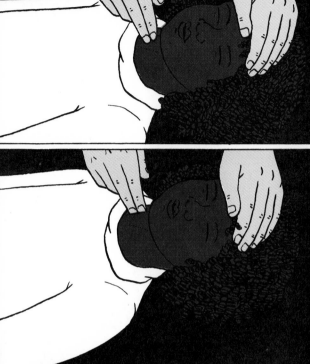

CHILD (OVER 1 YEAR OLD)

5 Check the child's **CIRCULATION** by checking her pulse: **For an infant under 1 year old,** continue to hold her head in the **neutral** position with your hand on her forehead, then **check the pulse slowly and carefully** by placing the fingertips of your other hand (but **not** your thumb) on the inside of her upper arm between the elbow and shoulder. **For a child over 1 year old, check the pulse slowly and carefully** at the large artery of the neck. Place your first two fingers on the child's Adam's apple (about halfway between the chin and the collarbone). Slide your fingers into the groove next to the windpipe on the side nearest you, then press gently. **It is extremely important to find the pulse if one is present. Take between 5 and 10 seconds to find it. Do not rush.** It is easily missed under emergency conditions.

CONTINUED ON NEXT PAGE

6A **If the child has no pulse,** see **HEART FAILURE,** pages 303-323.

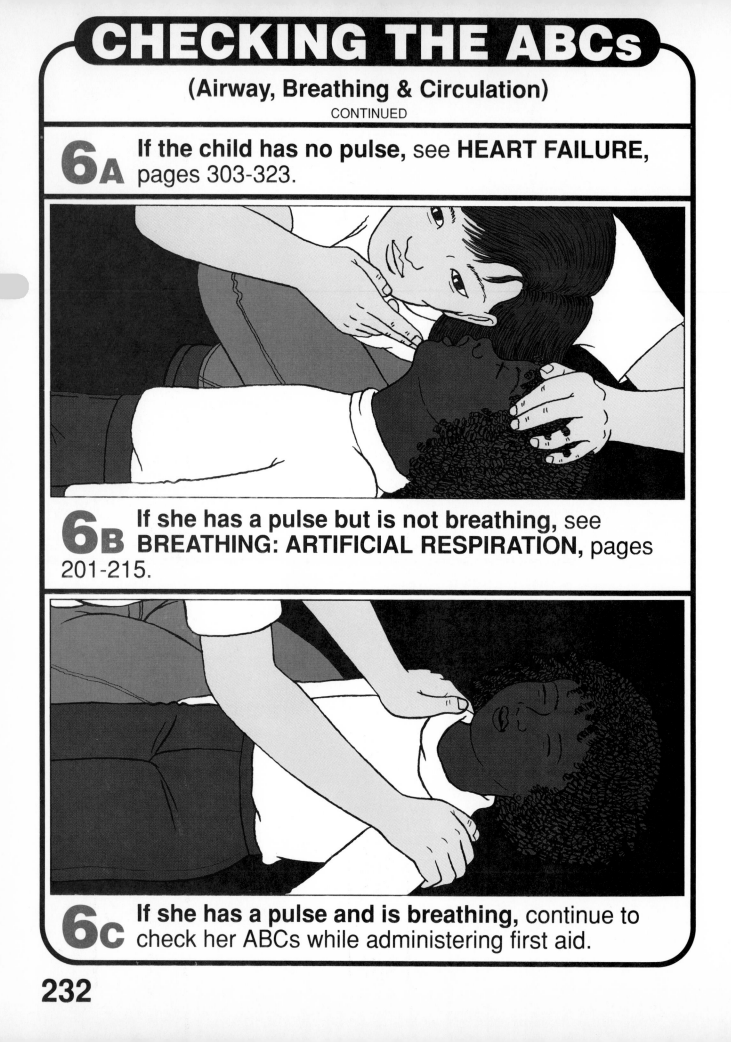

6B **If she has a pulse but is not breathing,** see **BREATHING: ARTIFICIAL RESPIRATION,** pages 201-215.

6C **If she has a pulse and is breathing,** continue to check her ABCs while administering first aid.

CHEST INJURIES

CRUSHED CHEST

IMPORTANT

- **Seek medical aid immediately.** Call 911 or Operator; see **EMS,** page 272.

- Check the child's ABCs (Airway, Breathing and Circulation); see **CHECKING THE ABCs,** pages 224-232.

- Observe for **SHOCK,** pages 354-356.

SIGNS & SYMPTOMS

Many broken ribs. The chest may collapse rather than expand when the child tries to inhale.

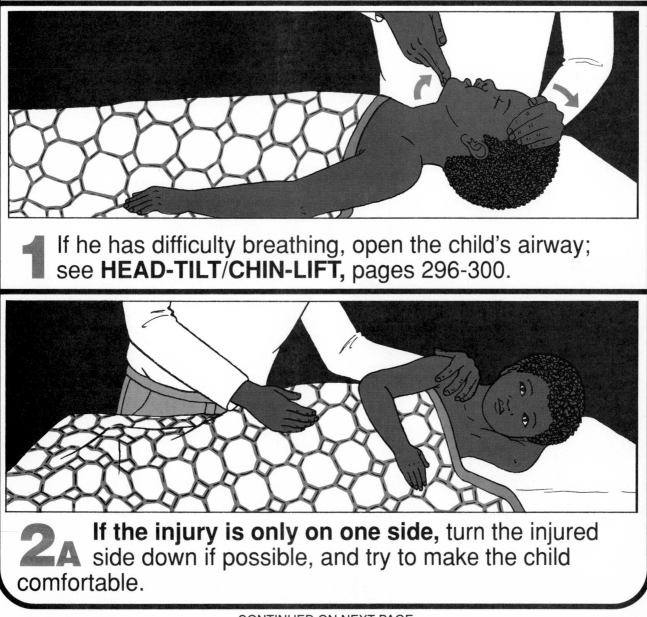

1 If he has difficulty breathing, open the child's airway; see **HEAD-TILT/CHIN-LIFT,** pages 296-300.

2A **If the injury is only on one side,** turn the injured side down if possible, and try to make the child comfortable.

CONTINUED ON NEXT PAGE

CRUSHED CHEST
CONTINUED

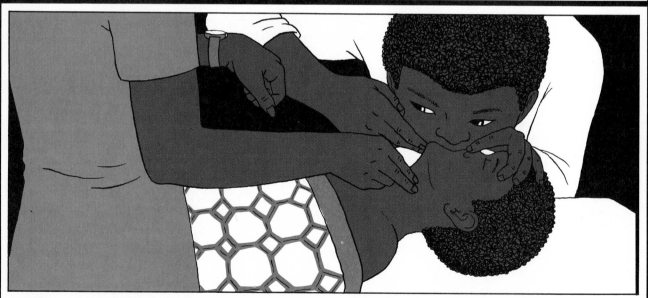

2B **If the injury is in the center or on both sides of the chest or if he has trouble breathing,** prop him up in a comfortable position. Place a pillow under **both** his head and his shoulders, **not** just his head.

3 If necessary, begin rescue breathing immediately; see **BREATHING: ARTIFICIAL RESPIRATION,** pages 201-215. Watch his pulse closely; see **TAKING THE PULSE,** pages 366-367. If it stops, treat for heart failure immediately; see **HEART FAILURE,** pages 303-323.

CHEST INJURIES

OPEN CHEST WOUNDS

IMPORTANT

- **Seek medical aid immediately.** Call 911 or Operator; see **EMS,** page 272.
- Check the child's ABCs (Airway, Breathing and Circulation); see **CHECKING THE ABCs,** pages 224-232.
- **Do not** move the child unless absolutely necessary.
- **Do not** give him anything to eat or drink.
- **Do not** place a pillow under his head if he is lying down.

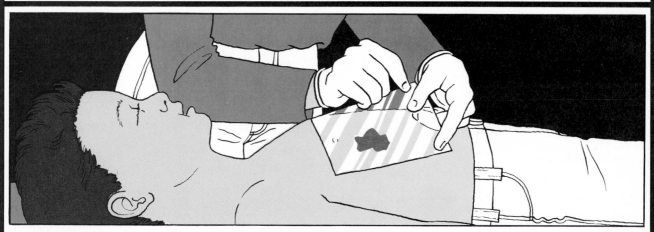

1 Seal the wound immediately with a nonporous dressing — plastic wrap, aluminum foil, etc. **Be sure** the seal extends beyond the edges of the wound.

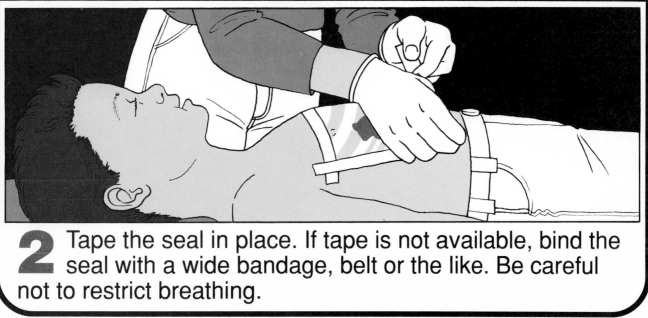

2 Tape the seal in place. If tape is not available, bind the seal with a wide bandage, belt or the like. Be careful not to restrict breathing.

CONTINUED ON NEXT PAGE

OPEN CHEST WOUNDS
CONTINUED

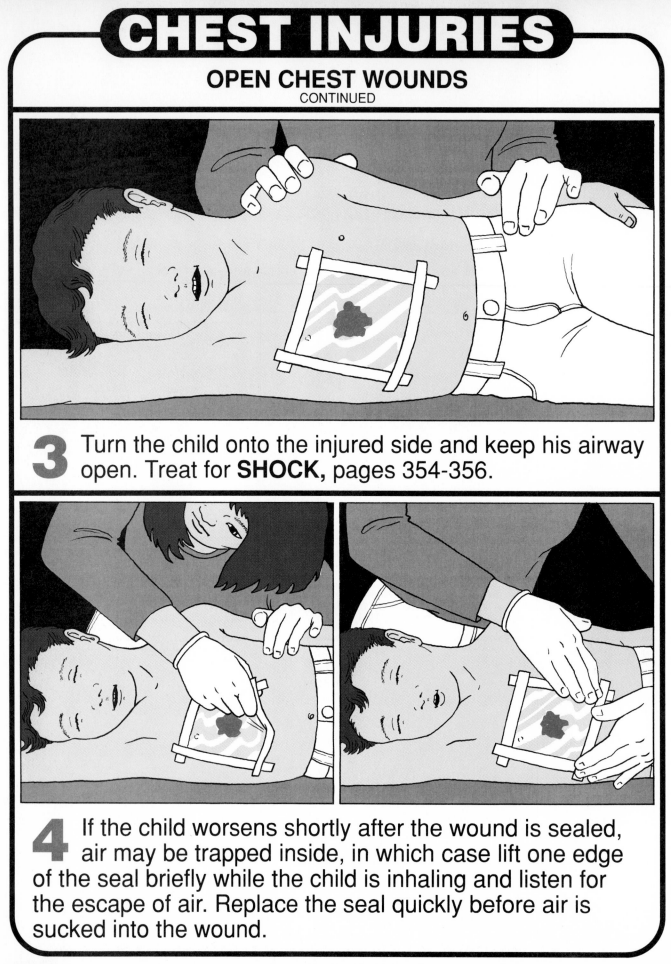

3 Turn the child onto the injured side and keep his airway open. Treat for **SHOCK,** pages 354-356.

4 If the child worsens shortly after the wound is sealed, air may be trapped inside, in which case lift one edge of the seal briefly while the child is inhaling and listen for the escape of air. Replace the seal quickly before air is sucked into the wound.

CHEST INJURIES

RIBS

IMPORTANT

- **Seek medical aid.** If necessary, call 911 or Operator; see **EMS,** page 272.
- Check the child's breathing. If necessary, see **BREATHING: ARTIFICIAL RESPIRATION,** pages 201-215.

SIGNS & SYMPTOMS

The child feels pain when he inhales or when the rib area is touched.

IF MEDICAL AID WILL ARRIVE WITHIN 1 HOUR

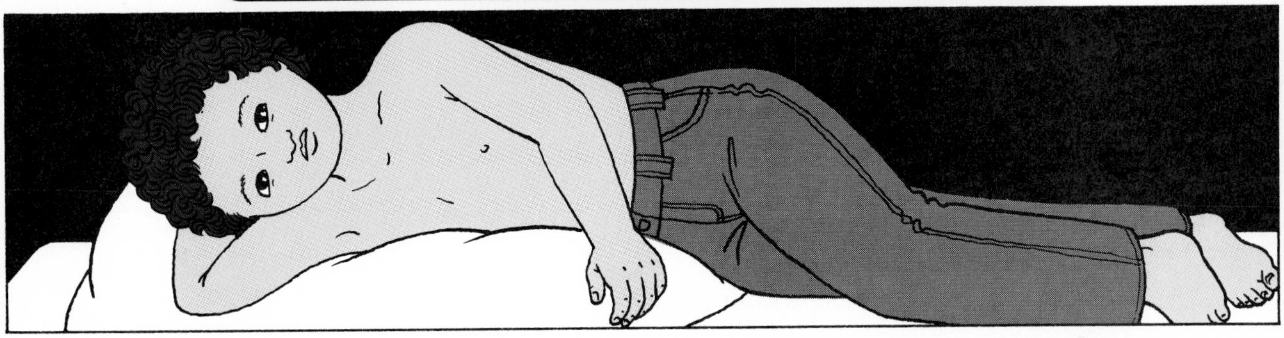

Place the child, injured side down, on a pillow or folded blanket.

IF MEDICAL AID WILL NOT ARRIVE WITHIN 1 HOUR OR YOU MUST TRANSPORT THE CHILD

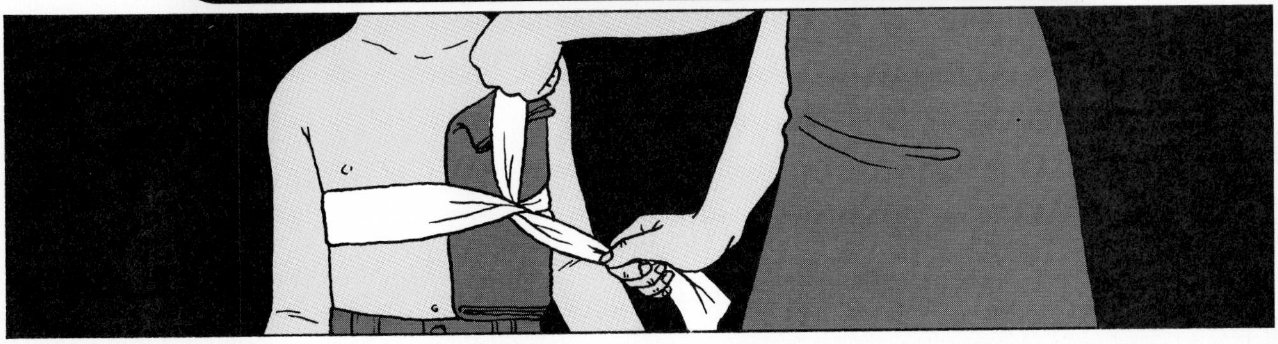

1 Restrict the movement of the chest by binding it with three wide cloth bandages. Place the first bandage around the center of the chest and bring the ends together in a loose half-knot on the uninjured side of the body. Slip a handkerchief or other folded cloth under the bandage to prevent discomfort from the knots.

CONTINUED ON NEXT PAGE

237

RIBS
CONTINUED

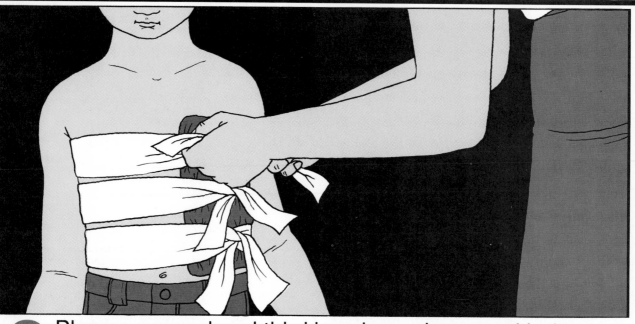

2 Place a second and third bandage above and below the first one. Then gently tie the half-knots. **Do not** tie too tightly. The bandages should apply gentle pressure to the injured area.

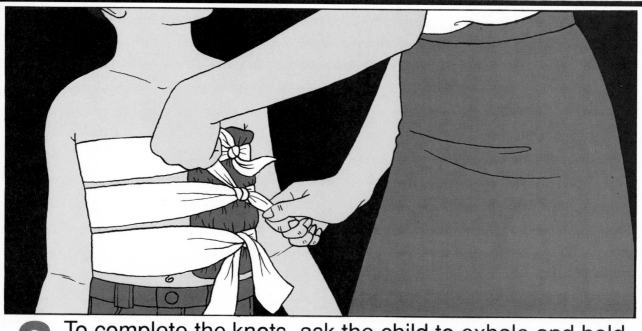

3 To complete the knots, ask the child to exhale and hold his breath. Then take out the slack and finish tying the knots before he starts his next breath.

CHOKING

CONSCIOUS INFANT (TO 1 YEAR OLD)

IMPORTANT

- **If the infant is unconscious,** see **CHOKING: UNCONSCIOUS INFANT (TO 1 YEAR OLD),** pages 242-245.

- **Seek medical aid immediately if the infant cannot breathe, cough or cry.** Have someone call 911 or Operator; see **EMS,** page 272. If necessary, see **BREATHING: ARTIFICIAL RESPIRATION,** pages 201-205.

- **Do not** interfere with the infant's own efforts to free the obstruction if he can breathe, cough or cry. If he cannot free the obstruction, follow first aid below.

- After all choking episodes, have the infant checked by a doctor.

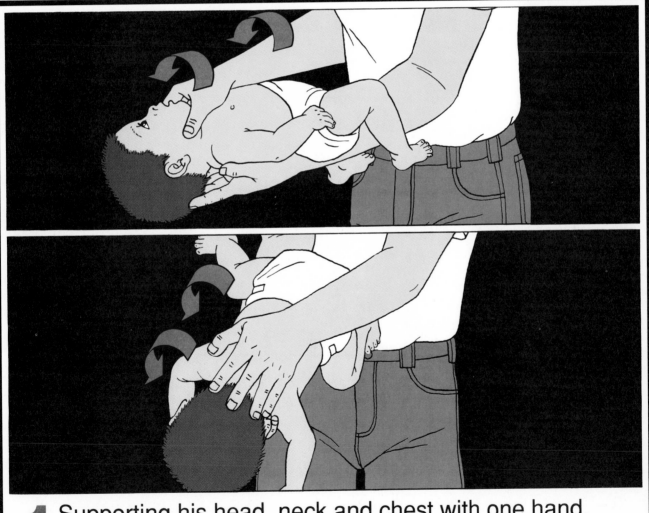

1 Supporting his head, neck and chest with one hand, place the infant facedown on your forearm with his head lower than the rest of his body.

CONTINUED ON NEXT PAGE

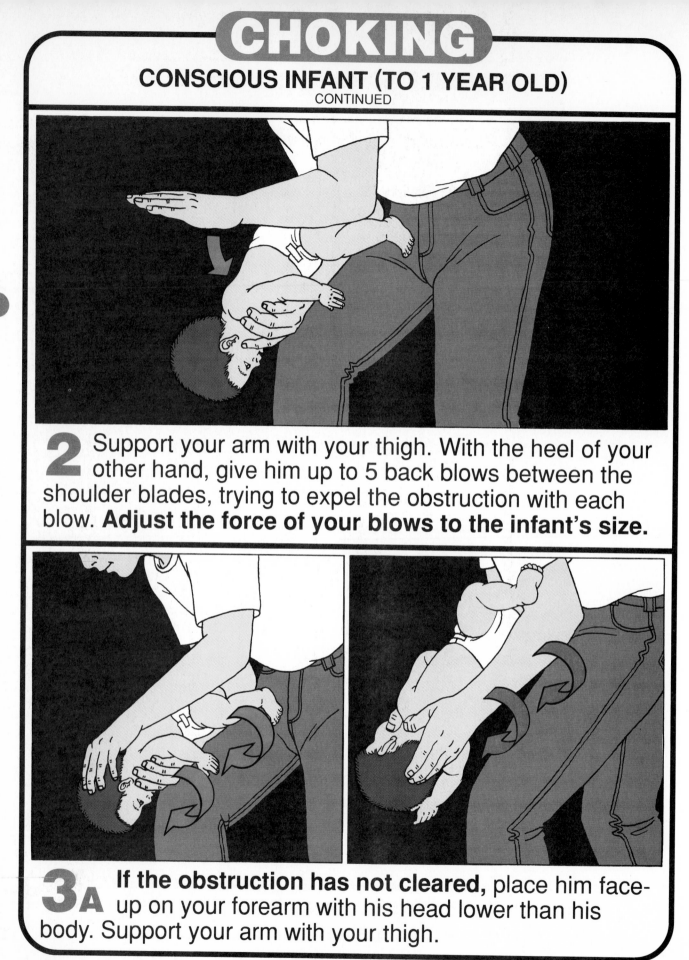

2 Support your arm with your thigh. With the heel of your other hand, give him up to 5 back blows between the shoulder blades, trying to expel the obstruction with each blow. **Adjust the force of your blows to the infant's size.**

3A **If the obstruction has not cleared,** place him face-up on your forearm with his head lower than his body. Support your arm with your thigh.

CONTINUED ON NEXT PAGE

CONSCIOUS INFANT (TO 1 YEAR OLD)
CONTINUED

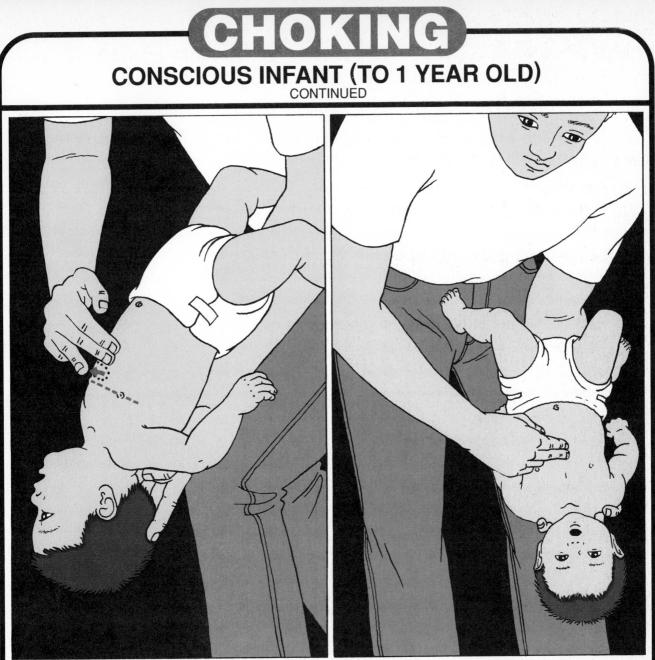

3B Place the pad of your ring finger just below the imaginary line between the infant's nipples. Then place the pads of your middle and index fingers next to the ring finger. Now lift your ring finger and make up to 5 quick thrusts downward toward his chest ½ to 1 inch deep, trying to expel the obstruction with each thrust. **Do not** thrust to either side. **Adjust the force of your thrusts to the infant's size.** Continue the series of up to 5 back blows and up to 5 chest thrusts until the object is dislodged. Watch breathing closely. If necessary, see **BREATHING: ARTIFICIAL RESPIRATION,** pages 201-205.

CHOKING

UNCONSCIOUS INFANT (TO 1 YEAR OLD)

IMPORTANT

- **Determine if the infant is responsive by calling her loudly, tapping her on the shoulder or shaking her gently.**

- **If she is responsive,** see **CHOKING: CONSCIOUS INFANT (TO 1 YEAR OLD),** pages 239-241.

- **If she is unresponsive, seek medical aid immediately.** Yell for help and have someone call 911 or Operator; see **EMS,** page 272. If no one answers your repeated shouts for help, administer first aid for 1 minute, then call EMS yourself. Return immediately and continue first aid.

- Remove a foreign object from the infant's mouth only if you can see it and it is accessible.

- After all choking episodes, have the infant checked by a doctor.

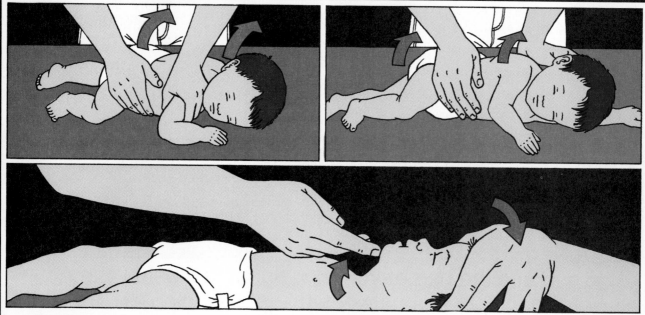

1 Moving her as a single unit, place the infant on her back on a firm surface and **open her airway** by using the **head-tilt/chin-lift:** Place your hand — the one closest to her head — on her forehead. Place 1 or 2 fingers (but **not** the thumb) of your other hand under the bony part of her jaw at the chin. Gently tilt back her head to a **neutral** position by applying gentle backward pressure on her forehead and lifting her chin. **Do not** press on the soft tissue under the chin or close her mouth completely.

CONTINUED ON NEXT PAGE

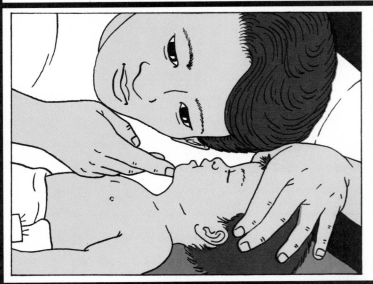

2 Taking 3 to 5 seconds, check for breathing by looking, listening and feeling for air leaving her lungs. (**Look** at her chest for movement. **Listen** for sounds of breathing. And **feel** for her breath on your cheek.)

3 If the infant is not breathing: Place your open mouth over the infant's nose and mouth, forming an airtight seal. Give 2 slow, gentle breaths (1 to 1½ seconds each). Remove your mouth between breaths and wait for her chest to fall before giving the next breath.

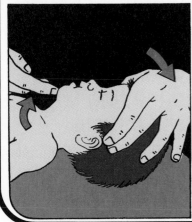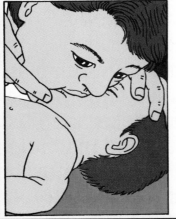

4 If breaths do not go in or the airway appears blocked: Reposition her head to the **neutral** position and once again try to give her 2 slow, gentle breaths.

CONTINUED ON NEXT PAGE

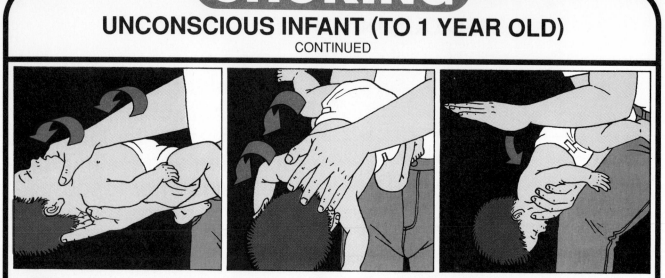

5 Supporting her head, neck and chest with one hand, place her facedown on your forearm with her head below the rest of her body. With the heel of your other hand, give her up to 5 blows between the shoulder blades, trying to dislodge the obstruction with each blow. **Adjust the force of your blows to the infant's size.**

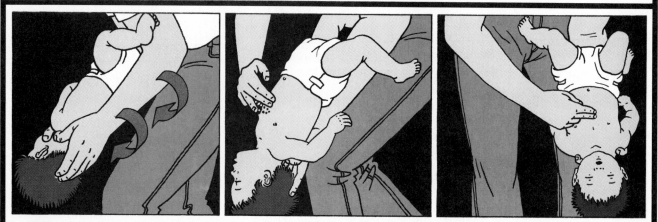

6 Immediately place her faceup on your forearm with her head below the rest of her body. Support your arm with your thigh. Place the pad of your ring finger just below the imaginary line between the infant's nipples. Then place the pads of your middle and index fingers next to the ring finger. Now lift your ring finger and make up to 5 quick thrusts downward toward her chest ½ to 1 inch deep, trying to expel the obstruction with each thrust. **Do not** thrust to either side. **Adjust the force of your thrusts to the infant's size.**

CONTINUED ON NEXT PAGE

UNCONSCIOUS INFANT (TO 1 YEAR OLD)
CONTINUED

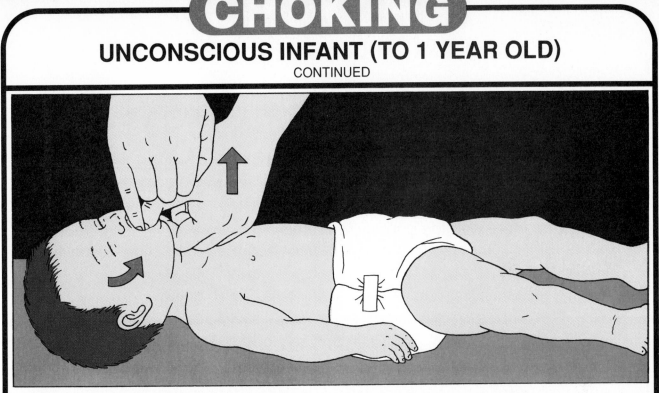

7 Look for the obstruction in the infant's mouth. If a foreign object is visible and accessible, clear it out with your little finger. Check her breathing. If necessary, continue rescue breaths until breathing is restored.

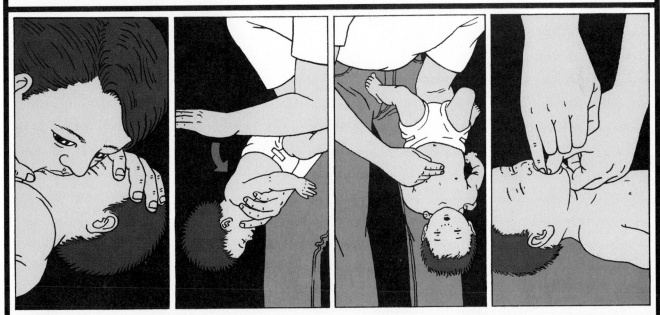

8 **If the obstruction has not cleared:** Continue series of 2 slow breaths followed by up to 5 back blows, up to 5 chest thrusts and a foreign object check until the object is dislodged or medical aid arrives.

CHOKING

CONSCIOUS CHILD (OVER 1 YEAR OLD)

IMPORTANT

- **If the child is unconscious,** see **CHOKING: UNCONSCIOUS CHILD (OVER 1 YEAR OLD),** pages 249-252.

- **Seek medical aid immediately if the child cannot breathe, speak or cough.** Have someone call 911 or Operator; see **EMS,** page 272. If necessary, see **BREATHING: ARTIFICIAL RESPIRATION,** pages 206-215.

- **Do not** interfere with the child's own efforts to free the obstruction if he can breathe, speak or cough. If he cannot free the obstruction, follow first aid below.

- After all choking episodes, have the child checked by a doctor.

IF HE IS STANDING OR SITTING

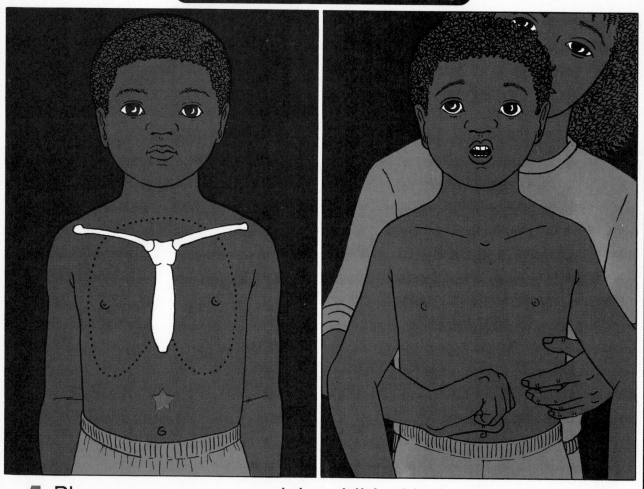

1 Place your arm around the child with the thumb side of your fist against his stomach above the navel and well below the sternum.

CONTINUED ON NEXT PAGE

246

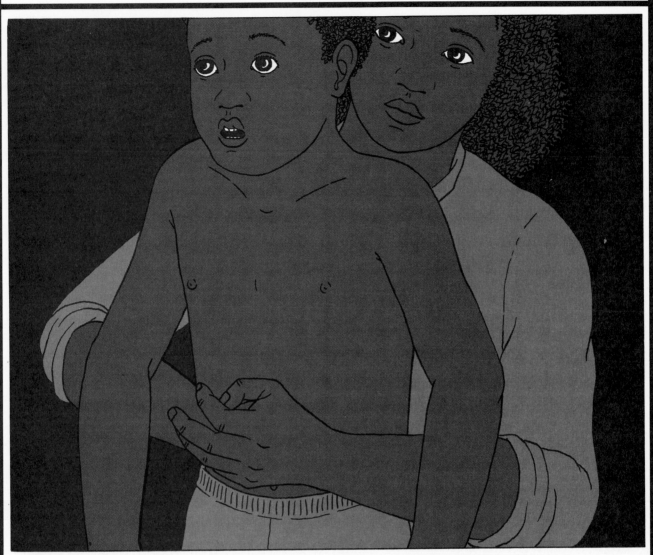

2 Grasp your fist with your other hand, and keeping your elbows pointed out, make a quick backward and upward thrust at the exact spot shown. **Do not** thrust to either side. **Adjust the force of your thrust to the child's size. Repeat up to 5 times if necessary, trying to dislodge the obstruction with each thrust.** If the obstruction has not yet cleared, reassess the situation: Recheck to make sure the child is still conscious and your hands are in the right position. Then repeat thrusts if necessary. Watch breathing closely. If necessary, see **BREATHING: ARTIFICIAL RESPIRATION,** pages 206-215.

CONTINUED ON NEXT PAGE

CHOKING

IF HE IS LYING DOWN

Roll him on his back and straddle his legs. Place the heel of one hand on his stomach above the navel and well below the sternum. Place your other hand on top of the first. Give up to 5 downward and forward thrusts, trying to expel the obstruction with each thrust. **Do not** thrust to either side. **Adjust the force of your thrusts to the child's size.** Between each thrust, check if the obstruction has been expelled. If the obstruction has not yet cleared, reassess the situation: Recheck to make sure the child is still conscious and your hands are in the right position. Then repeat thrusts if necessary. Watch breathing closely. If necessary, see **BREATHING: ARTIFICIAL RESPIRATION,** pages 206-215.

CHOKING

UNCONSCIOUS CHILD (OVER 1 YEAR OLD)

IMPORTANT

- **Determine if the child is responsive by calling her loudly, tapping her on the shoulder or shaking her gently.**

- **If she is responsive,** see **CHOKING: CONSCIOUS CHILD (OVER 1 YEAR OLD),** pages 246-248.

- **If she is unresponsive, seek medical aid immediately.** Yell for help and have someone call 911 or Operator; see **EMS,** page 272. **If the child is under 8 and no one answers your repeated shouts for help,** administer first aid for 1 minute, then call EMS yourself. Return immediately and continue first aid. **If the child is over 8 and no one responds,** call EMS yourself without waiting any longer, then return immediately and begin first aid.

- Remove a foreign object from the child's mouth only if you can see it and it is accessible.

- After all choking episodes, have the child checked by a doctor.

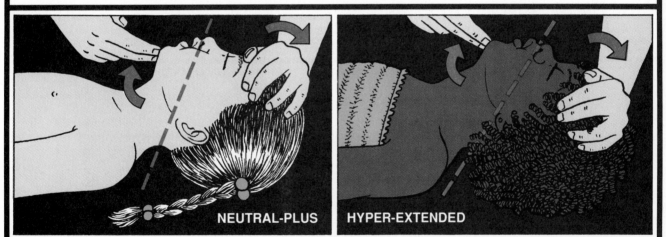

NEUTRAL-PLUS   HYPER-EXTENDED

1 Place the child on her back on a firm surface and **open her airway** by using the **head-tilt/chin-lift:** Place your hand — the one closest to her head — on her forehead. Place 2 or 3 fingers (but **not** the thumb) of your other hand under the bony part of her jaw at the chin. **If the child is under 8 years old,** gently tilt her head back to the **neutral-plus** position by applying gentle backward pressure on her forehead and lifting her chin. **Do not** close the child's mouth completely. **If she is over 8 years old,** use the **hyper-extended** position.

CONTINUED ON NEXT PAGE

UNCONSCIOUS CHILD (OVER 1 YEAR OLD)
CONTINUED

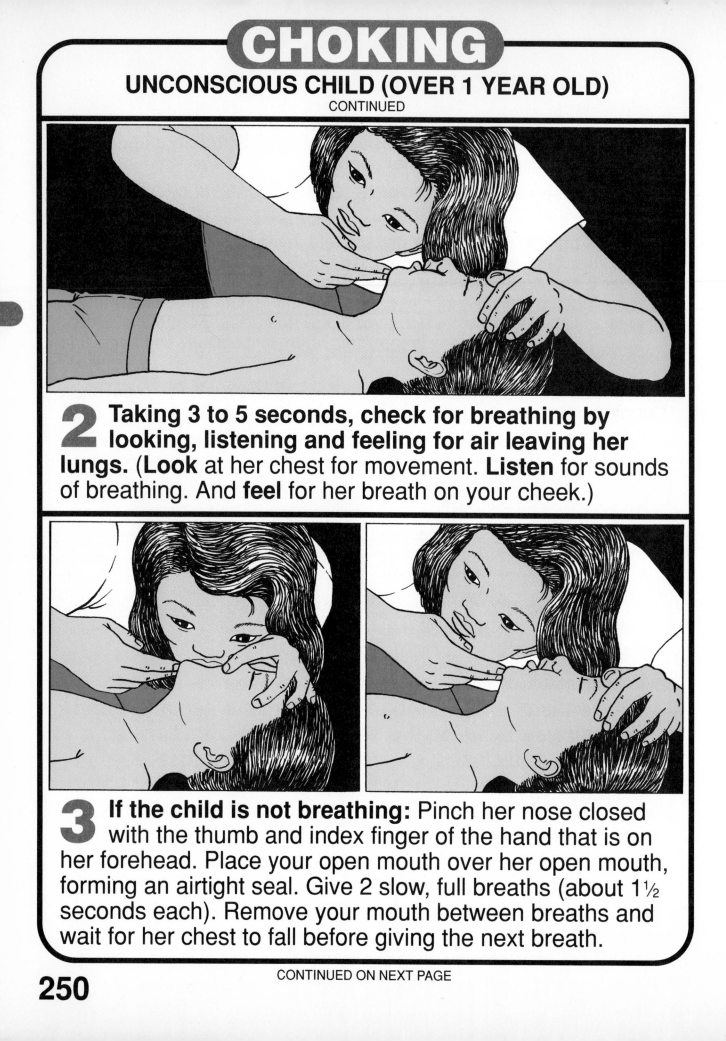

2 Taking 3 to 5 seconds, check for breathing by looking, listening and feeling for air leaving her lungs. (**Look** at her chest for movement. **Listen** for sounds of breathing. And **feel** for her breath on your cheek.)

3 If the child is not breathing: Pinch her nose closed with the thumb and index finger of the hand that is on her forehead. Place your open mouth over her open mouth, forming an airtight seal. Give 2 slow, full breaths (about 1½ seconds each). Remove your mouth between breaths and wait for her chest to fall before giving the next breath.

CONTINUED ON NEXT PAGE

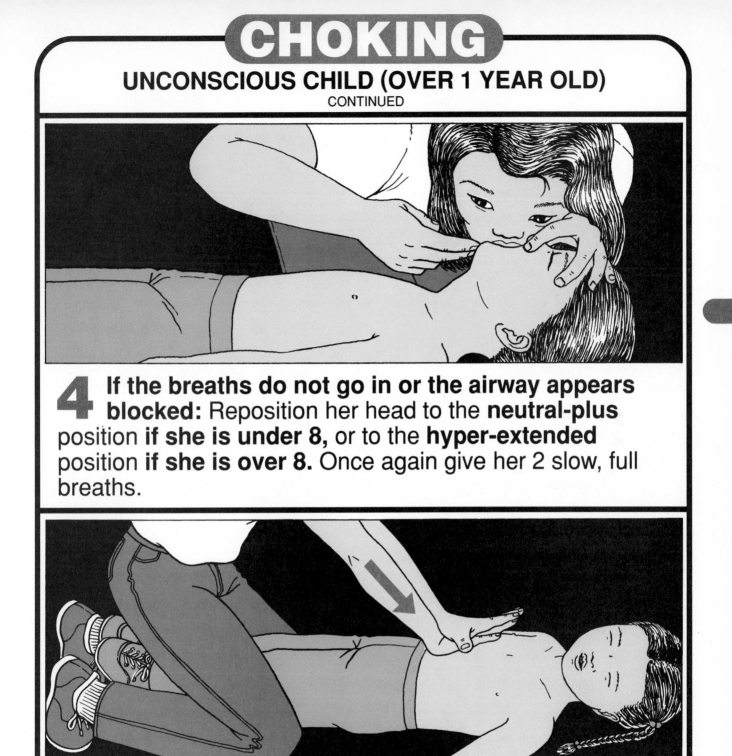

4 **If the breaths do not go in or the airway appears blocked:** Reposition her head to the **neutral-plus** position **if she is under 8,** or to the **hyper-extended** position **if she is over 8.** Once again give her 2 slow, full breaths.

5 Straddle the child's thighs. Place the heel of one hand on her stomach above the navel and well below the sternum, and put your other hand on top of the first. Then give up to 5 quick thrusts, pressing downward and forward, trying to expel the obstruction with each thrust. **Do not** thrust to either side. **Adjust the force of your thrusts to the child's size.**

CONTINUED ON NEXT PAGE

UNCONSCIOUS CHILD (OVER 1 YEAR OLD)
CONTINUED

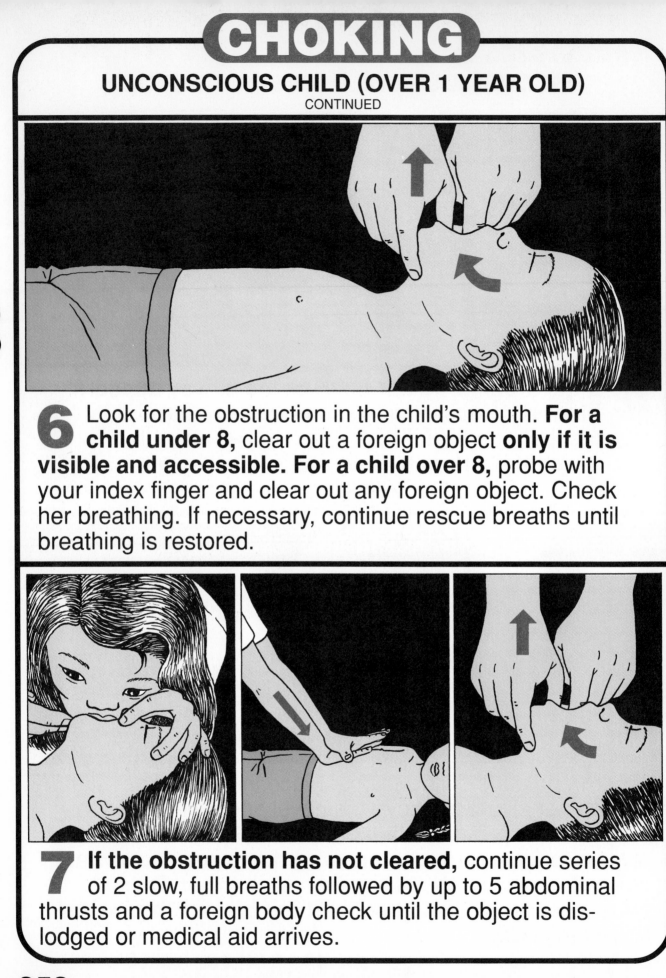

6 Look for the obstruction in the child's mouth. **For a child under 8,** clear out a foreign object **only if it is visible and accessible. For a child over 8,** probe with your index finger and clear out any foreign object. Check her breathing. If necessary, continue rescue breaths until breathing is restored.

7 **If the obstruction has not cleared,** continue series of 2 slow, full breaths followed by up to 5 abdominal thrusts and a foreign body check until the object is dislodged or medical aid arrives.

IMPORTANT

- **Seek medical aid for all convulsions and seizures, no matter how brief.** If necessary, call 911 or Operator; see **EMS,** page 272.

- Catch the child if she starts to fall, and lay her down gently.

- **Do not** give her anything to drink during the convulsion or place anything between her teeth.

- Check for injuries when the convulsion is over.

- For a seizure caused by a high fever, see **FEVER,** pages 284-285.

SIGNS & SYMPTOMS

Falling. Drooling. Frothing at the mouth. Stiffening of the body. Jerky, uncontrollable movements. Unconsciousness.

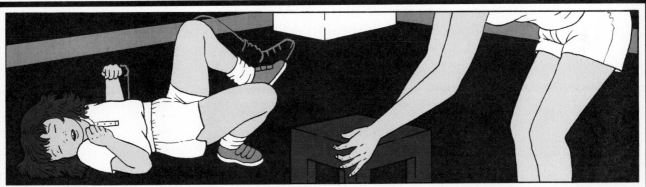

1 Clear the area of hard or sharp objects that might cause harm. Try to loosen tight clothing, particularly around the neck, but **do not** restrain the child.

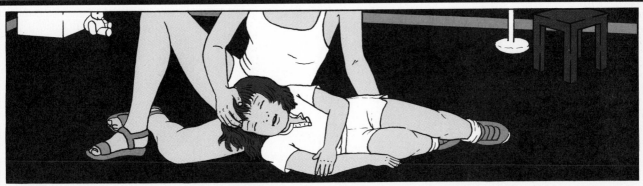

2 When the convulsion subsides, turn the child onto her side to prevent choking. Watch breathing closely. If necessary, see **BREATHING: ARTIFICIAL RESPIRATION,** pages 201-215.

DEHYDRATION

IMPORTANT

- **Dehydration, the excessive loss of body fluids, can be life-threatening, especially in infants.** If necessary, call 911 or Operator; see **EMS,** page 272.

- **Seek medical aid immediately** if an infant or very young child has a rapid pulse, sunken fontanel (the soft spot on top of the head) or is listless.

- A child who has diarrhea or a fever, or is sweating profusely or vomiting, may become dehydrated. **Seek medical aid immediately** if he also develops any of the signs and symptoms listed below.

- Consult your doctor if symptoms persist.

SIGNS & SYMPTOMS

Decreased intake of fluids. Extreme thirst. Dark yellow urine. Decreased frequency or amount of urine. Dry mouth and tongue. Sunken eyes. Sunken fontanel. Pale, dry skin. Rapid pulse. Cramps. Listlessness. Drowsiness. Irritability. Weight loss. Blood in the vomit or stool.

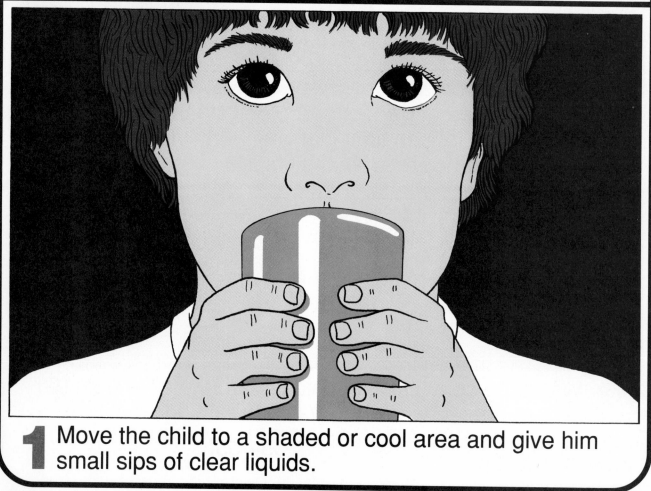

1 Move the child to a shaded or cool area and give him small sips of clear liquids.

CONTINUED ON NEXT PAGE

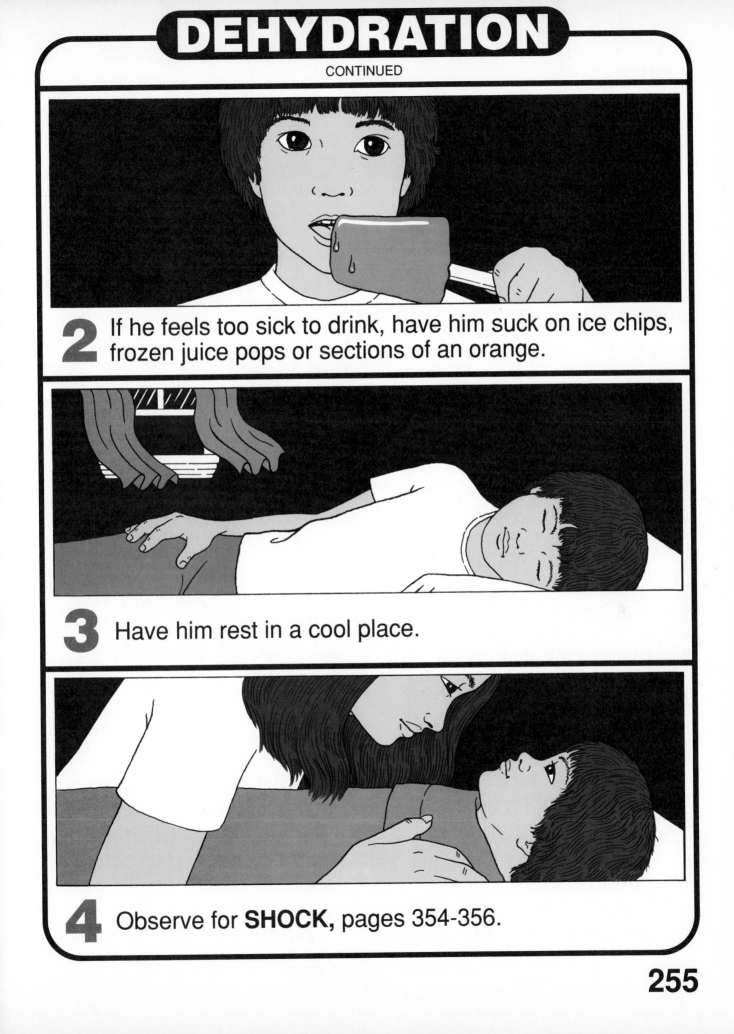

2 If he feels too sick to drink, have him suck on ice chips, frozen juice pops or sections of an orange.

3 Have him rest in a cool place.

4 Observe for **SHOCK,** pages 354-356.

IMPORTANT

- **Send for help immediately.** Call 911 or Operator; see **EMS,** page 272.

- **Do not** swim to the child unless you cannot use reaching assists from land or a boat and it is a matter of life or death.

- **Try to touch the child's hand or body with the reaching assist.** He may be too panicked to realize the assist is there if it doesn't touch him directly.

- When you have returned the child to safety, see **DROWNING: FIRST AID,** pages 259-260.

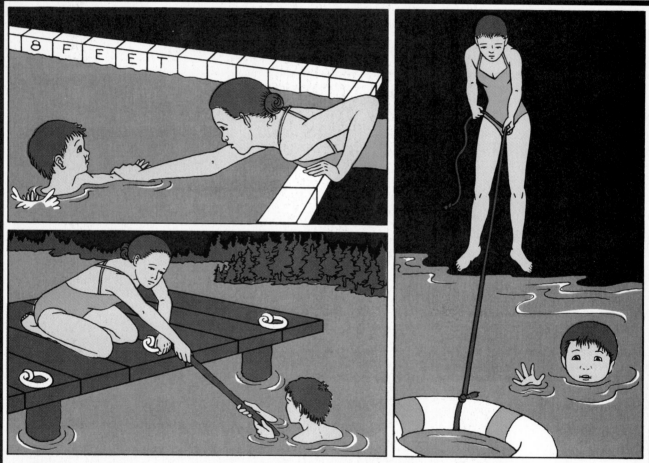

1A Try to reach the child from land with a hand, leg, clothing, pole, rope, etc. Always hold onto something with your other hand. **Do not** let the child grab you. Or throw him a buoy, board or anything that floats. Take care not to hit him; you may accidentally knock him unconscious. Ropes or objects attached to ropes should be thrown beyond the child, then pulled directly into his grasp.

CONTINUED ON NEXT PAGE

CONTINUED

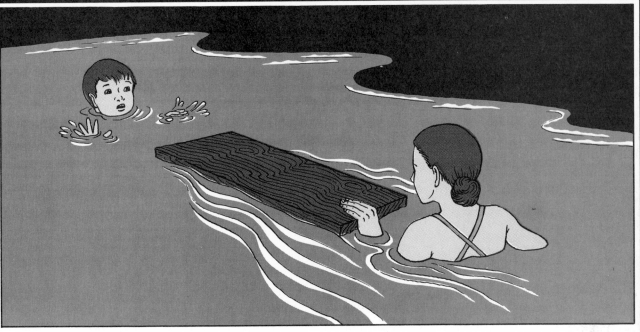

1B If he is too far to reach, **wade in closer with reaching assists.**

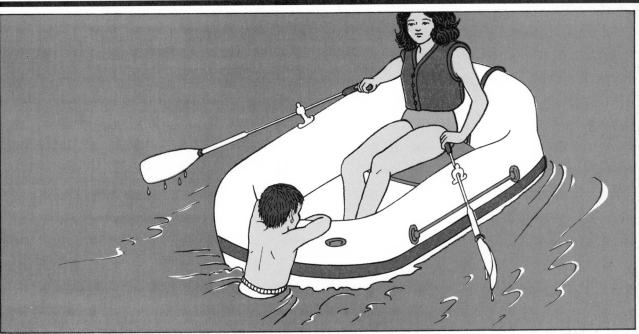

1C Or if a rowboat is available, row out to him, then hand him a reaching assist and pull him toward you. If possible, have him hang onto the rear of the boat while you row back to shore. If this isn't possible, pull him aboard carefully from the rear of the boat, so you don't capsize.

CONTINUED ON NEXT PAGE

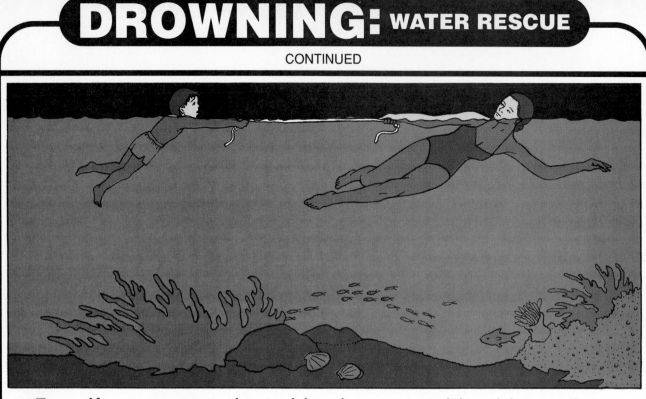

1D If you must swim to him, keep watching him or the spot you saw him last. Bring something for the child to hold onto and tow him to shore. **Do not** let him grab you.

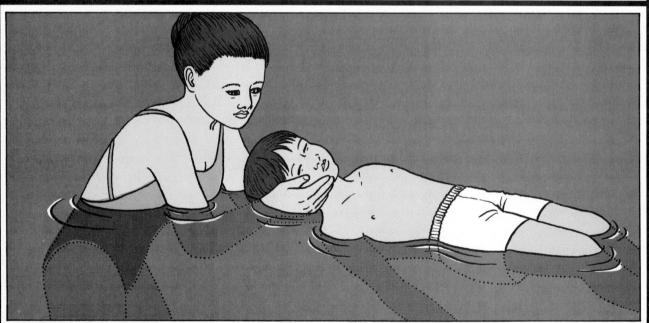

1E **If you suspect a neck or back injury (as in a diving or surfboard accident):** Turn him over gently if he is lying facedown, taking care to keep his head, neck and back in alignment. **Do not** remove him from the water until professional help arrives.

DROWNING: FIRST AID

IMPORTANT

- To rescue a drowning child, see **DROWNING: WATER RESCUE,** pages 256-258, or **ICE RESCUE,** pages 336-337.

- **Seek medical aid immediately.** Have someone call 911 or Operator; see **EMS,** page 272.

- If the child is obviously not breathing, begin rescue breathing immediately, even before leaving the water; see **BREATHING: ARTIFICIAL RESPIRATION,** pages 201-215.

- **Do not** delay rescue breathing by trying to drain water from the child's lungs.

- If the child has been in cold water, it may be necessary to continue rescue breathing or CPR for an extended period of time. **Do not** stop until she revives or professional help arrives.

- After the child has revived, **do not** let her get up and walk around or have anything to eat or drink. Wait for medical assistance to arrive.

- Have the child checked by a doctor for possible complications.

SIGNS & SYMPTOMS

No breathing. Bluish face, especially the lips and ears. Cold skin. Pale appearance.

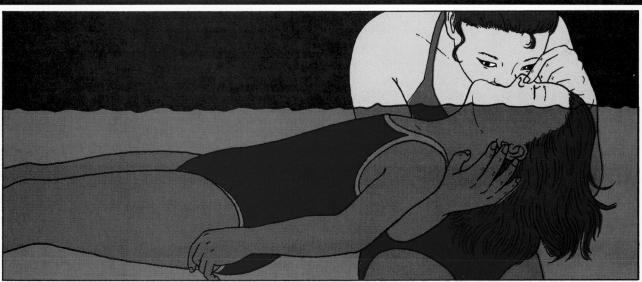

1 Check the child's ABCs (Airway, Breathing and Circulation); see **CHECKING THE ABCs,** pages 224-232. If necessary, begin rescue breathing or CPR immediately and continue until she revives.

CONTINUED ON NEXT PAGE

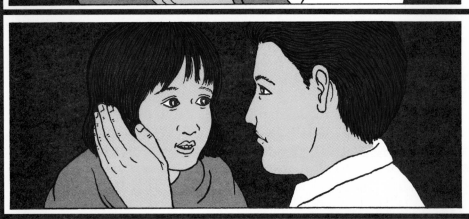

2 Remove wet clothing and warm her with blankets, a sleeping bag, etc. Observe for **HYPOTHERMIA (COLD EXPOSURE)**; see pages 332-335.

3 Calm and reassure the child, especially if she is coughing or still having difficulty breathing.

4 If you do not suspect an injury to the neck or spine, place her in the **RECOVERY POSITION**; see page 353. Observe for **SHOCK**; see pages 354-356.

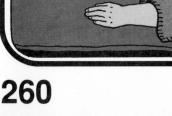

DRUG OVERDOSE

IMPORTANT

- **Seek medical aid immediately.** Call 911 or Operator; see **EMS,** page 272.

- Try to find out what drug the child has taken, how much he took, and how and when he took it. If possible, bring a sample of the drug to the hospital. If he vomits, also bring along a specimen for analysis.

- Call your local Poison Control Center for advice about what to do until medical help arrives. Make sure to ask whether you should induce vomiting or allow the child to fall asleep.

- **Do not** panic or threaten the child. Be supportive, tolerant and gentle. Keep the environment quiet and peaceful.

- Anyone who has injected a drug with a shared or used needle should be tested for hepatitis and AIDS.

- Habitual drug users require ongoing professional help. Consult your doctor, local Poison Control Center or drug hotline about the rehabilitation programs that are available in your community.

- To keep your child from becoming involved with drugs, teach him about the dangerous consequences to help lessen the temptation. If you suspect he is already using something, discuss the matter with him openly, then seek out the appropriate help.

SIGNS & SYMPTOMS OF DRUG ABUSE & OVERDOSE

Vary greatly according to the kind of drug that has been taken as well as the dosage, potency and individual reaction.

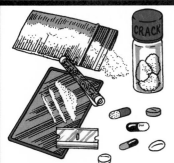

STIMULANTS ("UPPERS")

Amphetamine pills and powders, smokable amphetamine ("ice"), cocaine powder, smokable cocaine ("freebase" and "crack"): Hyperactivity. Insomnia. Headache. Extreme irritability and restlessness. Mood swings. Loss of balance and coordination. Speech problems. Rapid pulse. Elevated blood pressure. Fever. Sweating. Chills. Nausea and vomiting. Ringing in the ears. Chest pain. Fainting. Enlarged pupils. Impaired judgment. Hysterical outbursts. Erratic or violent behavior. Trembling. Muscle spasms. Heart palpitations. Extreme weight loss. Confusion. Anxiety. Deep depression. Fearfulness. Paranoia. Hallucinations. Psychosis. Difficulty breathing. Heart attack. Convulsions. Sudden collapse. Stroke. Coma. **All forms of cocaine and amphetamine are highly addictive.**

CONTINUED ON NEXT PAGE

DRUG OVERDOSE

DEPRESSANTS ("DOWNERS")

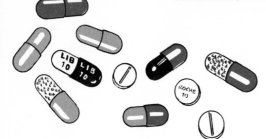

Sedatives, barbituates, hypnotics, tranquilizers: Drowsiness. Slurred speech. Loss of coordination. Confused thinking. Dulled reactions. Impaired memory. Delusions. Difficulty breathing. Unconsciousness. Coma. **Especially dangerous when taken with alcohol.**

OPIATES ("NARCOTICS")

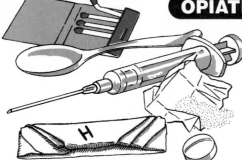

Heroin, morphine, opium, opium derivatives (codeine, Demerol, Dilaudid, etc.): Anxiety. Dizziness, nausea and vomiting. Itchiness. Sweating. Constipation. Loss of appetite and physical energy. Very small pupils. Disassociation. Sluggishness. Drowsiness. Slurred speech. Impaired memory and judgment. Slow pulse and respiration. Difficulty breathing. Lowered temperature. Weight loss and overall breakdown in health. Shock. Coma. **All opiates are highly addictive.**

HALLUCINOGENS ("PSYCHEDELICS")

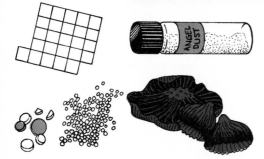

LSD, mescaline, peyote, "ecstacy," psilocybin ("mushrooms"), PCP ("angel dust"): Distorted perceptions of time and space. High blood pressure. Enlarged pupils. Dizziness. Nausea. Loss of coordination. Apathy. Anxiety. Depression. Hysterical outbursts. Erratic or violent behavior. Disorientation. Delusions. Impaired memory. Fearfulness. Hallucinations. Psychosis. Stupor. Convulsions. Coma.

CANNABIS ("GRASS")

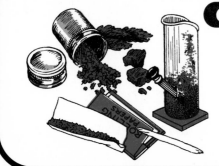

Marijuana, hashish, hash oil: Drowsiness. Reddened eyes. Distorted perceptions of time and space. Impaired coordination, concentration and memory. Irritability and nervousness. Fearfulness. Hallucinations. Paranoia.

CONTINUED ON NEXT PAGE

DRUG OVERDOSE

ALCOHOL

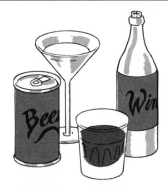

Drowsiness. Slurred speech. Dizziness, nausea and vomiting. Double vision. Loss of coordination. Uninhibited behavior. Impaired reactions and judgment. Aggressiveness. Stupor. Difficulty breathing. Convulsions. Unconsciousness. Coma. **Alcohol is highly addictive. Habitual use can damage the liver, brain, nervous system and heart.**

INHALANTS

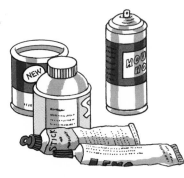

Aerosols, airplane glue, nitrous oxide ("laughing gas"), amyl nitrate, butyl nitrate: Severe headache. Loss of appetite. Dizziness, nausea and vomiting. Slurred speech. Impaired reactions and judgment. Loss of coordination. Blurred vision. Buzzing in the ears. Abdominal pain. Restlessness. Confusion. Incoherence. Excitability. Erratic or violent behavior. Hallucinations. Rapid pulse. Flushed skin. Weakness. Fatigue. Difficulty breathing. Unconsciousness. Heart failure. Coma. **Habitual use can damage the liver, kidneys, brain and nervous system.**

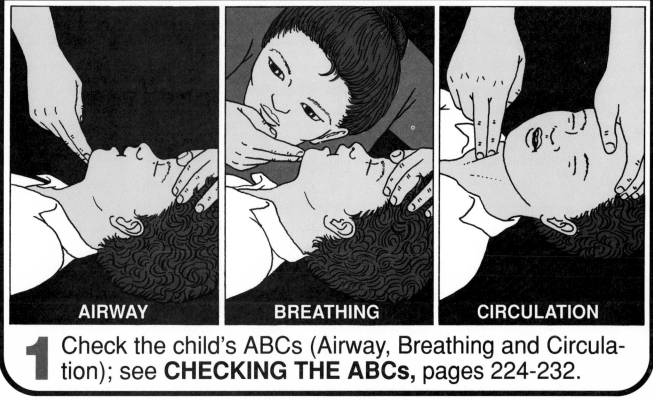

AIRWAY

BREATHING

CIRCULATION

1 Check the child's ABCs (Airway, Breathing and Circulation); see **CHECKING THE ABCs,** pages 224-232.

CONTINUED ON NEXT PAGE

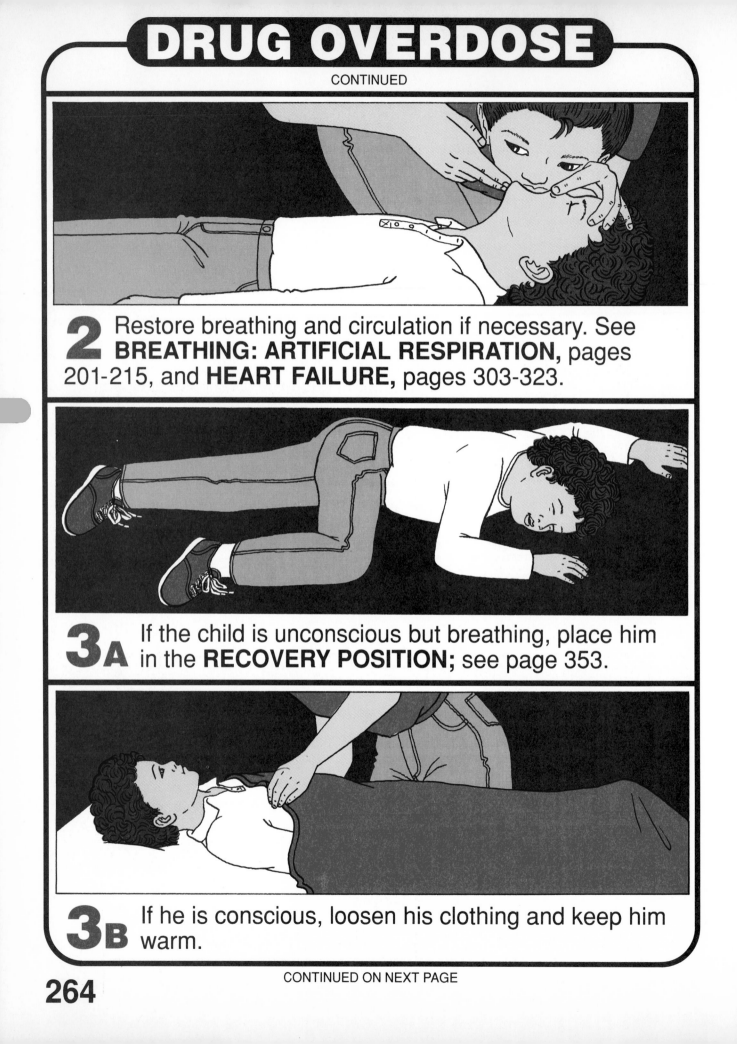

2 Restore breathing and circulation if necessary. See **BREATHING: ARTIFICIAL RESPIRATION,** pages 201-215, and **HEART FAILURE,** pages 303-323.

3A If the child is unconscious but breathing, place him in the **RECOVERY POSITION;** see page 353.

3B If he is conscious, loosen his clothing and keep him warm.

CONTINUED ON NEXT PAGE

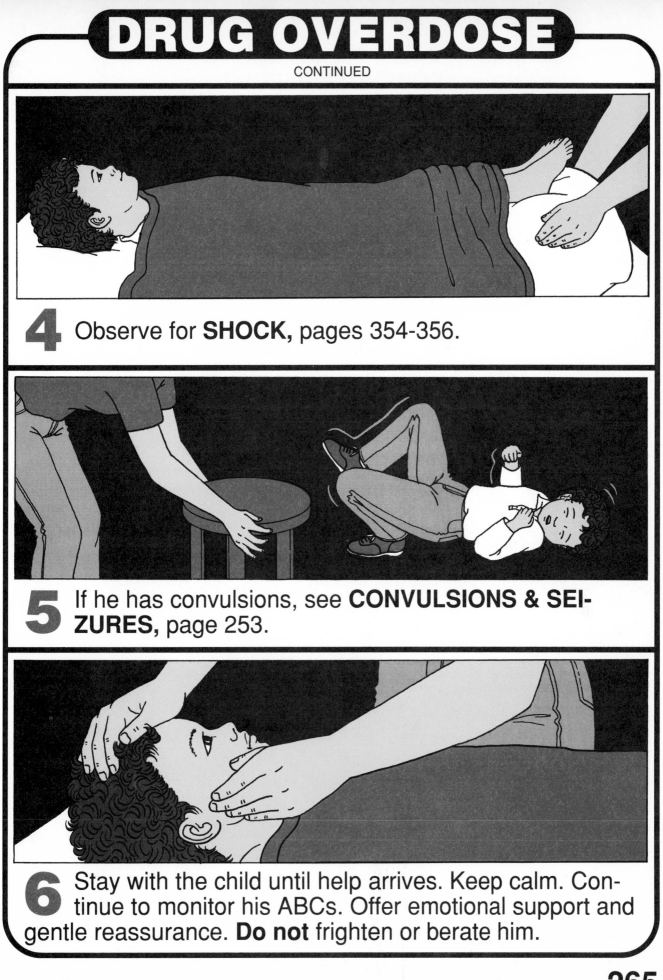

4 Observe for **SHOCK,** pages 354-356.

5 If he has convulsions, see **CONVULSIONS & SEIZURES,** page 253.

6 Stay with the child until help arrives. Keep calm. Continue to monitor his ABCs. Offer emotional support and gentle reassurance. **Do not** frighten or berate him.

EAR INJURIES

FOREIGN OBJECTS

- **Do not** try to flush out the object with water or oil.
- **Do not** try to remove anything **inside** the ear.

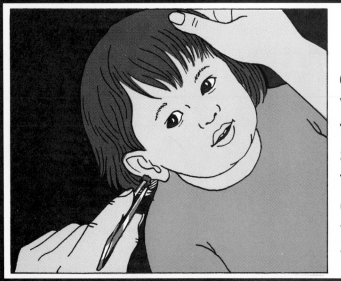

1A Calm and reassure the child. **If the foreign object is clearly visible at the entrance to the ear canal,** turn her head so her ear points down, then gently remove the object with tweezers. See your doctor to make sure you have gotten all of it out.

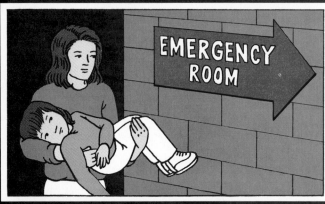

1B **If the foreign object is not visible or easily accessible,** turn the child's head onto the injured side and **seek medical aid immediately. Do not** try to remove it yourself.

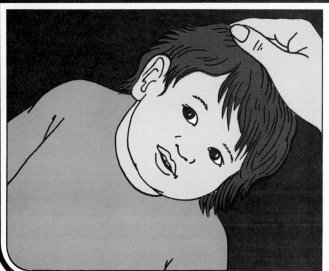

1C **If the child has an insect in her ear,** turn her head so her ear points up, and wait for the insect to crawl out. Make sure she keeps her hands away from her ear. If the insect doesn't crawl out after a few minutes, **seek medical aid.**

CUTS

IMPORTANT

- If the ear is severed, see **BLEEDING: CUTS & WOUNDS (AMPUTATIONS)**, pages 173-174.

- Blood or clear fluid coming from the ear suggests a serious injury to the head; see **HEAD INJURIES: CLOSED HEAD INJURIES**, page 289.

- Wash your hands thoroughly and, if possible, put on sterile latex gloves before beginning first aid.

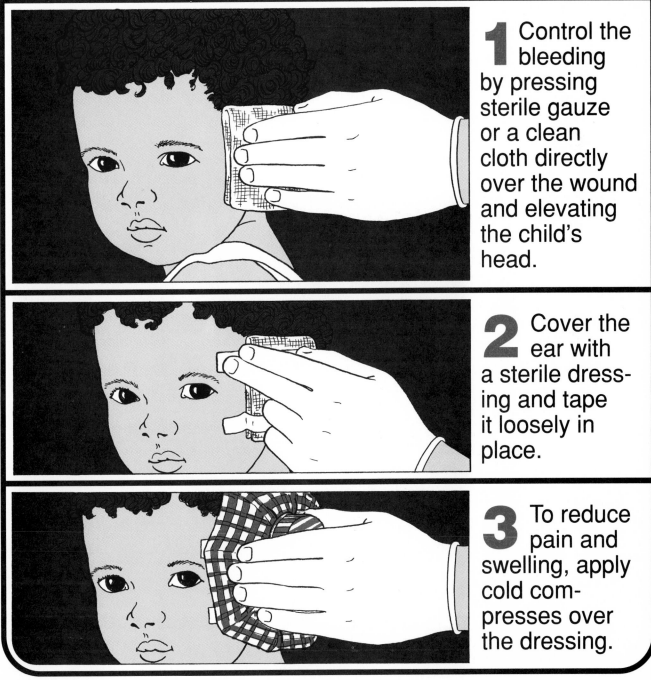

1 Control the bleeding by pressing sterile gauze or a clean cloth directly over the wound and elevating the child's head.

2 Cover the ear with a sterile dressing and tape it loosely in place.

3 To reduce pain and swelling, apply cold compresses over the dressing.

267

EAR INJURIES

PERFORATED EARDRUM

- **Seek medical aid immediately.**

- If the child has received a blow to the head, check for symptoms of serious head injuries before treating the ear; see **HEAD INJURIES: CLOSED HEAD INJURIES,** page 289.

- **Do not** insert drops, fingers or instruments into the ear if you suspect a perforated eardrum.

- **Do not** permit the child to hit the side of his head in an effort to restore lost hearing.

SIGNS & SYMPTOMS

Sudden severe pain. Reduction in hearing. Ringing in the ears. Possible dizziness. Possible blood or fluid draining from the ear.

IF PERFORATION HAS BEEN CAUSED BY A BLOW TO THE HEAD

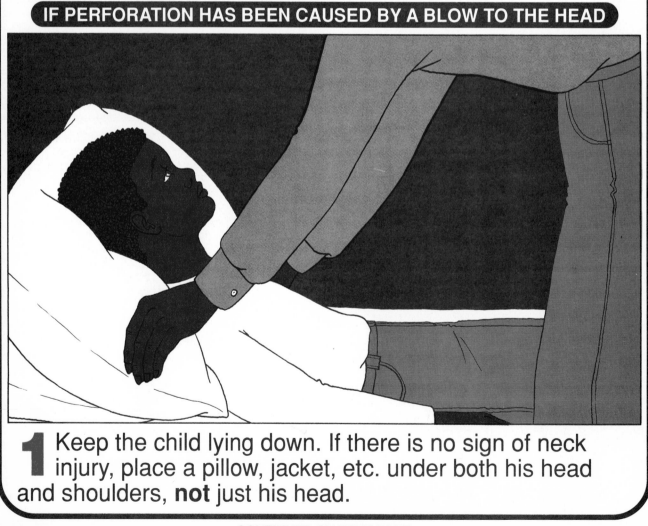

1 Keep the child lying down. If there is no sign of neck injury, place a pillow, jacket, etc. under both his head and shoulders, **not** just his head.

CONTINUED ON NEXT PAGE

PERFORATED EARDRUM
CONTINUED

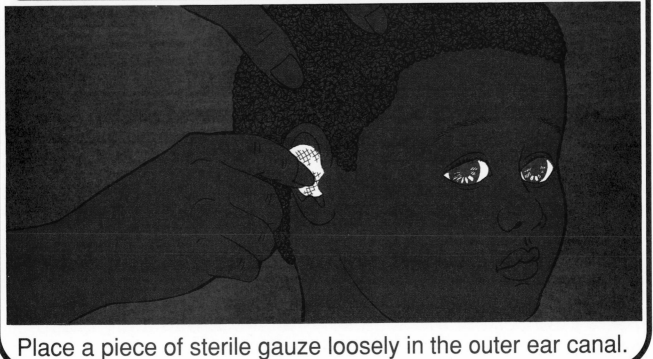

2 Turn the head toward the affected side so fluids may drain from the ear. **Do not** stop the flow of fluid or clean the ear canal.

IF PERFORATION HAS NOT BEEN CAUSED BY A BLOW TO THE HEAD

Place a piece of sterile gauze loosely in the outer ear canal.

ELECTRIC SHOCK

- **Do not** touch the child directly while she remains in contact with the current.

- After removing her from the current, call **EMS;** see page 272.

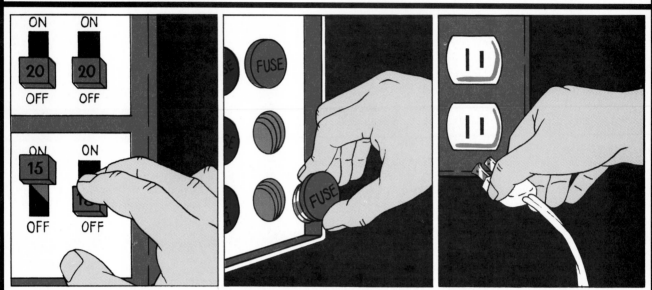

1A Try to break the contact by turning off the current, removing the fuse or unplugging the electrical cord from the outlet.

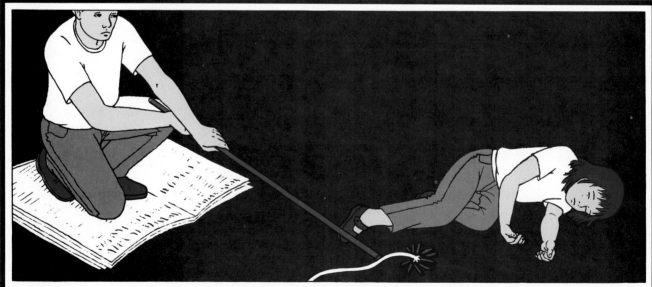

1B If that isn't possible, stand on something dry — a blanket, rubber mat, newspapers, etc. — and push away the child or the source of the shock with a dry board or wooden pole.

CONTINUED ON NEXT PAGE

CONTINUED

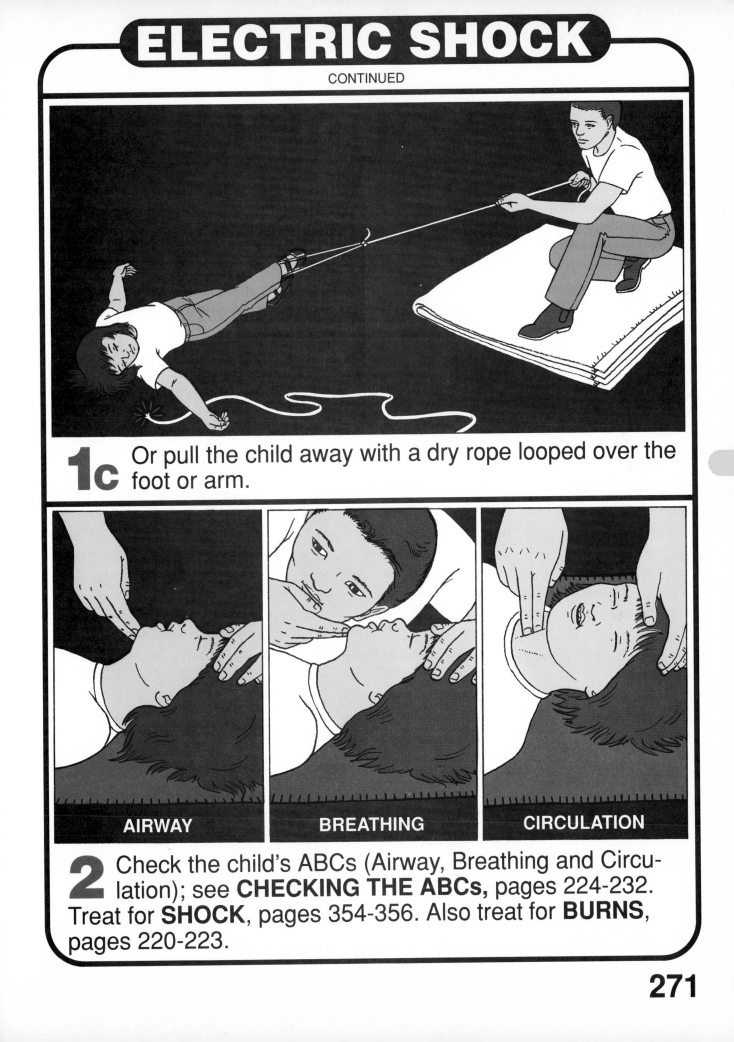

1c Or pull the child away with a dry rope looped over the foot or arm.

AIRWAY

BREATHING

CIRCULATION

2 Check the child's ABCs (Airway, Breathing and Circulation); see **CHECKING THE ABCs,** pages 224-232. Treat for **SHOCK**, pages 354-356. Also treat for **BURNS**, pages 220-223.

EMS (EMERGENCY MEDICAL SERVICES)

If an injury seems at all serious, send for medical aid immediately by calling Emergency Medical Services (EMS).

EMS is a coordinated community system that can dispatch police, fire department and medical ambulance personnel to the scene. **In most communities it is activated by calling 911 or "O" (Operator) and giving the following information:**

1. **What happened.**
2. **Location:** the exact address of the emergency, with cross streets or roads.
3. **The telephone number** you are calling from.
4. **Your name.**
5. **How many are injured.**
6. **The condition of the injured.**
7. **What help is being given.**

Stay on the line in case the EMS dispatcher has any further questions. ALWAYS BE THE LAST TO HANG UP.

EPIGLOTTITIS

IMPORTANT

- **Epiglottitis—a bacterial infection that causes a swelling of the tissue that covers the opening of the windpipe during swallowing—is a potentially life-threatening emergency. Seek medical aid immediately.** Call 911 or Operator; see **EMS,** page 272.

- **Do not** try to look down the child's throat or force her to change the position of her head.

- Antibiotics are recommended for other family members to keep the infection from spreading.

SIGNS & SYMPTOMS

Wakes up drooling. Wants to sit or be held up. Severe difficulty breathing, which causes the child to sit with her jaw pointed out, mouth open and tongue protruding. Difficulty swallowing. High fever. Severe sore throat. Anxiety. Irritability. Restlessness. May eventually become pale, turn blue and lose consciousness. Symptoms may appear very suddenly.

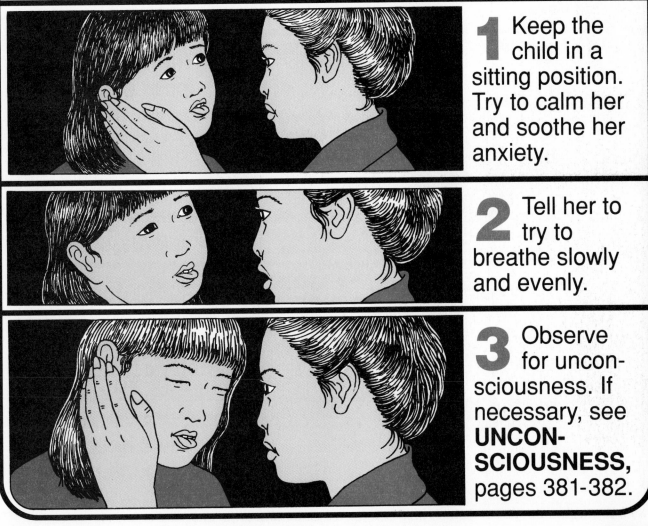

1 Keep the child in a sitting position. Try to calm her and soothe her anxiety.

2 Tell her to try to breathe slowly and evenly.

3 Observe for unconsciousness. If necessary, see **UNCONSCIOUSNESS,** pages 381-382.

273

EYE INJURIES

FOREIGN OBJECTS

IMPORTANT

- **Seek medical aid immediately** if the foreign object is on the iris or pupil or seems embedded in the eye. See **EYE INJURIES: IMPALED OBJECTS,** pages 280-281.

- **Seek medical aid** if the child is wearing contact lenses. **Do not** try to remove them yourself unless there is rapid swelling or no medical aid is available.

- Wash your hands thoroughly before beginning first aid.

- **Do not** press on the affected eye or allow the child to rub it.

- **Do not** try to remove the object with tweezers, cotton balls or a cotton-tipped swab.

SIGNS & SYMPTOMS

Pain. Burning, itching sensation. Tearing. Reddened eye. Sensitivity to light. Blurred vision.

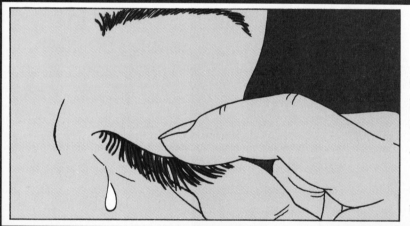

1 Gently pull the upper eyelid down over the lower eyelid and hold it there a moment until the flow of tears has a chance to wash the object away.

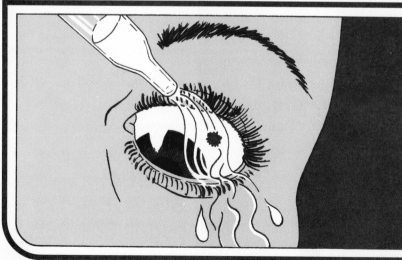

2 If that doesn't work, try to flush it out with warm water from a medicine dropper or glass, or by holding the child's head under a gentle stream of running water.

CONTINUED ON NEXT PAGE

FOREIGN OBJECTS
CONTINUED

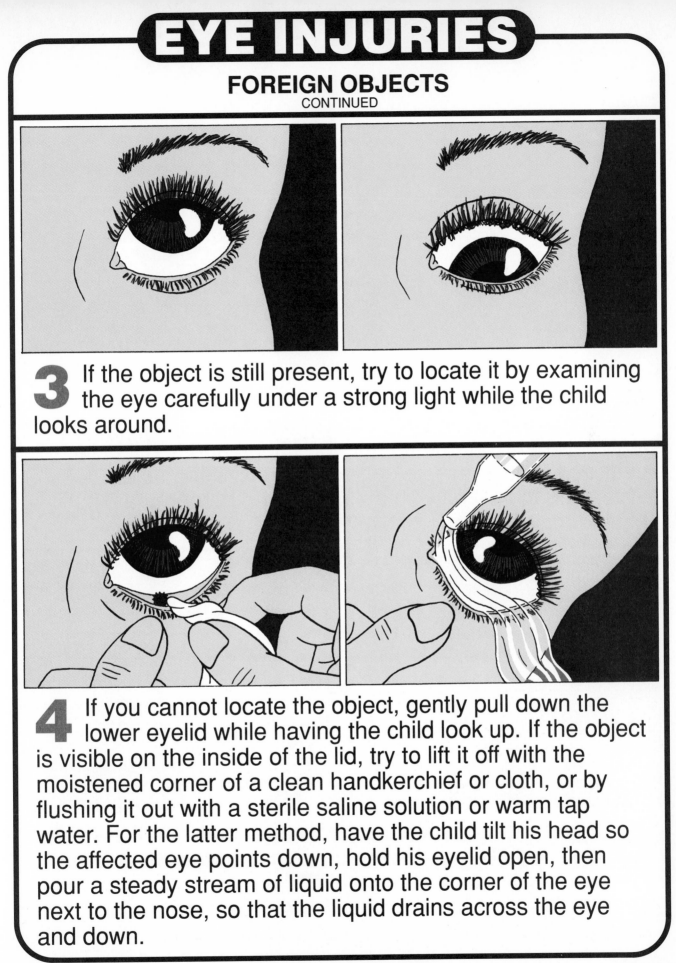

3 If the object is still present, try to locate it by examining the eye carefully under a strong light while the child looks around.

4 If you cannot locate the object, gently pull down the lower eyelid while having the child look up. If the object is visible on the inside of the lid, try to lift it off with the moistened corner of a clean handkerchief or cloth, or by flushing it out with a sterile saline solution or warm tap water. For the latter method, have the child tilt his head so the affected eye points down, hold his eyelid open, then pour a steady stream of liquid onto the corner of the eye next to the nose, so that the liquid drains across the eye and down.

CONTINUED ON NEXT PAGE

FOREIGN OBJECTS
CONTINUED

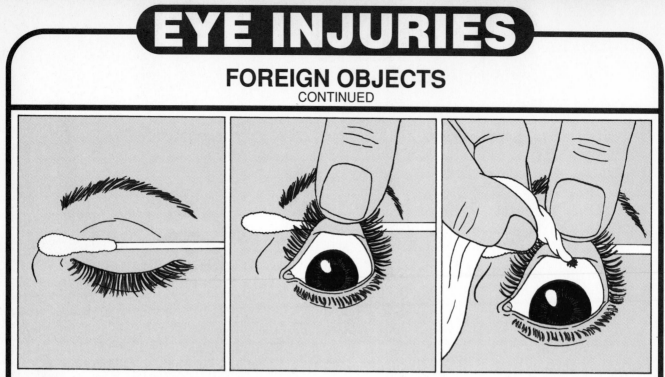

5 If the object is not visible on the lower eyelid, check the upper eyelid. Have the child look down, clasp the upper lash between your thumb and forefinger, and fold it back over an applicator swab, matchstick, etc. If the object is visible, try to lift it off with the moistened corner of a clean handkerchief or cloth, or by flushing it out as in Step 4.

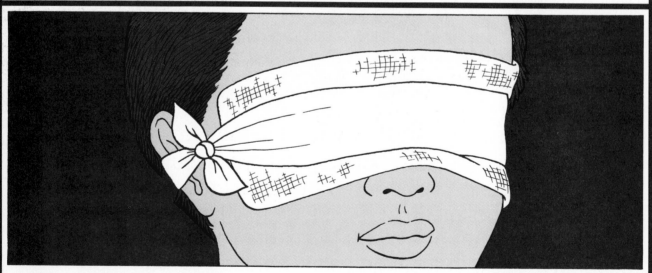

6 If you cannot locate or remove the object, or if the child continues to feel discomfort after the object has been taken out, calm and reassure him, cover both his eyes with a sterile dressing or clean cloth, and **seek medical aid immediately.**

EYE INJURIES

CHEMICALS IN THE EYE

IMPORTANT

- **Harmful chemicals in the eye can cause permanent damage within 1 to 5 minutes. Begin first aid immediately, even before seeking medical assistance.**

- After administering first aid, call the Poison Control Center for further advice, then get the child to a hospital emergency room. If necessary, call 911 or Operator; see **EMS,** page 272.

- **Do not** press on the injured eye or allow the child to rub it.

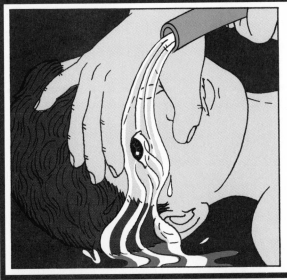

1A If one eye is affected: Holding the eyelids open, flush the eye immediately in a steady stream of gently running water for at least 5 minutes (15 minutes if the chemical is a strong alkali). Tilt the child's head so the affected eye points down, taking care that the water does not run into the other eye.

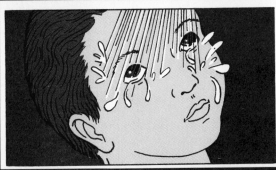

1B If both eyes are affected: Let the water flow over both eyes, quickly alternate from one eye to the other, or stand him under a shower until both eyes have been thoroughly flushed.

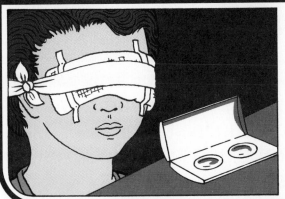

2 Remove contact lenses. Have him close both his eyes, then cover them with a sterile dressing or clean cloth. Hold it in place with a loosely fastened bandage. **Seek medical aid immediately.**

EYE INJURIES

BLACK EYE

IMPORTANT

- **Seek medical aid immediately for a lacerated eyeball or eyelid;** see **EYE INJURIES: LACERATIONS,** page 279.

- Consult a doctor to determine if there is a more serious injury, especially if the child is wearing contact lenses. **Do not** try to remove contact lenses yourself.

- **Do not** press on the eye or allow the child to rub it.

SIGNS & SYMPTOMS

Pain following a blow to the area around the eye. Rapid swelling and dark discoloration of the eyelid or skin around the eye. Discoloration may last 2 to 3 weeks.

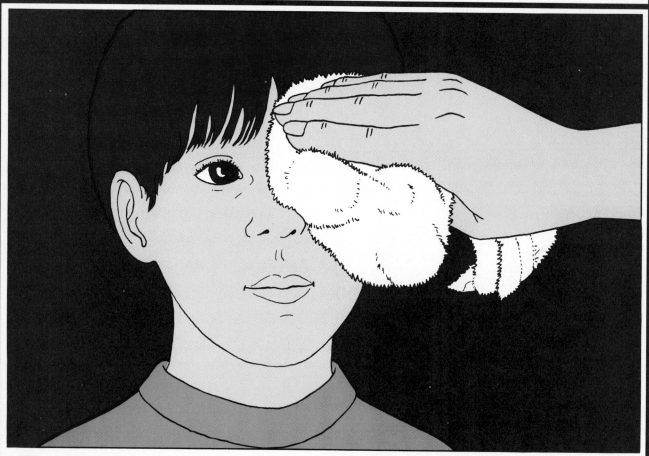

To minimize swelling, gently apply an ice bag covered with a towel to the affected area. If an ice bag isn't available, use ice cubes wrapped in a cloth. **Do not** place ice directly on the skin or eye. **Do not** apply raw steak.

EYE INJURIES

LACERATIONS

IMPORTANT

- **Seek medical aid immediately for a lacerated eyeball or eyelid, especially if the child is wearing contact lenses.** If necessary, call 911 or Operator; see **EMS,** page 272. **Do not** try to remove contact lenses yourself.

- Wash your hands thoroughly and, if possible, put on sterile latex gloves before starting first aid.

- **Do not** wash out the eye.

- **Do not** press on the eye or allow the child to rub it.

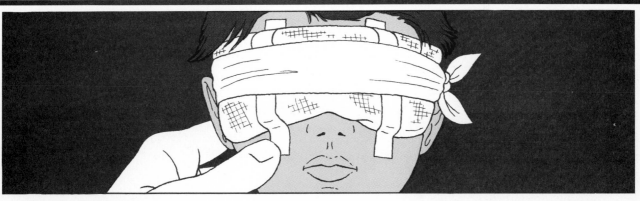

1 Cover **both** eyes loosely with sterile gauze or a clean cloth. **Do not** apply pressure. Secure it in place with a bandage.

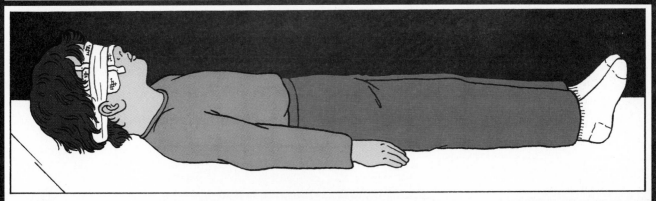

2 Keep the child lying down flat on his back until medical aid arrives. If you must take the child to the hospital yourself, use a stretcher. See **TRANSPORTING THE INJURED: PULLS, CARRIES & STRETCHERS,** pages 377-380.

IMPALED OBJECTS

IMPORTANT

- **Seek medical aid immediately.** Call 911 or Operator; see **EMS,** page 272.

- Wash your hands thoroughly and, if possible, put on sterile latex gloves before starting first aid.

- **Do not** try to remove the impaled object.

- **Do not** wash out the eye.

- **Do not** touch the eye or allow the child to rub it.

- **Do not** try to remove contact lenses.

- Keep the child lying down flat on her back. If you must move her, use a stretcher. See **TRANSPORTING THE INJURED: PULLS, CARRIES & STRETCHERS,** pages 377-380.

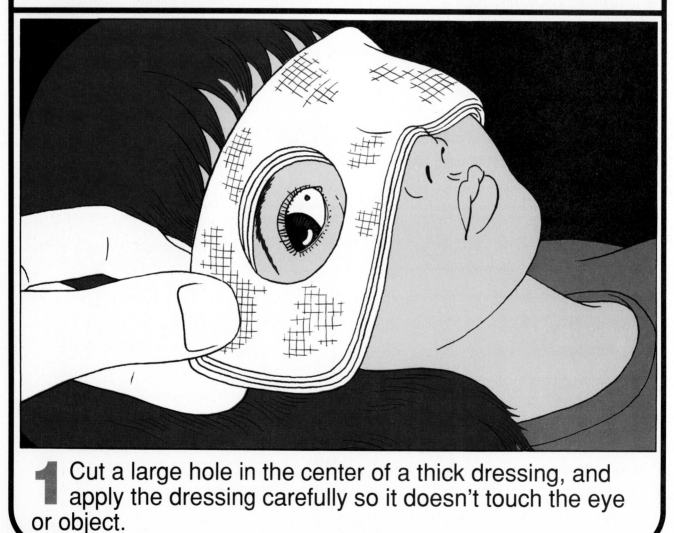

1 Cut a large hole in the center of a thick dressing, and apply the dressing carefully so it doesn't touch the eye or object.

CONTINUED ON NEXT PAGE

IMPALED OBJECTS
CONTINUED

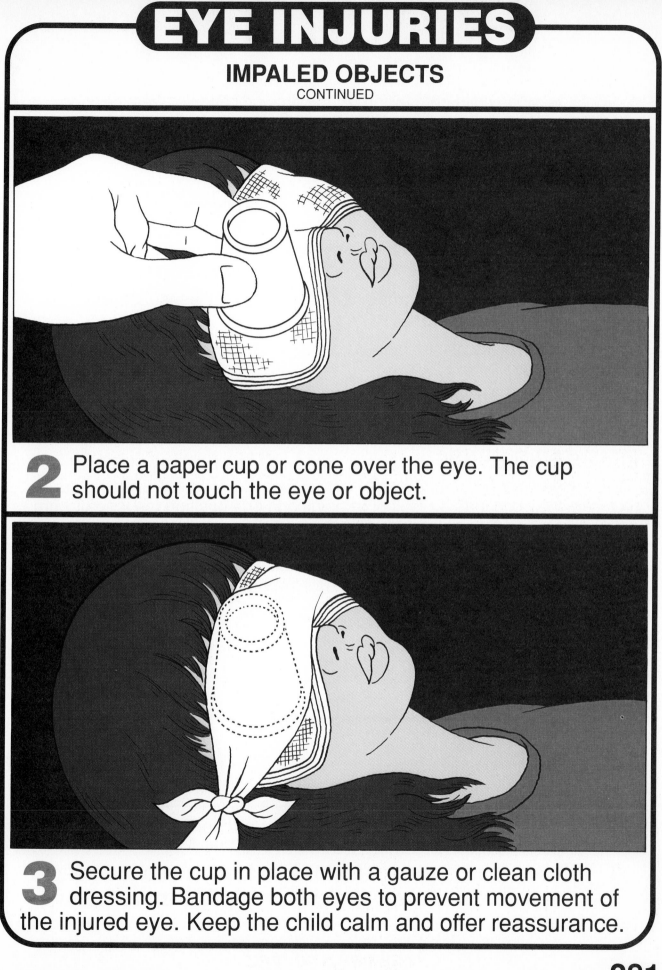

2 Place a paper cup or cone over the eye. The cup should not touch the eye or object.

3 Secure the cup in place with a gauze or clean cloth dressing. Bandage both eyes to prevent movement of the injured eye. Keep the child calm and offer reassurance.

FAINTING

IMPORTANT

- Try to keep the child from falling. At the first indication of weakness or faintness, help him sit down with his head between his knees.

- **Seek medical aid.** Tell your doctor about all periods of unconsciousness, no matter how brief.

- Check the child's ABCs (Airway, Breathing and Circulation); see **CHECKING THE ABCs,** pages 224-232.

- **If the child is unconscious, do not** give him anything to drink, or try to rouse him by slapping or shaking him or throwing water in his face.

- If the child has fallen, check for injuries that may have resulted; see **ASSESSING THE EMERGENCY,** pages 127-128.

- If he vomits, place him on his side or turn his head sideways to keep him from choking.

- If he does not recover fully in 5 minutes or feels ill, call 911 or Operator; see **EMS,** page 272.

SIGNS & SYMPTOMS

Brief, sudden, partial or total loss of consciousness, followed by complete recovery. May occur as a result of remaining in one position too long or from pain, illness, anxiety or other emotional stress. **Early symptoms may include:** Paleness. Sweating. Nausea. Dizziness.

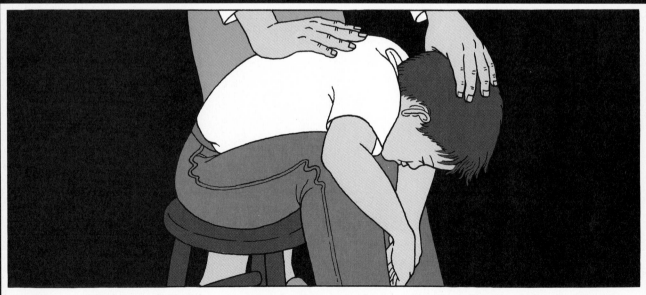

1A If the child is conscious and seated, place his head between his knees. Watch him closely to make sure he doesn't fall.

CONTINUED ON NEXT PAGE

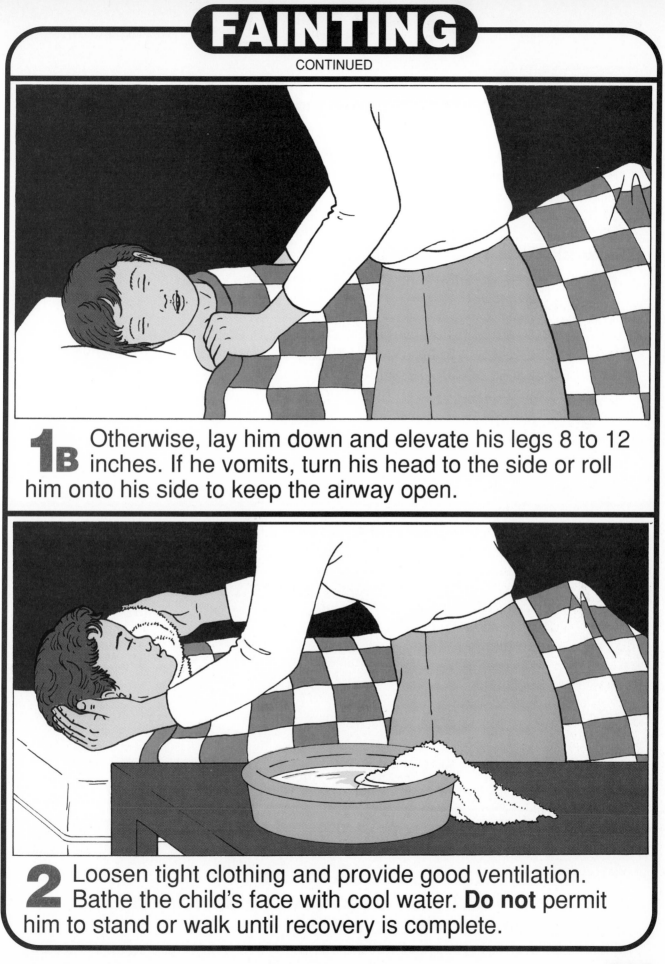

1B Otherwise, lay him down and elevate his legs 8 to 12 inches. If he vomits, turn his head to the side or roll him onto his side to keep the airway open.

2 Loosen tight clothing and provide good ventilation. Bathe the child's face with cool water. **Do not** permit him to stand or walk until recovery is complete.

FEVER

- To determine if the child has a fever, see **TAKING THE TEMPERATURE**, pages 368-373.

- Fever is part of the body's way of fighting off infections and other illnesses. A low-grade fever does not necessarily indicate that something is wrong, and children can run high fevers without being seriously ill. However, you should call your doctor if an infant under 3 months old has a temperature over 100.2°F (37.9°C), or a child over 3 months old has a temperature over 101°F (38.3°C), particularly if he does not seem well.

- **Do not** use medication, enemas, or alcohol or ice water rubs unless your doctor so advises.

- High fevers can bring on febrile seizures in children. These seizures, which resemble shivering, do not usually last long but should always be reported to your doctor. Take the child's temperature after the febrile seizure passes, and if his temperature is still high, gently cool him as described below.

- If a fever reaches 103°F (39.4°C) or higher in a younger child, or 102°F (38.8°C) in an older child and you cannot reach your doctor, begin gently cooling the child as described below.

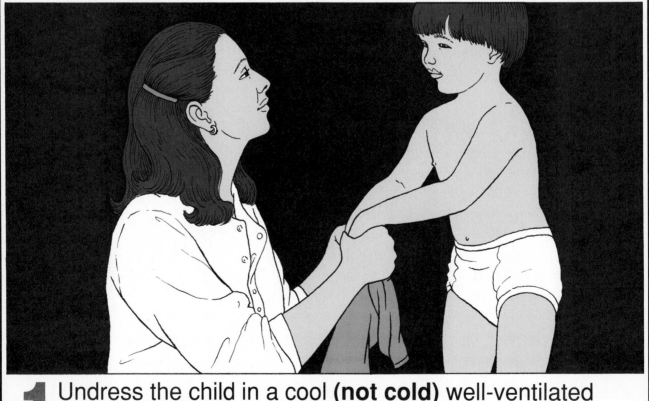

1 Undress the child in a cool (**not cold**) well-ventilated room. Avoid drafts and chilling.

CONTINUED ON NEXT PAGE

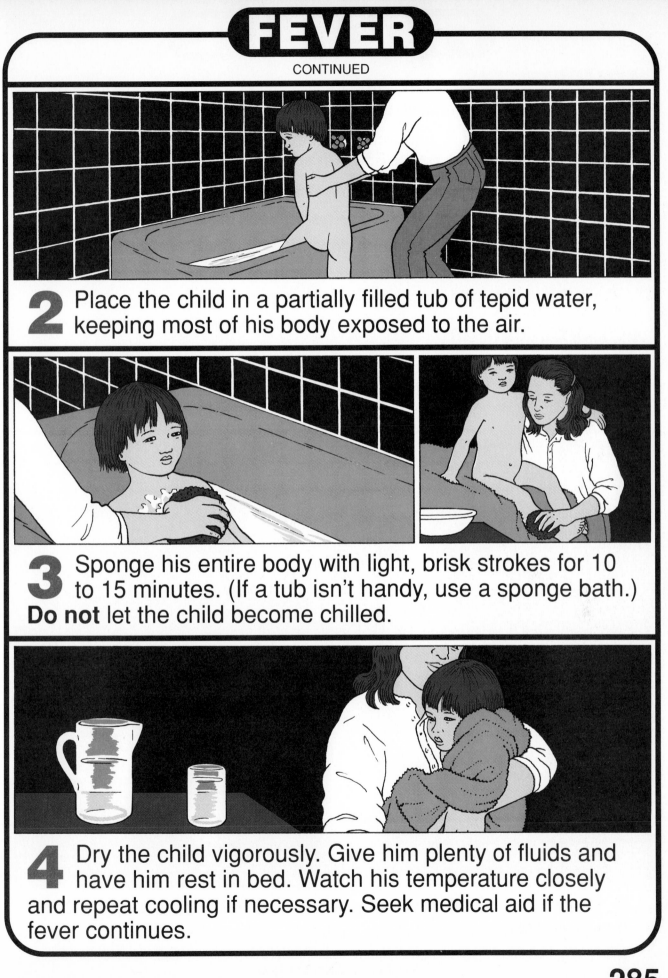

2 Place the child in a partially filled tub of tepid water, keeping most of his body exposed to the air.

3 Sponge his entire body with light, brisk strokes for 10 to 15 minutes. (If a tub isn't handy, use a sponge bath.) **Do not** let the child become chilled.

4 Dry the child vigorously. Give him plenty of fluids and have him rest in bed. Watch his temperature closely and repeat cooling if necessary. Seek medical aid if the fever continues.

FROSTBITE

IMPORTANT

- **Seek medical aid immediately. If severe,** call **EMS;** see page 272.
- If the child also has hypothermia, treat that first; see **HYPOTHERMIA (COLD EXPOSURE),** pages 332-335.
- **Do not** warm the affected parts if you can't keep them thawed.
- **Do not** rub or massage affected areas or break blisters.
- **Do not** apply hot water or strong heat; no heat lamps, hot-water bottles, etc.
- **Do not** give the child anything alcoholic to drink.

SIGNS & SYMPTOMS

Usually affects the fingers, toes, ears, nose or cheeks. At first the skin is red, then glossy and white or grayish yellow and hard to the touch. Blisters may develop. Pain, changing to feeling of intense cold and numbness.

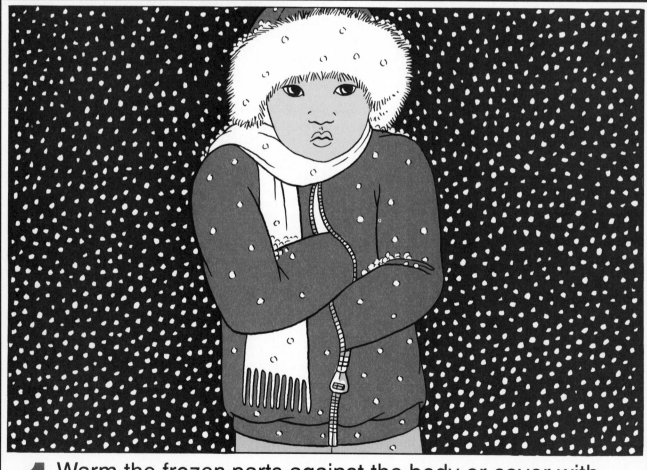

1 Warm the frozen parts against the body or cover with extra clothing.

CONTINUED ON NEXT PAGE

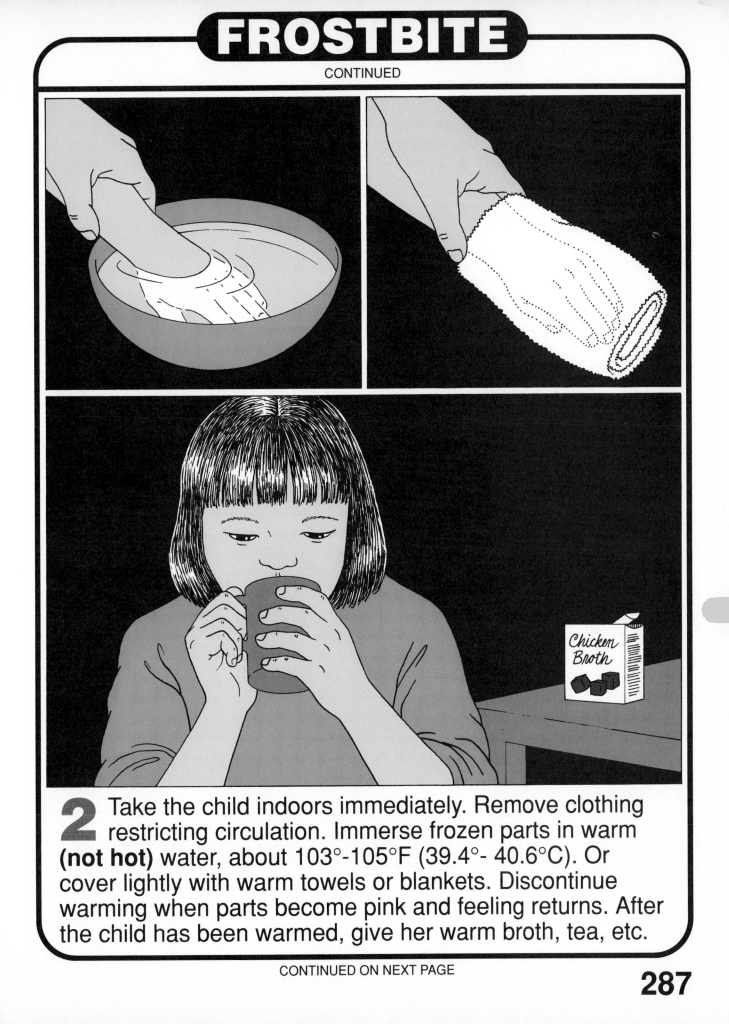

Chicken
Broth

2 Take the child indoors immediately. Remove clothing restricting circulation. Immerse frozen parts in warm **(not hot)** water, about 103°-105°F (39.4°- 40.6°C). Or cover lightly with warm towels or blankets. Discontinue warming when parts become pink and feeling returns. After the child has been warmed, give her warm broth, tea, etc.

CONTINUED ON NEXT PAGE

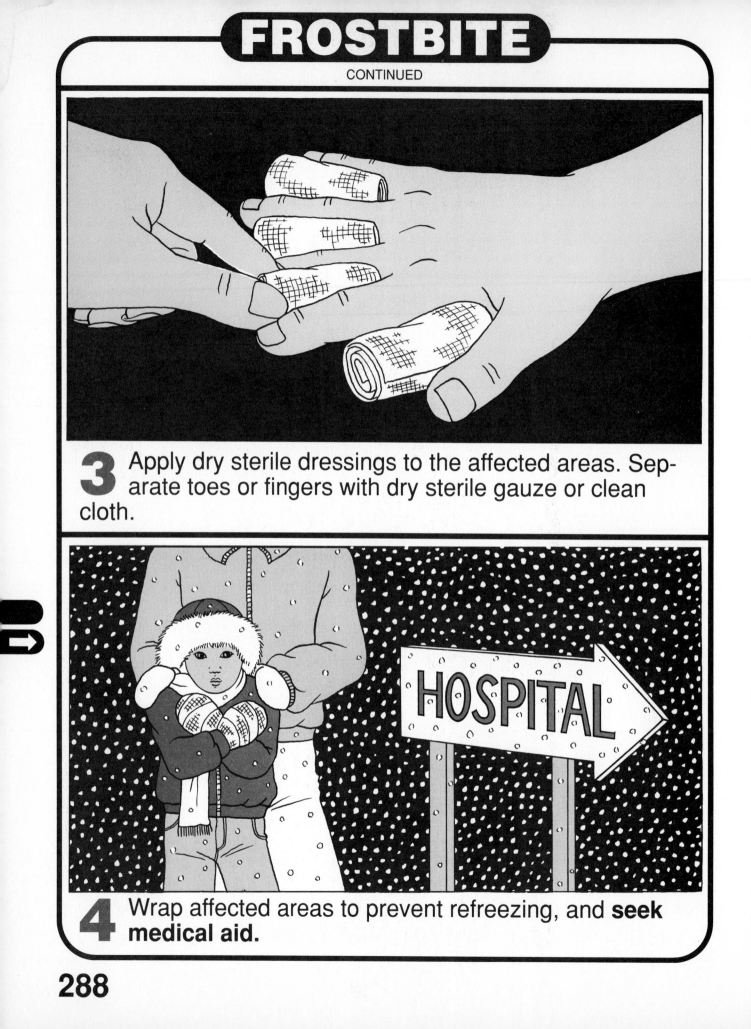

3 Apply dry sterile dressings to the affected areas. Separate toes or fingers with dry sterile gauze or clean cloth.

4 Wrap affected areas to prevent refreezing, and **seek medical aid.**

HEAD INJURIES

CLOSED HEAD INJURIES

IMPORTANT

- Head injuries may be more severe than they seem. **To be safe, call your doctor immediately.** If necessary, call **EMS;** see page 272.

- Check the child's ABCs (Airway, Breathing and Circulation); see **CHECKING THE ABCs,** pages 224-232.

- **Do not** pick up or move the child unless absolutely necessary. If you must move him, see **TRANSPORTING THE INJURED,** pages 374-380.

- If the child is unconscious, assume there is a neck injury. See **BACK & NECK INJURIES,** pages 135-136. Note how long he remains unconscious.

- Observe closely for several days for delayed symptoms.

SIGNS & SYMPTOMS OF SERIOUS HEAD INJURIES

Unconsciousness. Confusion. Difficulty breathing. Vomiting. Convulsions. Clear fluid or blood running from ears, nose or mouth. Paralysis of any part of the body. Loss of bladder or bowel control. Unequal pupils. Skull deformity.

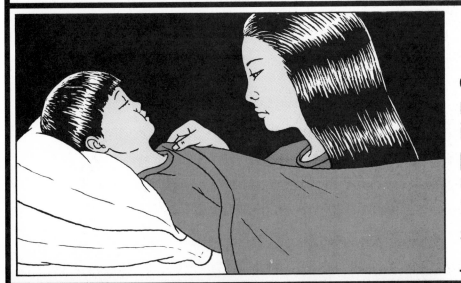

1 Keep the child lying down. If there is no sign of neck injury, place a pillow, jacket, etc. under **both** his head and his shoulders, **not** just his head.

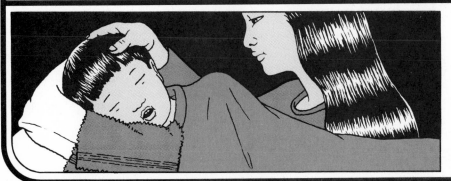

2 Turn him onto his side so fluids may drain from his mouth. **Seek medical aid immediately.**

HEAD INJURIES

OPEN HEAD INJURIES

IMPORTANT

- **Seek medical aid immediately.** Head injuries may be more severe than they seem. If necessary, call **EMS;** see page 272.

- Check the child's ABCs (Airway, Breathing and Circulation); see **CHECKING THE ABCs,** pages 224-232.

- Wash your hands thoroughly and, if possible, put on sterile latex gloves before starting first aid.

- **Do not** attempt to clean deep scalp wounds or remove any foreign matter.

- Observe for **VOMITING.** If necessary, see page 123.

- Check with your doctor to make sure the child's tetanus immunization is still current.

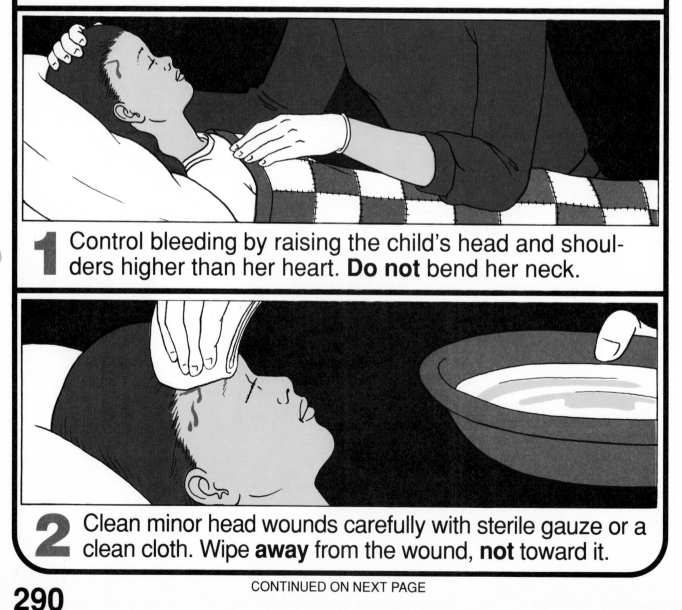

1 Control bleeding by raising the child's head and shoulders higher than her heart. **Do not** bend her neck.

2 Clean minor head wounds carefully with sterile gauze or a clean cloth. Wipe **away** from the wound, **not** toward it.

CONTINUED ON NEXT PAGE

OPEN HEAD INJURIES
CONTINUED

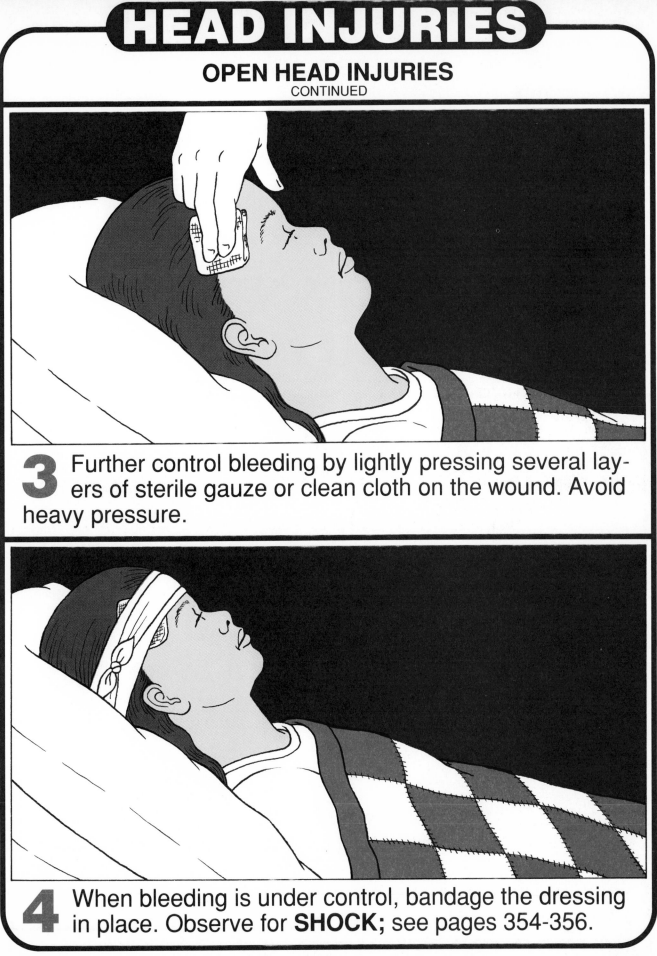

3 Further control bleeding by lightly pressing several layers of sterile gauze or clean cloth on the wound. Avoid heavy pressure.

4 When bleeding is under control, bandage the dressing in place. Observe for **SHOCK;** see pages 354-356.

HEAD INJURIES

FACE & JAW

IMPORTANT

- **Seek medical aid.** If necessary, call **EMS;** see page 272.

- Check the child's ABCs (Airway, Breathing and Circulation); see **CHECKING THE ABCs,** pages 224-232.

- Wash your hands thoroughly and, if possible, put on sterile latex gloves before starting first aid.

- Remove all broken teeth and foreign matter from the child's mouth. Wrap the teeth in a cool, moist cloth, and bring them to the doctor or dentist for possible replanting.

- Observe for **SHOCK,** pages 354-356.

- Check with your doctor to make sure the child's tetanus immunization is still current.

FACE

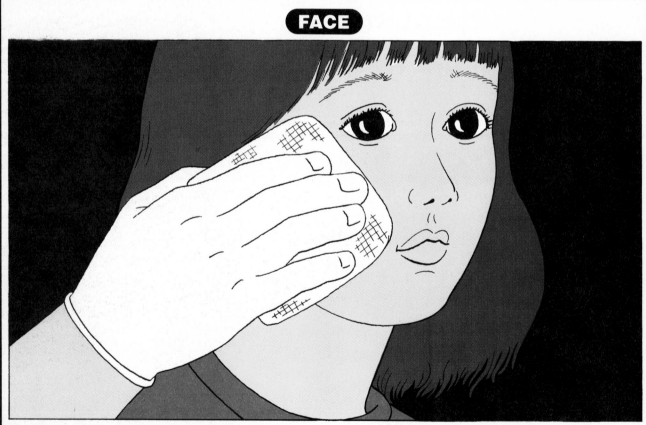

1 Raise the head higher than the heart and control bleeding through direct pressure with sterile gauze or a clean cloth. Apply pressure gently if you suspect broken facial bones.

CONTINUED ON NEXT PAGE

FACE & JAW
CONTINUED

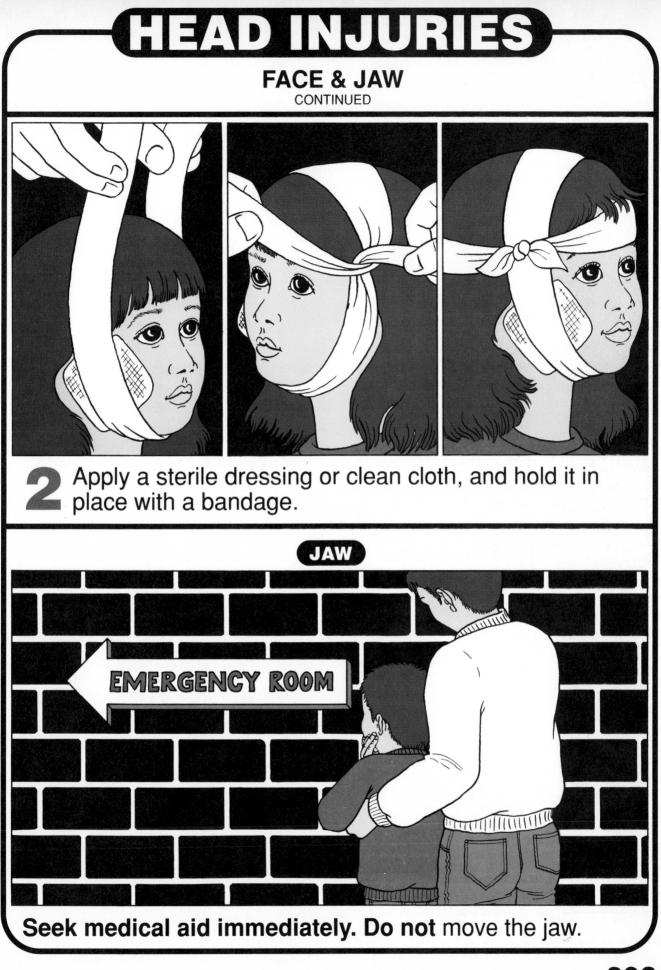

2 Apply a sterile dressing or clean cloth, and hold it in place with a bandage.

JAW

Seek medical aid immediately. Do not move the jaw.

HEAD LICE

IMPORTANT

- Head lice are not the result of personal uncleanliness or unclean homes, as is sometimes believed, and should never cause any embarrassment. They are common among schoolchildren, and though very communicable, are easily treated. If your child has head lice, notify his school, camp or day-care center immediately, as well as the families of his playmates.

- To discover if your child has become infested, examine his head and hair carefully in bright natural light, using a magnifying glass. Lice are tiny parasitic insects, usually brown in color, and are very hard to find. Their eggs, called nits, are tear-shaped, whitish specks that can be more easily discovered attached to the hair shafts, especially around the ears and the nape of the neck.

- If head lice are found on your child, everyone in the family should also be examined, and all those who are infested, treated at the same time.

- Consult your doctor before using any medication, especially if you are pregnant or nursing, or your child is under 6 years old, has numerous cuts or scratches on his head or neck, or is taking other medications. Head lice medications should never be used on infants.

- To help prevent your child from becoming infested, teach him not to share his hat, clothing, comb or other personal articles with other children.

SIGNS & SYMPTOMS

Severe itching on the head and neck. Frequent scratching. Red bite or scratch marks on the scalp and neck. **May lead to:** Swollen glands in the neck or under the arms. Skin infections.

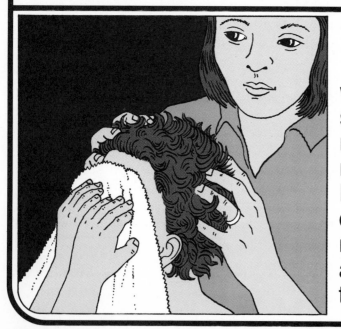

1 Remove the child's shirt, have him cover his eyes with a towel, then treat his scalp and neck with the medicated shampoo or lotion recommended by your doctor. Follow the accompanying directions very carefully. Administer the medication over a sink, not while the child is taking a bath or shower.

CONTINUED ON NEXT PAGE

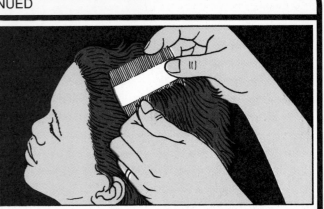

2 Dry his hair thoroughly, then remove the nits with a special nit comb, tweezers or your fingernails, examining each strand of hair separately under a bright light. After the nits have been removed, have him change into clean clothing.

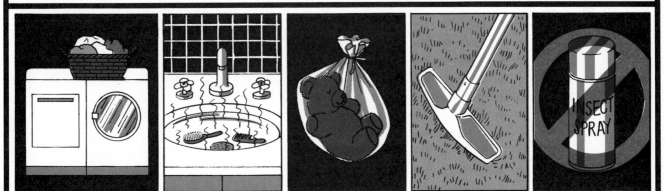

3 Wash all the clothes, linens and towels that he has recently used in soapy hot water, then dry them in a hot dryer. Soak his comb and hairbrush in very hot water for at least 20 minutes. Dry-clean or vacuum non-washables, including stuffed animals, or place them in airtight plastic bags for several weeks. Vacuum all rugs, mattresses and upholstered furniture. **Do not** use insecticidal sprays; they are ineffective against head lice and may be harmful to family members and pets.

4 Continue to check for nits daily for at least 10 days after first applying the medication. If infestation recurs, consult your doctor.

HEAD-TILT/CHIN-LIFT

INFANT (TO 1 YEAR OLD)

IMPORTANT

- When an infant loses consciousness and is lying on her back, her tongue may fall backward into her throat and block her airway, making it impossible for her to breathe. The head-tilt/chin-lift raises the tongue away from the throat and usually opens the airway.

- The procedure should be used whenever you check an infant's ABCs (Airway, Breathing and Circulation) and before you administer first aid if she is unconscious, as long as there is no neck or back injury.

- **Do not use the head-tilt/chin-lift if you suspect an injury to the neck or back.** To open the infant's airway, gently move her jaw forward **without** tilting or moving her head.

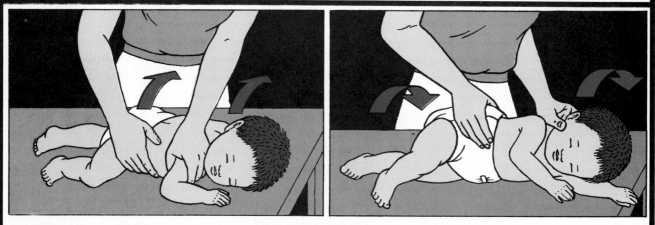

1 Moving her as a single unit, place the infant on her back on a firm surface with her head at the same level as her heart.

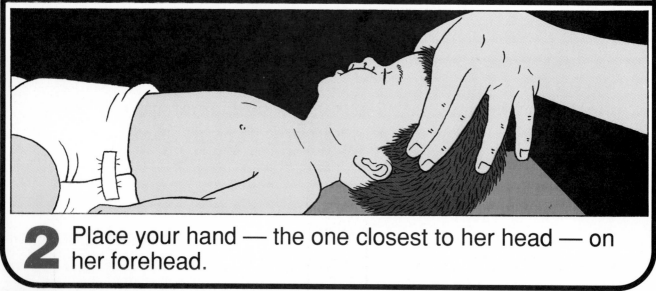

2 Place your hand — the one closest to her head — on her forehead.

CONTINUED ON NEXT PAGE

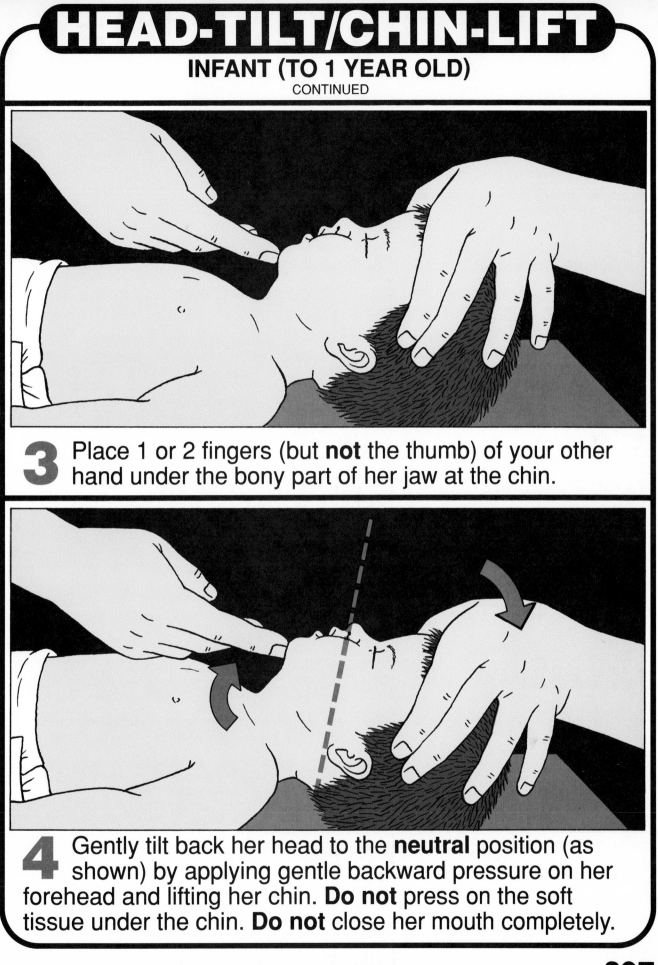

3 Place 1 or 2 fingers (but **not** the thumb) of your other hand under the bony part of her jaw at the chin.

4 Gently tilt back her head to the **neutral** position (as shown) by applying gentle backward pressure on her forehead and lifting her chin. **Do not** press on the soft tissue under the chin. **Do not** close her mouth completely.

HEAD-TILT/CHIN-LIFT

CHILD (OVER 1 YEAR OLD)

IMPORTANT

- When a child loses consciousness and is lying on his back, his tongue may fall backward into his throat and block his airway, making it impossible for him to breathe. The head-tilt/chin-lift raises the tongue away from the throat and usually opens the airway.

- The procedure should be used whenever you check a child's ABCs (Airway, Breathing and Circulation) and before you administer first aid if he is unconscious, as long as there is no neck or back injury.

- **Do not use the head-tilt/chin-lift if you suspect an injury to the neck or back.** To open the child's airway, gently move his jaw forward **without** tilting or moving his head.

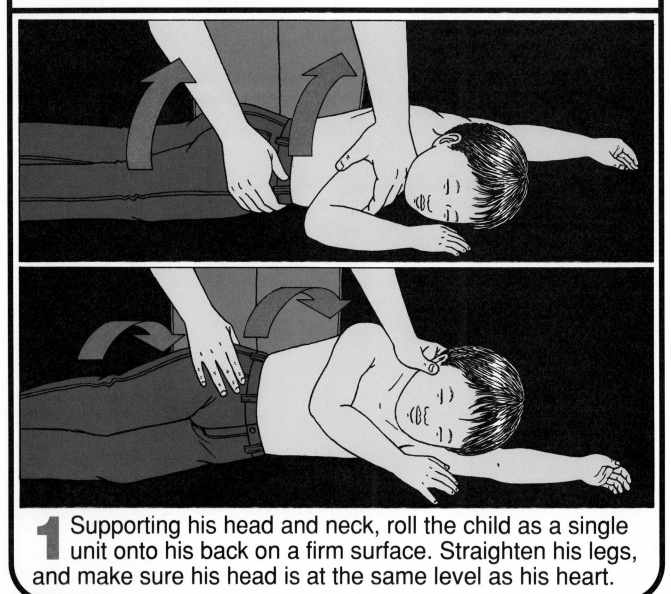

1 Supporting his head and neck, roll the child as a single unit onto his back on a firm surface. Straighten his legs, and make sure his head is at the same level as his heart.

CONTINUED ON NEXT PAGE

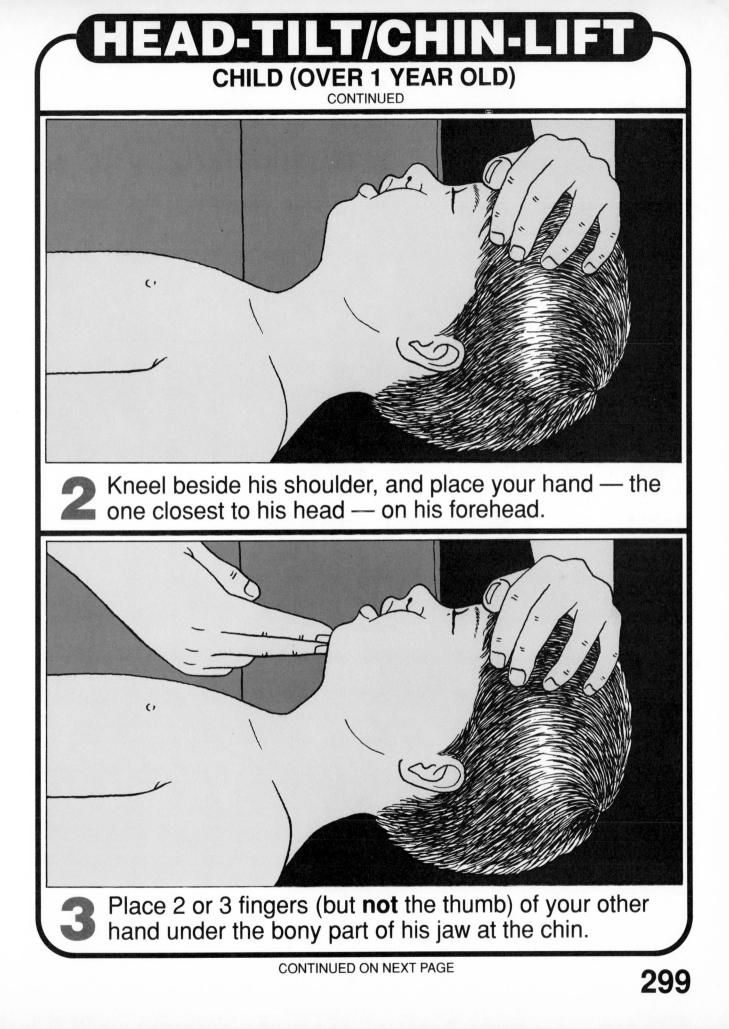

2 Kneel beside his shoulder, and place your hand — the one closest to his head — on his forehead.

3 Place 2 or 3 fingers (but **not** the thumb) of your other hand under the bony part of his jaw at the chin.

CONTINUED ON NEXT PAGE

CHILD (OVER 1 YEAR OLD)
CONTINUED

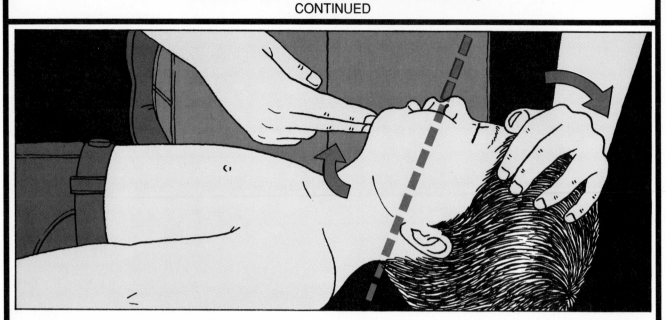

4A **If he is under 8 years old:** Gently tilt back his head to the **neutral-plus** position (as shown) by applying gentle backward pressure on his forehead and lifting his chin. **Do not** close his mouth completely.

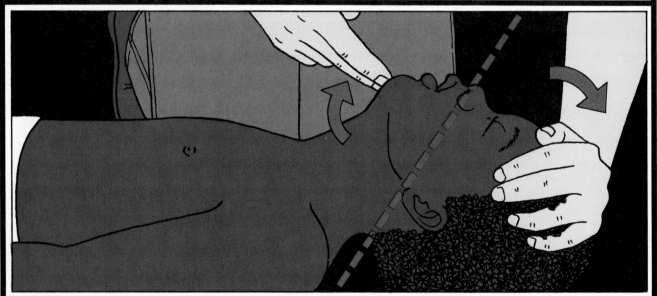

4B **If he is over 8 years old:** Gently tilt back his head to the **hyper-extended** position (with his chin pointing straight up, as shown) by applying gentle backward pressure on his forehead and lifting his chin. **Do not** close his mouth completely.

HEART ATTACK

IMPORTANT

- **Send for an ambulance and oxygen immediately.** Call 911 or Operator; see **EMS,** page 272.

- Check the child's ABCs (Airway, Breathing and Circulation); see **CHECKING THE ABCs,** pages 224-232.

- If the child has prescribed heart medication, help him take it, but **do not** give him anything to eat or drink.

- Calm and reassure the child.

- Observe for **SHOCK,** pages 354-356.

SIGNS & SYMPTOMS

Persistent pain at the center of the chest, which may radiate to the shoulders, neck or jaw. (May be mistaken for indigestion.) Extreme shortness of breath. Anxiety. Weakness. Profuse sweating. Dizziness. Nausea and vomiting. Cold, clammy skin. Pale or bluish lips, skin and fingernails. Unconsciousness.

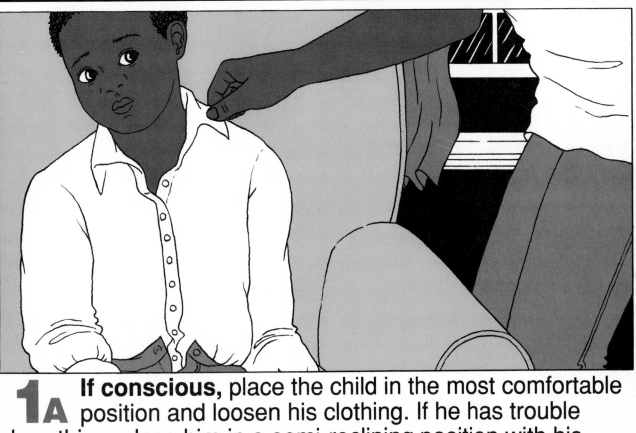

1A **If conscious,** place the child in the most comfortable position and loosen his clothing. If he has trouble breathing, place him in a semi-reclining position with his head and shoulders propped up. Provide good ventilation but keep him warm.

CONTINUED ON NEXT PAGE

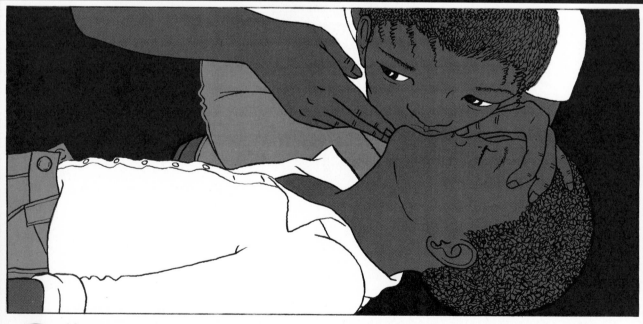

1B **If unconscious,** place him on his back and loosen his clothing. (To check unconsciousness, tap him on the shoulder or shake him gently.) Open his airway; see **HEAD-TILT/CHIN-LIFT,** pages 296-300.

2 If necessary, start rescue breathing immediately; see **BREATHING: ARTIFICIAL RESPIRATION,** pages 201-215. If he is not breathing and has no pulse, see **HEART FAILURE,** pages 303-323.

HEART FAILURE: CPR

INFANT (TO 1 YEAR OLD)

SIGNS & SYMPTOMS

Unconsciousness. No breathing. No pulse.

IMPORTANT

- **Waste no time, but be certain each sign is present before starting first aid.** To check unconsciousness, call the infant loudly, tap him on the shoulder or shake him gently.

- **Seek medical aid immediately.** Yell for help and have someone call 911 or Operator; see **EMS,** page 272. **If no one responds to your repeated shouts for help, administer first aid for 1 minute, then call EMS yourself.** Return immediately and continue first aid.

- **Because first aid for heart failure is difficult and potentially dangerous, it is best administered by someone who has been fully trained in the procedure. However, if a trained person is not present, you must begin first aid immediately since the alternative is death.**

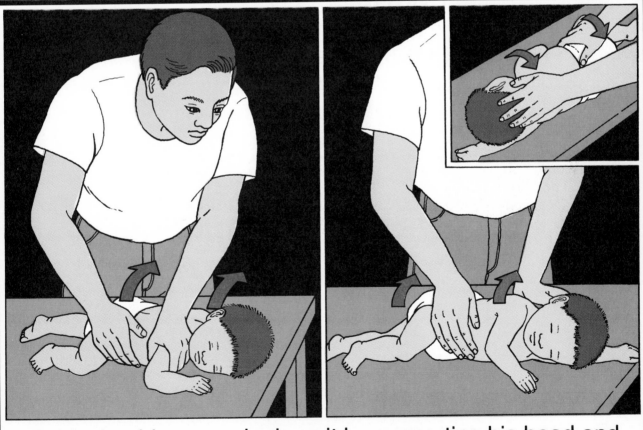

1 Moving him as a single unit by supporting his head and neck, roll the infant onto his back on a firm surface. Stand or kneel facing him from the side.

CONTINUED ON NEXT PAGE

INFANT (TO 1 YEAR OLD)
CONTINUED

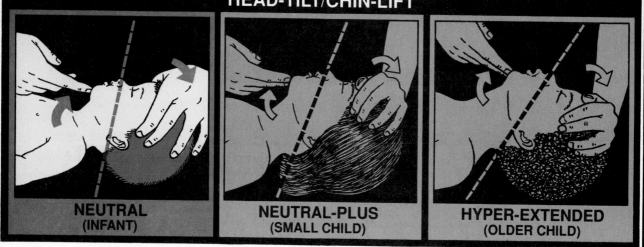

HEAD-TILT/CHIN-LIFT

NEUTRAL
(INFANT)

NEUTRAL-PLUS
(SMALL CHILD)

HYPER-EXTENDED
(OLDER CHILD)

2A **If there is no neck or back injury, open the airway** by using the **head-tilt/chin-lift:** Place your hand — the one closest to his head — on his forehead. Place 1 or 2 fingers (but **not** the thumb) of your other hand under the bony part of his jaw at the chin. Gently tilt his head back to the **neutral** position (as shown) by applying gentle backward pressure on his forehead and lifting his chin. **Do not** close his mouth completely.

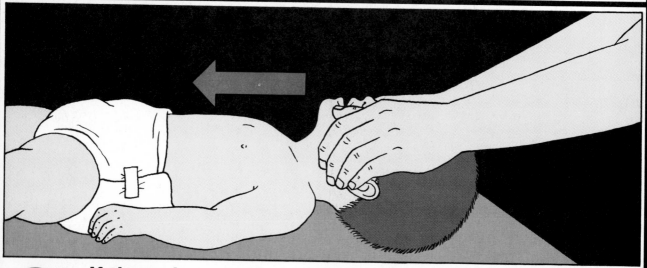

2B **If there is a neck or back injury, open the airway** by gently moving his jaw forward **without** tilting or moving his head.

CONTINUED ON NEXT PAGE

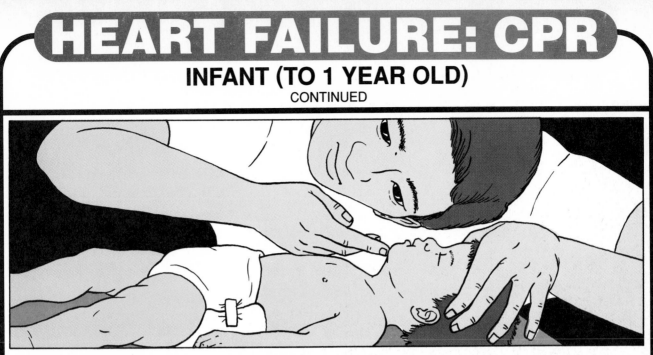

3 Taking 3 to 5 seconds, check for breathing by looking, listening and feeling for air leaving his lungs. (**Look** at his chest for movement. **Listen** for sounds of breathing. And **feel** for his breath on your cheek.)

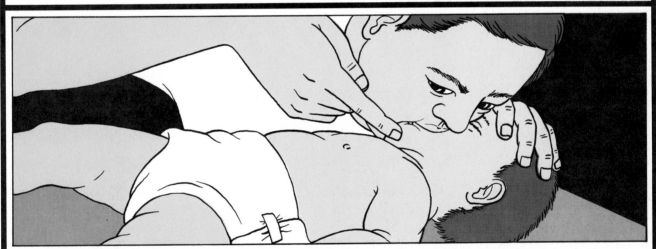

4 **If the infant is not breathing:** Put your open mouth over his nose and mouth, forming an airtight seal, and give 2 slow, gentle breaths (1 to 1½ seconds each), allowing the lungs to deflate fully between each breath. **If the entry or return of air seems blocked, or his chest does not rise, try again to open his airway** (see Step 2A or 2B) and give 2 slow, gentle breaths. **If the airway still seems blocked,** see **CHOKING,** pages 239-245. When the obstruction is cleared, continue on to Step 5.

CONTINUED ON NEXT PAGE

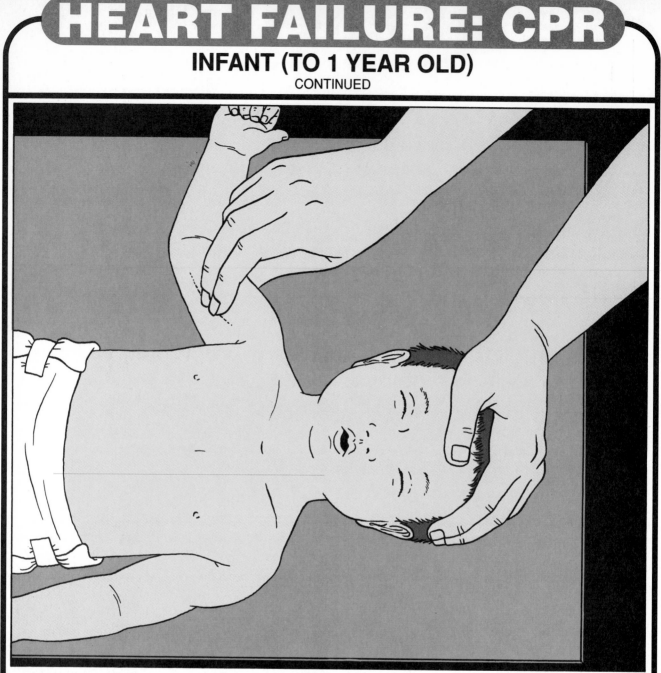

5 Continue to hold the infant's head in the **neutral** position with your hand on his forehead. **Check the pulse slowly and carefully** by placing the fingertips of your other hand (but **not** your thumb) on the inside of his upper arm between the elbow and shoulder. **It is extremely important to find the pulse if one is present. Take between 5 and 10 seconds to find it. Do not rush.** It is easily missed under emergency conditions. **If a pulse is present**, see **BREATHING: ARTIFICIAL RESPIRATION,** pages 201-205.

CONTINUED ON NEXT PAGE

INFANT (TO 1 YEAR OLD)
CONTINUED

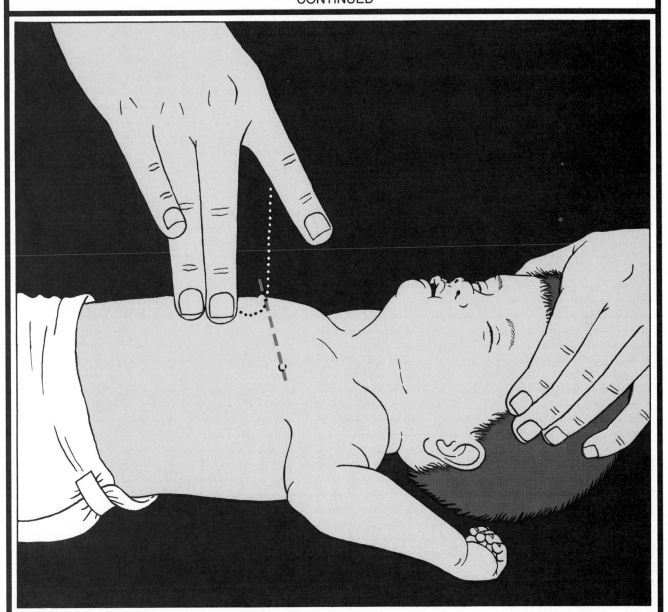

6 **If no pulse is present:** Place the pad of your index finger just below the imaginary line between the infant's nipples. Then place the pads of your middle and ring fingers next to the index finger. Now lift your index finger. Your other 2 fingers should be in the correct position for compressions (as shown). **Do not press the lower end of the breastbone.** If you feel the tip of the sternum, move your 2 fingers up toward the infant's head until they are off the tip.

CONTINUED ON NEXT PAGE

INFANT (TO 1 YEAR OLD)
CONTINUED

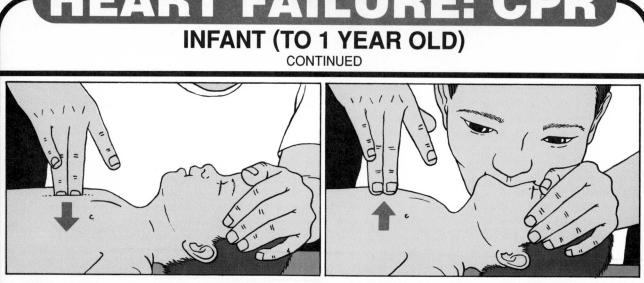

7 Make 5 short, smooth compressions directly downward about ½ to 1 inch, taking about ½ second for each compression (at a rate of about 100 to 120 per minute). **Do not remove your fingertips between compressions.** Then, keeping your fingertips in place, stop and give the infant a slow, gentle breath (1 to 1½ seconds). Continue the process of 5 compressions and 1 breath. **Establish the correct rate and rhythm by quickly counting out loud: "1, 2, 3, 4, 5, breathe."**

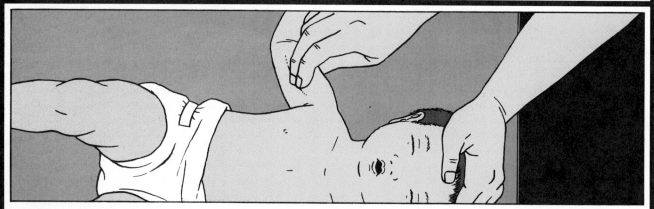

8 After one minute or 10 cycles of 5 compressions and 1 breath, recheck the pulse and breathing for 3 to 5 seconds, then recheck every few minutes thereafter. If the airway is blocked, see **CHOKING,** pages 239-245, then resume first aid. **Discontinue compressions when the pulse is restored; continue rescue breathing until the infant breathes on his own or professional help arrives.**

HEART FAILURE: CPR

SMALL CHILD (1 TO 8 YEARS OLD)

SIGNS & SYMPTOMS

Unconsciousness. No breathing. No pulse.

IMPORTANT

- **Waste no time, but be certain each sign is present before starting first aid.** To check unconsciousness, call the child loudly, tap her on the shoulder or shake her gently.

- **Seek medical aid immediately.** Yell for help and have someone call 911 or Operator; see **EMS**, page 272. **If no one responds to your repeated shouts for help, administer first aid for 1 minute, then call EMS yourself.** Return immediately and continue first aid.

- **Because first aid for heart failure is difficult and potentially dangerous, it is best administered by someone who has been fully trained in the procedure. However, if a trained person is not present, you must begin first aid immediately since the alternative is death.**

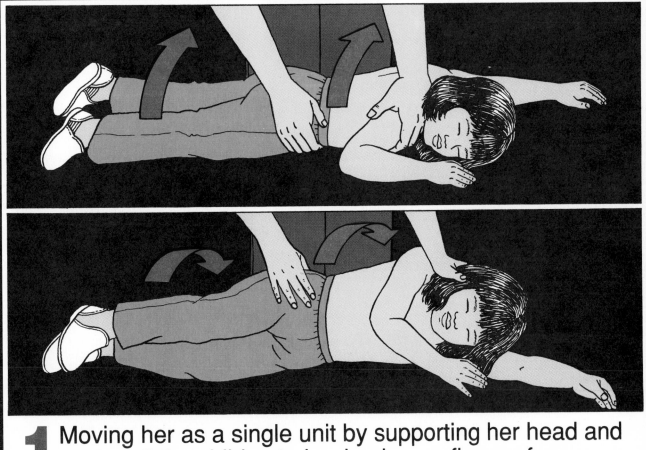

1 Moving her as a single unit by supporting her head and back, roll the child onto her back on a firm surface. Kneel beside her chest.

CONTINUED ON NEXT PAGE

SMALL CHILD (1 TO 8 YEARS OLD)
CONTINUED

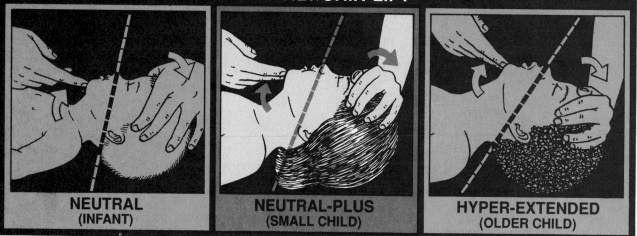

HEAD-TILT/CHIN-LIFT

NEUTRAL
(INFANT)

NEUTRAL-PLUS
(SMALL CHILD)

HYPER-EXTENDED
(OLDER CHILD)

2A **If there is no neck or back injury, open the airway** by using the **head-tilt/chin-lift:** Place your hand — the one closest to her head — on her forehead. Place 2 or 3 fingers (but **not** the thumb) of your other hand under the bony part of her jaw at the chin. Gently tilt her head back to the **neutral-plus** position (as shown) by applying gentle backward pressure on her forehead and lifting her chin. **Do not** close her mouth completely.

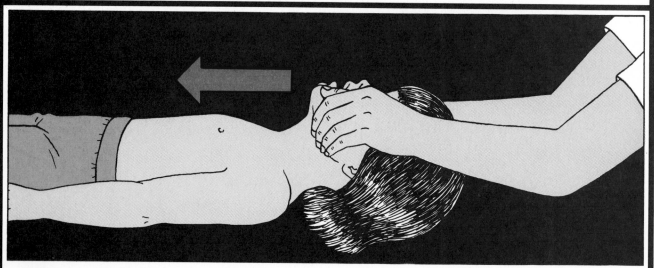

2B **If there is a neck or back injury, open the airway** by gently moving her jaw forward **without** tilting or moving her head.

CONTINUED ON NEXT PAGE

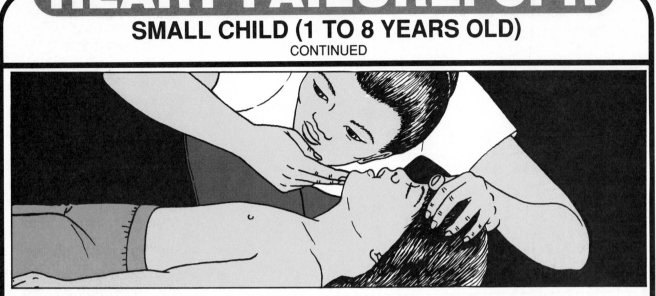

3 Taking 3 to 5 seconds, check for breathing by looking, listening and feeling for air leaving her lungs. (**Look** at her chest for movement. **Listen** for sounds of breathing. And **feel** for her breath on your cheek.)

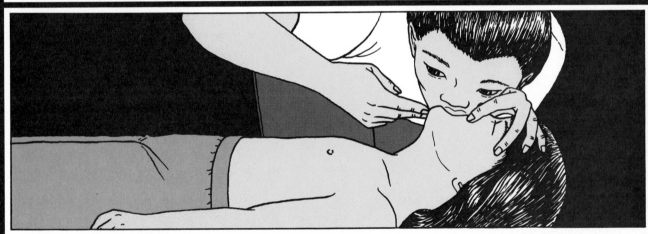

4 **If the child is not breathing:** Pinch her nose closed with the thumb and index finger of the hand that is on her forehead. Place your open mouth over her open mouth, forming an airtight seal. Give 2 slow, gentle breaths (1 to 1½ seconds each), allowing the lungs to deflate fully between each breath. **If the entry or return of air seems blocked, or her chest does not rise, try again to open her airway** (see Step 2A or 2B) and give 2 slow, gentle breaths. **If the airway still seems blocked,** see **CHOKING,** pages 246-252. When the obstruction is cleared, continue on to Step 5.

CONTINUED ON NEXT PAGE

SMALL CHILD (1 TO 8 YEARS OLD)
CONTINUED

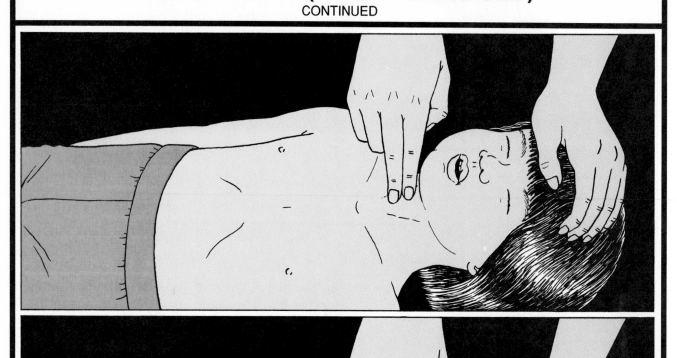

5 **Check the pulse slowly and carefully** at the large artery of the neck. Place your first two fingers on the child's Adam's apple (about halfway between the chin and the collarbone). Slide your fingers into the groove next to the windpipe on the side nearest you, then press gently. **It is extremely important to find the pulse if one is present. Take between 5 and 10 seconds to find it. Do not rush.** It is easily missed under emergency conditions. **If a pulse is present,** see **BREATHING: ARTIFICIAL RESPIRATION,** pages 206-210.

CONTINUED ON NEXT PAGE

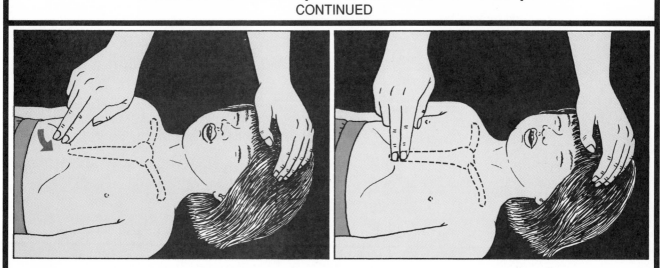

6 **If no pulse is present:** Maintain the **neutral-plus head-tilt** position with your hand on the child's forehead. Move the index and middle fingers of your other hand up along the lower edge of her rib cage (on the side closest to you) until your middle finger locates the notch above the tip of the breastbone. Put your middle finger in the notch and your index finger beside it (as shown).

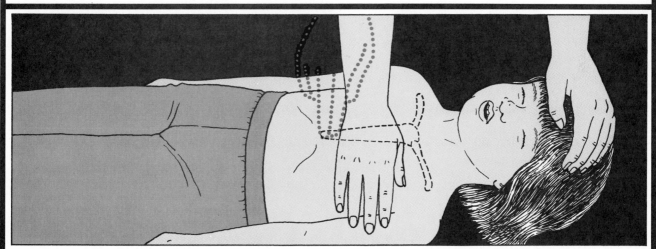

7 Lift your fingers off the breastbone and place the heel of the **same** hand just above the point where the top of your index finger was resting (2 finger-widths above the notch on the breastbone). **Do not** press the **tip** of the breastbone. Your fingertips should be pointing directly across the child's body but not pressing against the ribs.

CONTINUED ON NEXT PAGE

SMALL CHILD (1 TO 8 YEARS OLD)
CONTINUED

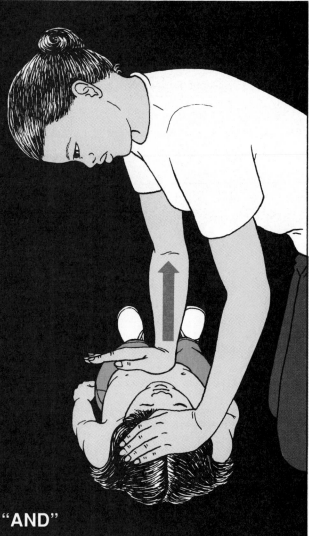

"1"   "AND"

8 Continue to maintain the **neutral-plus head-tilt** position with your hand on her forehead. With your shoulder directly over your other hand on the child's chest, make 5 short, smooth compressions straight downward (**do not** rock back and forth) about 1 to 1½ inches deep, taking about ¾ second for each compression (at a rate of about 80 to 100 per minute). Establish the correct rate and rhythm by counting out loud: "1 and 2 and 3 and 4 and 5 and breathe." Push down as you say the number and come up as you say the "and." **Do not remove your hand between compressions,** but allow the chest to return to its normal position.

CONTINUED ON NEXT PAGE

SMALL CHILD (1 TO 8 YEARS OLD)
CONTINUED

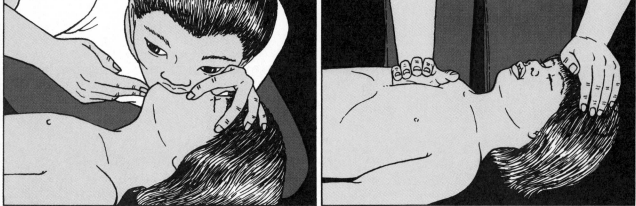

9 Stop after every 5 compressions, remove your hand from her chest and lift her chin. Pinch her nose closed with the hand that is on her forehead and give her a slow, gentle breath (1 to 1½ seconds). Now replace the heel of the hand that is under her chin back on her chest in the **exact** position as before. Continue the process of 5 compressions and 1 breath.

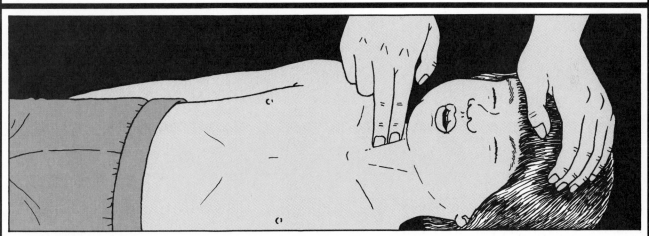

10 After 1 minute or 10 cycles of 5 compressions and 1 breath, recheck the pulse and breathing for 5 seconds, then recheck every few minutes thereafter. If the airway is blocked, see **CHOKING,** pages 246-252, then resume first aid. **Discontinue compressions when the pulse is restored; continue rescue breathing until the child breathes on her own or professional help arrives.**

HEART FAILURE: CPR

OLDER CHILD (8 YEARS & OLDER)

SIGNS & SYMPTOMS

Unconsciousness. No breathing. No pulse.

IMPORTANT

- **Waste no time, but be certain each sign is present before starting first aid.** To check unconsciousness, call the child loudly, tap him on the shoulder or shake him gently.

- **Seek medical aid immediately.** Yell for help and have someone call 911 or Operator; see **EMS,** page 272. **If no one is available, call EMS yourself, then return immediately and begin first aid.**

- **Because first aid for heart failure is difficult and potentially dangerous, it is best administered by someone who has been fully trained in the procedure. However, if a trained person is not present, you must begin first aid immediately since the alternative is death.**

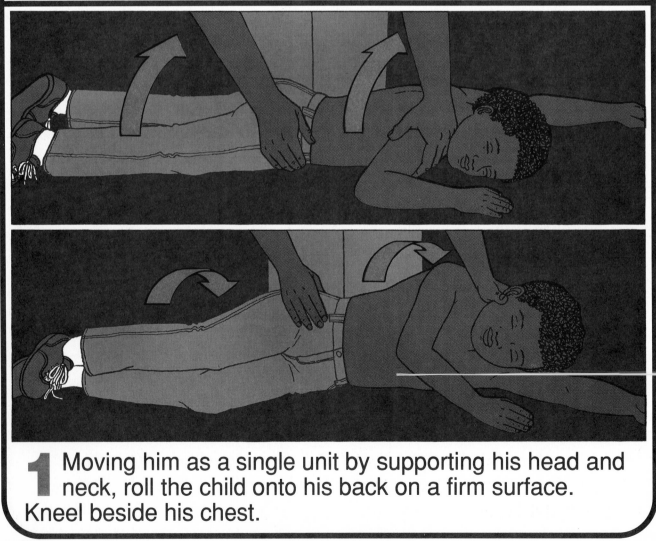

1 Moving him as a single unit by supporting his head and neck, roll the child onto his back on a firm surface. Kneel beside his chest.

CONTINUED ON NEXT PAGE

HEART FAILURE: CPR

OLDER CHILD (8 YEARS & OLDER)
CONTINUED

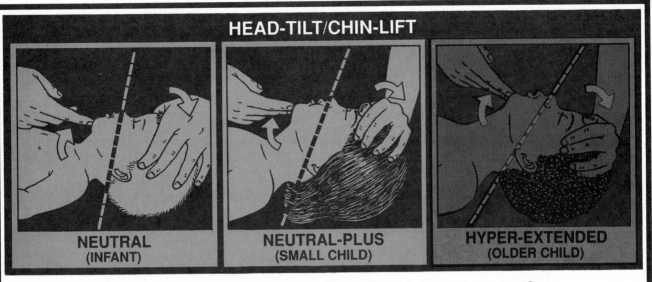

HEAD-TILT/CHIN-LIFT

NEUTRAL
(INFANT)

NEUTRAL-PLUS
(SMALL CHILD)

HYPER-EXTENDED
(OLDER CHILD)

2A **If there is no neck or back injury, open the airway** by using the **head-tilt/chin-lift:** Place your hand — the one closest to his head — on his forehead. Place 2 or 3 fingers (but **not** the thumb) of your other hand under the bony part of his jaw at the chin. Gently tilt his head back to the **hyper-extended** position (with his chin pointing straight up, as shown) by applying gentle backward pressure on his forehead and lifting his chin. **Do not** close his mouth completely.

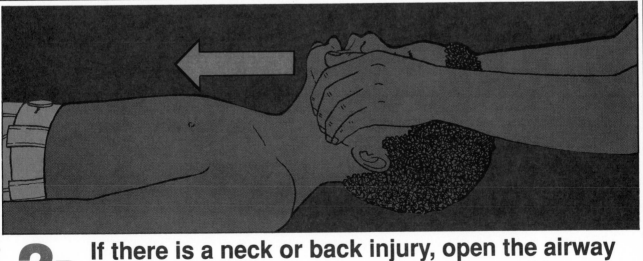

2B **If there is a neck or back injury, open the airway** by gently moving his jaw forward **without** tilting or moving his head.

CONTINUED ON NEXT PAGE

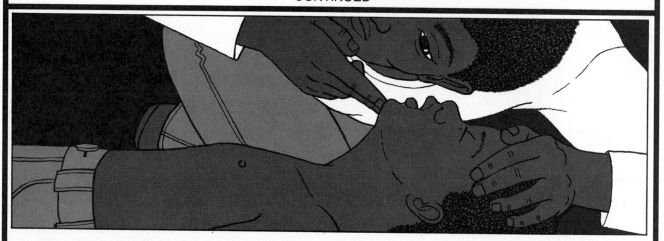

3 Taking 3 to 5 seconds, check for breathing by looking, listening and feeling for air leaving his lungs. (**Look** at his chest for movement. **Listen** for sounds of breathing. And **feel** for his breath on your cheek.)

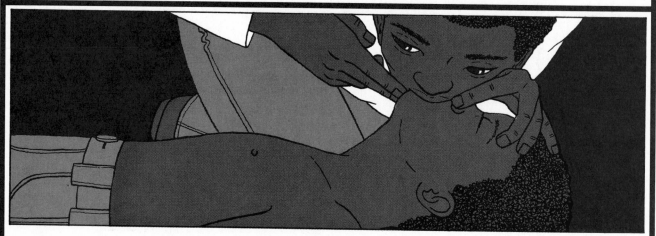

4 **If the child is not breathing:** Pinch his nose closed with the thumb and index finger of the hand that is on his forehead. Place your open mouth over his open mouth, forming an airtight seal. Give 2 slow, full breaths (1½ to 2 seconds each), allowing the lungs to deflate fully between each breath. **If the entry or return of air seems blocked, or his chest does not rise, try again to open his airway** (see Step 2A or 2B) and give 2 slow, full breaths. **If the airway still seems blocked,** see **CHOKING,** pages 246-252. When the obstruction is cleared, continue on to Step 5.

CONTINUED ON NEXT PAGE

OLDER CHILD (8 YEARS & OLDER)
CONTINUED

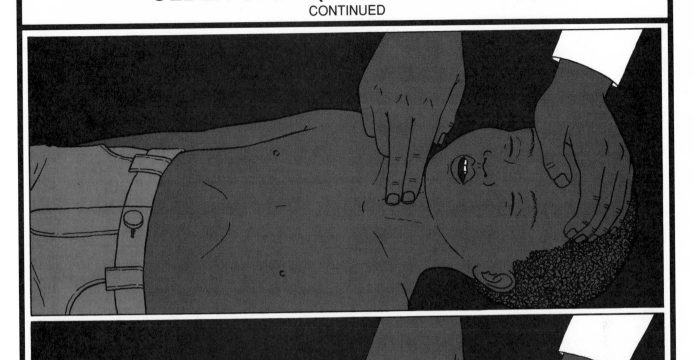

5 **Check the pulse slowly and carefully** at the large artery of the neck. Place your first two fingers on the child's Adam's apple (about halfway between the chin and the collarbone). Slide your fingers into the groove next to the windpipe on the side nearest you, then press gently. **It is extremely important to find the pulse if one is present. Take between 5 and 10 seconds to find it. Do not rush.** It is easily missed under emergency conditions. **If a pulse is present,** see **BREATHING: ARTIFICIAL RESPIRATION,** pages 211-215.

CONTINUED ON NEXT PAGE

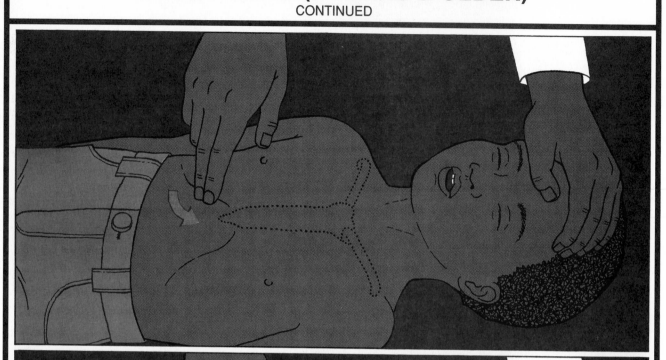

6 **If no pulse is present:** Using the hand nearest the child's legs, find the lower edge of his rib cage (on the side closest to you). Move your index and middle fingers up along the edge of his rib cage until your middle finger locates the notch above the tip of the breastbone. Put your middle finger in the notch and your index finger beside it (as shown).

CONTINUED ON NEXT PAGE

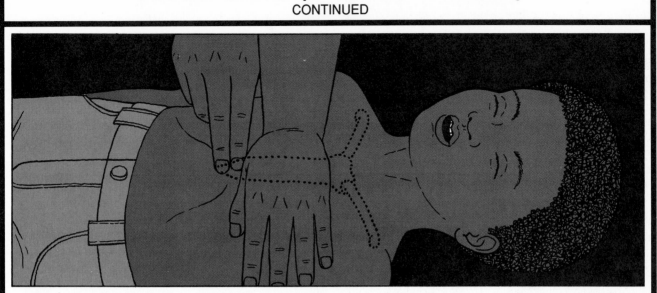

7 Place the heel of your other hand on the child's breast-bone, just above the point where the top of your index finger is resting (2 finger-widths above the notch on the breastbone). **Do not** press the **tip** of the breastbone. Your fingertips should be pointing directly across his body, but not pressing against his ribs.

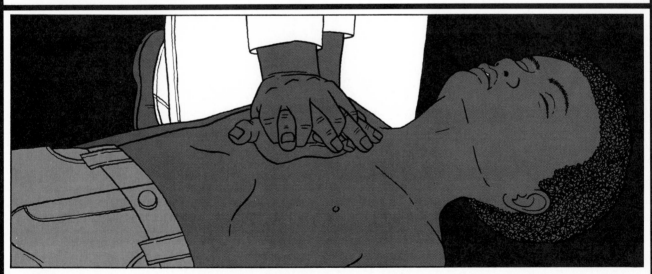

8 Now remove your hand from the notch and place it on top of the hand resting on the breastbone (as shown). With your fingertips still pointing directly across the child's body, interlace the fingers of both hands (as shown). Press down with the heel only and **never press on the ribs.**

CONTINUED ON NEXT PAGE

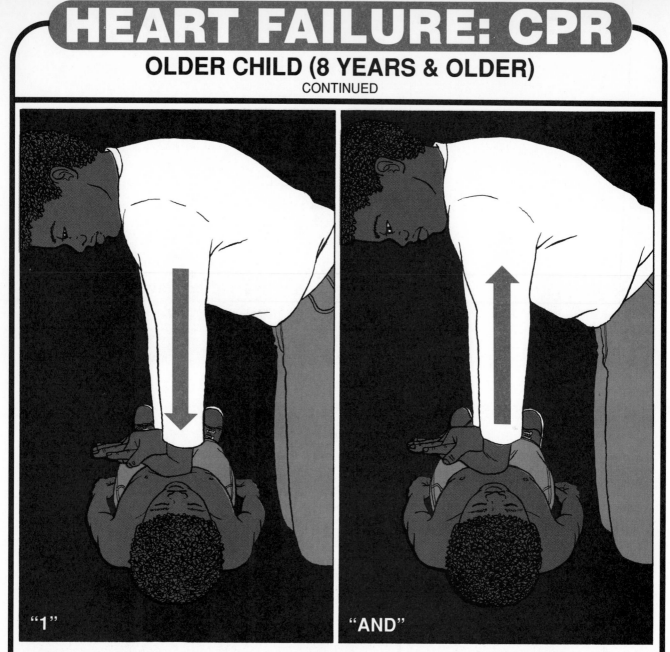

"1"   "AND"

9 Keeping your elbows straight and your shoulders directly over your interlaced hands, make 15 smooth compressions directly downward (**do not** rock back and forth) about 1½ to 2 inches deep, taking about ¾ second for each compression (at a rate of about 80 to 100 per minute). Establish the correct rate and rhythm by counting out loud: "1 and 2 and 3 and 4 and 5 and 6 and 7 and 8 and 9 and 10 and 11 and 12 and 13 and 14 and 15." Push down as you say the number and come up as you say the "and." **Do not remove your hands between compressions,** but allow the chest to return to its normal position.

CONTINUED ON NEXT PAGE

OLDER CHILD (8 YEARS & OLDER)
CONTINUED

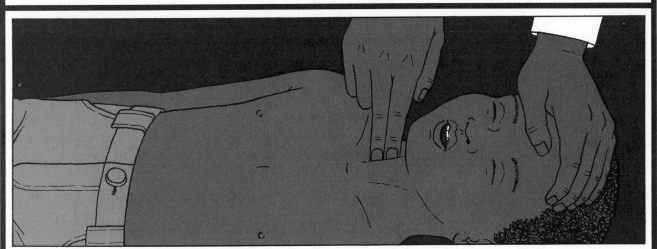

10 Stop after every 15 compressions, remove your hands from his chest and using the **hyper-extended head-tilt/chin-lift** position, give the child 2 slow, full breaths (1½ to 2 seconds each). Then place your hands back on his chest in the **exact** position as before. Continue the process of 15 compressions and 2 breaths.

11 After 1 minute or 4 cycles of 15 compressions and 2 breaths, recheck the pulse and breathing for 5 seconds, then recheck every few minutes thereafter. If the airway is blocked, see **CHOKING,** pages 246-252, then resume first aid. **Discontinue compressions when the pulse is restored; continue rescue breathing until the child breathes on his own or professional help arrives.**

HEAT CRAMPS

IMPORTANT

- **Seek medical aid.** Heat cramps may occur alone or occasionally as one of the early symptoms of sunstroke or heat exhaustion; see **SUNSTROKE (HEATSTROKE),** pages 364-365, and **HEAT EXHAUSTION,** page 326.

- **Do not** give the child salt tablets, aspirin or other medications commonly used to reduce fever, or drinks that contain alcohol or caffeine.

SIGNS & SYMPTOMS

Sudden onset of severe intermittent muscle pain or spasm following strenuous exertion in high heat and humidity. Often affects the calf, thigh or abdomen, but may be felt elsewhere. **May include:** Pale, moist skin. Profuse sweating. Weakness.

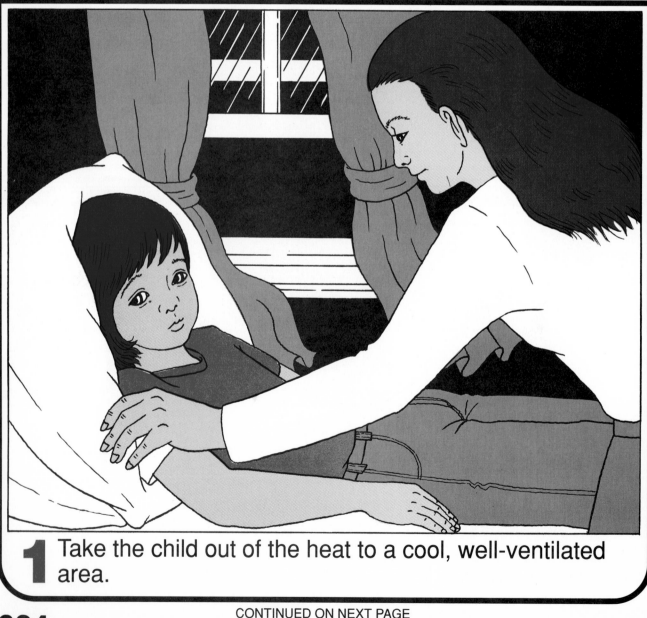

1 Take the child out of the heat to a cool, well-ventilated area.

CONTINUED ON NEXT PAGE

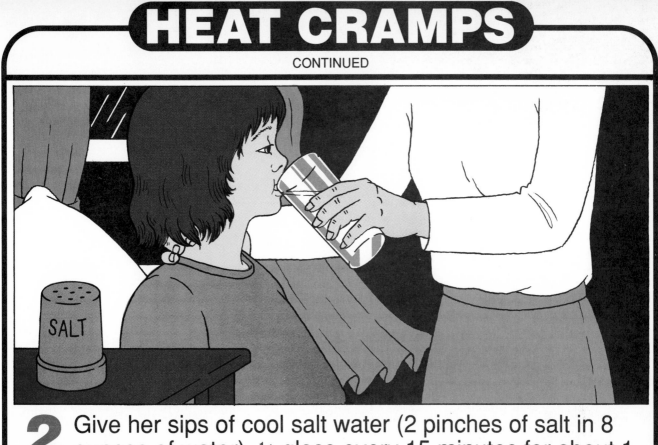

2 Give her sips of cool salt water (2 pinches of salt in 8 ounces of water), ½ glass every 15 minutes for about 1 hour. **Do not** use more than the recommended dosage of salt. Discontinue water if she vomits.

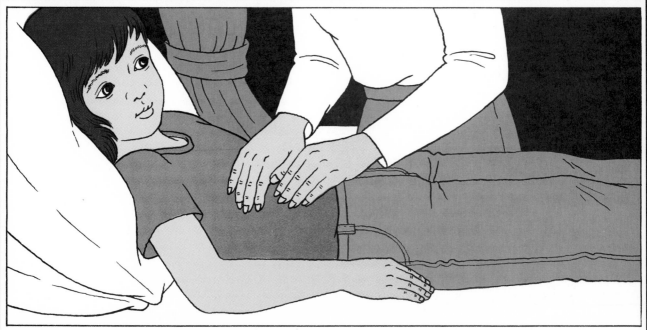

3 To help relieve muscle cramps, apply warm packs, then gently massage the affected area or apply pressure with your hands.

325

HEAT EXHAUSTION

IMPORTANT

- **Consult your doctor if the child does not respond to first aid.**

- **Do not** give her aspirin or other medications commonly used to reduce fever, or drinks that contain alcohol or caffeine.

- Observe for **SHOCK** (pages 354-356), **SEIZURES** (page 253) and **UNCONSCIOUSNESS** (pages 381-382).

SIGNS & SYMPTOMS

Pale, cold and moist skin. Profuse sweating. Extreme thirst. Body temperature is about normal. **Early symptoms may also include:** Muscle cramps. Nausea. Vomiting. Weakness. Dizziness. Fainting.

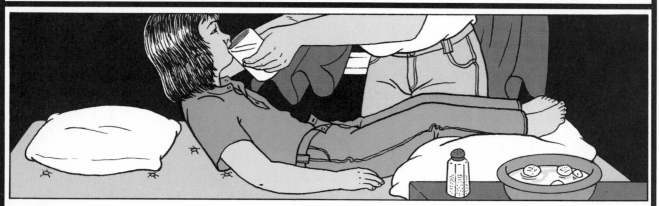

1 Take the child to a cool, shaded, well-ventilated room. Loosen her clothing and have her lie down. Elevate her feet 8 to 12 inches. Cool her off with cool, moist cloths.

2 Give her sips of cool salt water (2 pinches of salt in 8 ounces of water) or plain tap water, ½ glass every 15 minutes for about 1 hour. **Do not** use more than the recommended dosage of salt. Discontinue water if she vomits.

HEAT RASH (PRICKLY HEAT)

SIGNS & SYMPTOMS

Burning, prickling sensation around the underarm, thigh or groin. May affect other parts of the body. Sometimes accompanied by itching. Usually occurs in high heat and humidity or when a child is overdressed. Progresses to tiny red and pink pinpoints or blisters. The affected area may become inflamed. Commonly affects infants.

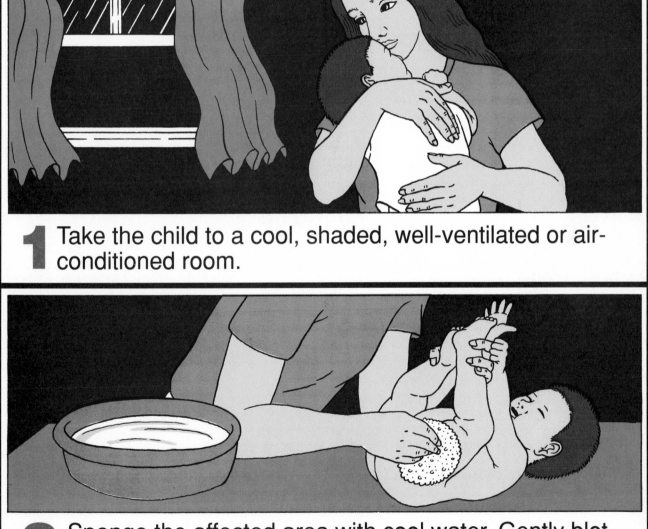

1 Take the child to a cool, shaded, well-ventilated or air-conditioned room.

2 Sponge the affected area with cool water. Gently blot dry.

CONTINUED ON NEXT PAGE

CONTINUED

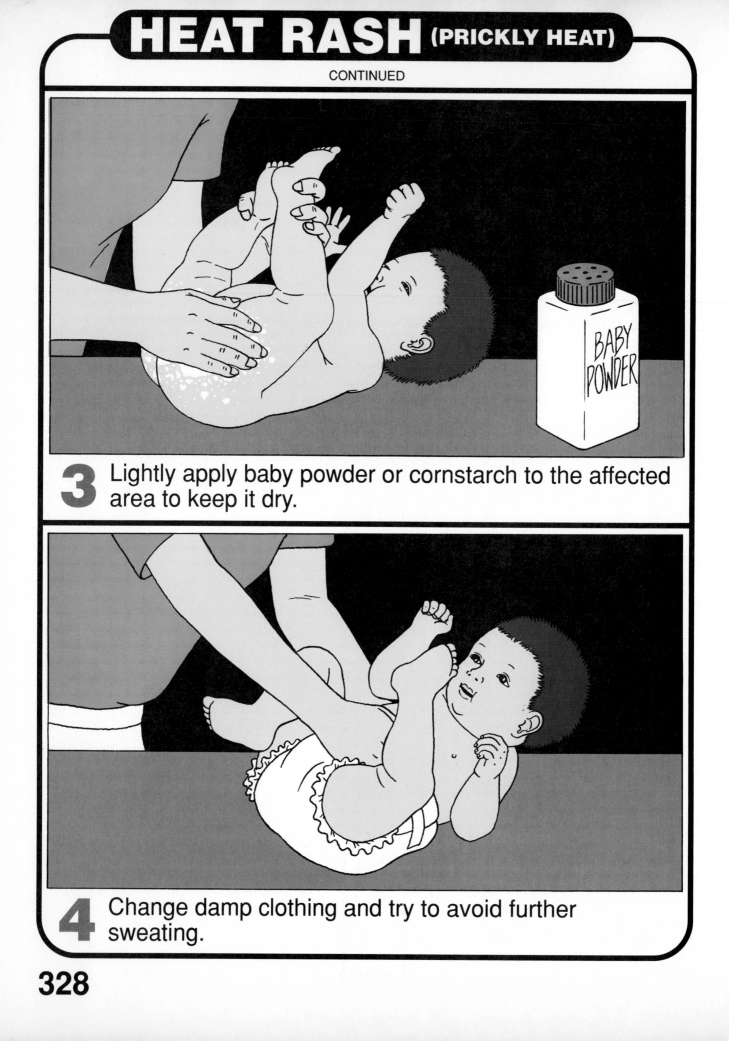

3 Lightly apply baby powder or cornstarch to the affected area to keep it dry.

4 Change damp clothing and try to avoid further sweating.

HYPERVENTILATION

- **Seek medical aid** if breathing does not return to normal after first aid or if the child hyperventilates frequently. Hyperventilation is usually caused by anxiety or excessive exercise, but it can also be the result of illness or injury or an adverse reaction to medication.

SIGNS & SYMPTOMS

Rapid breathing. Anxiety. **May lead to:** Dizziness. Fainting.

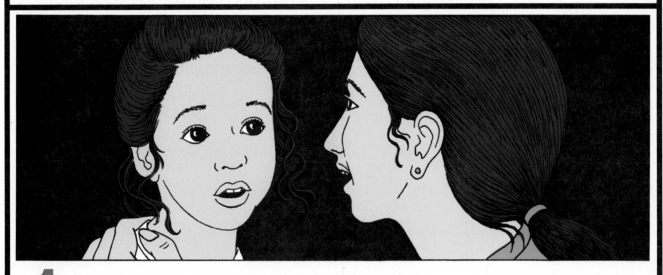

1 Try to calm and reassure the child.

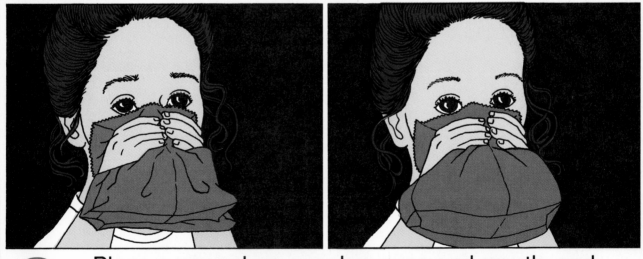

2A Place a paper bag over her nose and mouth, and have her breathe in and out of it for a few breaths. Tell her to try to breathe normally and not sigh or take frequent deep breaths.

CONTINUED ON NEXT PAGE

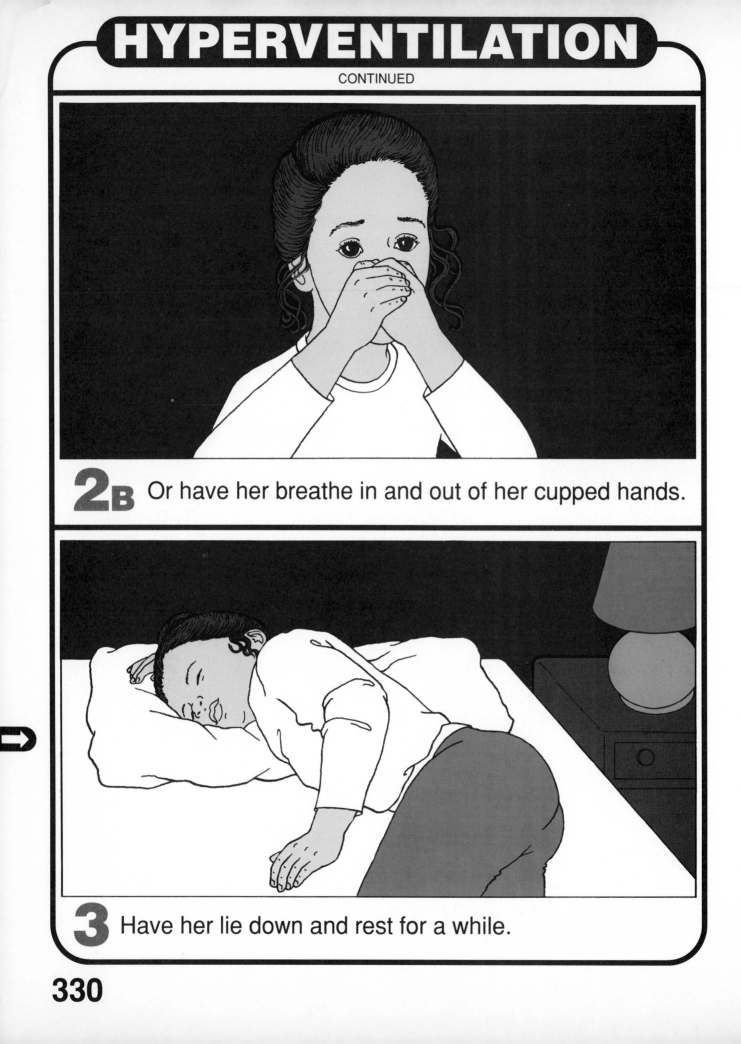

2B Or have her breathe in and out of her cupped hands.

3 Have her lie down and rest for a while.

HYPOGLYCEMIA (LOW BLOOD SUGAR)

IMPORTANT

- **If the child is unconscious, seek medical aid immediately.** Call 911 or Operator; see **EMS,** page 272.

- Treat for **SHOCK,** pages 354-356.

- **Do not** give the child anything to drink if he is unconscious or has difficulty swallowing.

SIGNS & SYMPTOMS

May affect anyone, though especially common in diabetics who are reacting to an excessive dose of insulin or who have taken a prescribed dose of insulin, then engaged in excessive exercise or have missed a meal. **Sudden appearance of:** Moist, clammy, ashen or pale skin. Profuse cold sweat. **May include:** Hunger. Shallow breathing. Confusion. Trembling hands. Shaking. Anxiety. Weakness. Dizziness. Personality change. **May progress to:** Convulsions. Coma.

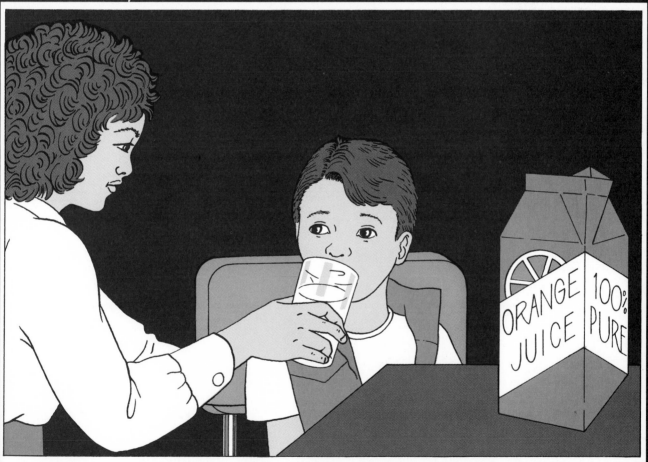

Give the child orange juice, soft drinks containing sugar, candy or sugar in any form. If he doesn't improve in 10 minutes, seek medical aid.

HYPOTHERMIA (COLD EXPOSURE)

IMPORTANT

- **Hypothermia is a life-threatening emergency caused by the lowering of the body core temperature.** It is usually caused by cold or cool air, wind, immersion in water, or wet clothing. Hypothermia may become extremely serious in a matter of minutes or develop slowly over the course of hours or even days.

- **Seek medical aid immediately.** Call 911 or Operator; see **EMS,** page 272. A child who has received emergency first aid for hypothermia should be examined by a doctor even if he appears to have recovered fully.

- Check the child's ABCs (Airway, Breathing and Circulation); see **CHECKING THE ABCs,** pages 224-232.

- If symptoms are present, treat for hypothermia even if the child claims to be fine.

- **Do not** let the child walk if his feet are frostbitten.

- **Do not** give him anything to drink if he is semiconscious, unconscious or has difficulty swallowing.

- **Do not** rub the child's body. **Handle him very gently.** Unnecessary manipulation may cause heart failure.

SIGNS & SYMPTOMS

May include: Persistent or violent shivering. Slow or slurred speech. Personality change. Loss of control over hands. Stumbling. Drowsiness. Impaired reasoning. Confusion. The child may fail to acknowledge symptoms. **In advanced stages:** Muscle spasms and rigidity. Inability to use the arms or legs. Unconsciousness that may mimic death.

In all cases, it is extremely important to reach medical aid as quickly as possible.

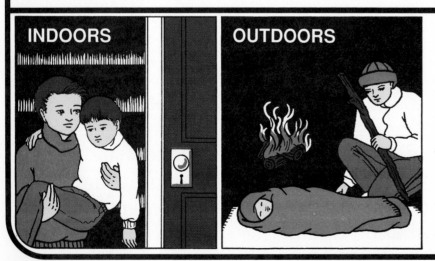

INDOORS OUTDOORS

1 Gently carry the child out of the wind and cold to a warm place, preferably indoors. If that isn't possible, start a fire and improvise a shelter.

CONTINUED ON NEXT PAGE

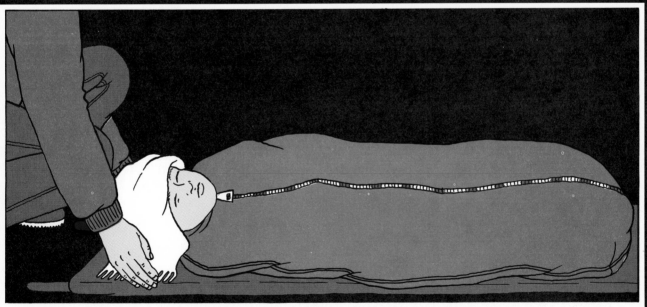

2 Gently remove his wet clothing and change to dry clothes if available. (If outdoors, place a folded blanket under him to insulate him from the cold.) Wrap him in a blanket and cover his head with a scarf, towel, etc.

3A **If hypothermia has developed quickly** (as in the case of immersion in cold water): Gently place him in a sleeping bag or several blankets, cover his head, and **transport him to medical aid immediately;** see **TRANSPORTING THE INJURED,** pages 377-380.

CONTINUED ON NEXT PAGE

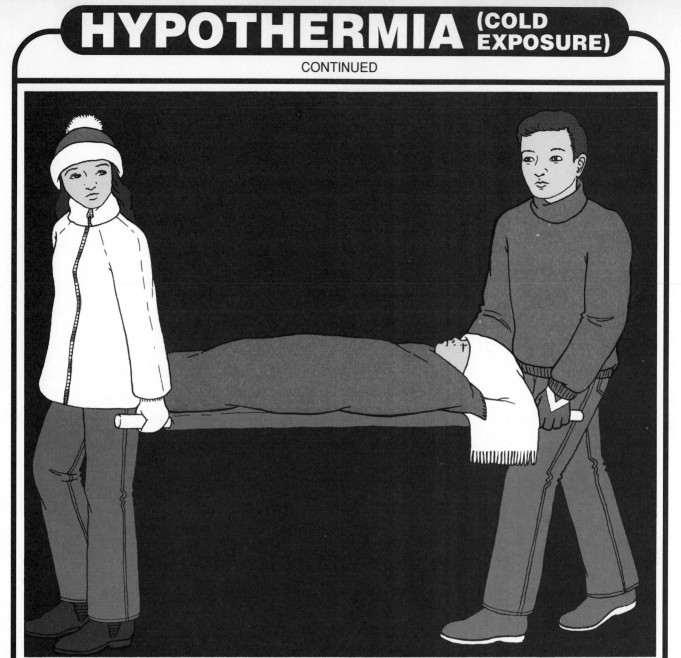

3B **If hypothermia has developed slowly over several hours or days** (as in the case of a lost child or the failure of a home heating system): Protect the child from further heat loss by gently wrapping him in a blanket. Loosely cover his head with a scarf or other suitable cloth to conserve heat further and pre-warm the air he breathes. If possible, further insulate the child from wind and cold by placing him in a sleeping bag or wrapping him in a sheet of plastic or plastic garbage bags. **(Do not** cover his face.) **Transport him to medical aid immediately;** see **TRANS-PORTING THE INJURED,** pages 377-380.

CONTINUED ON NEXT PAGE

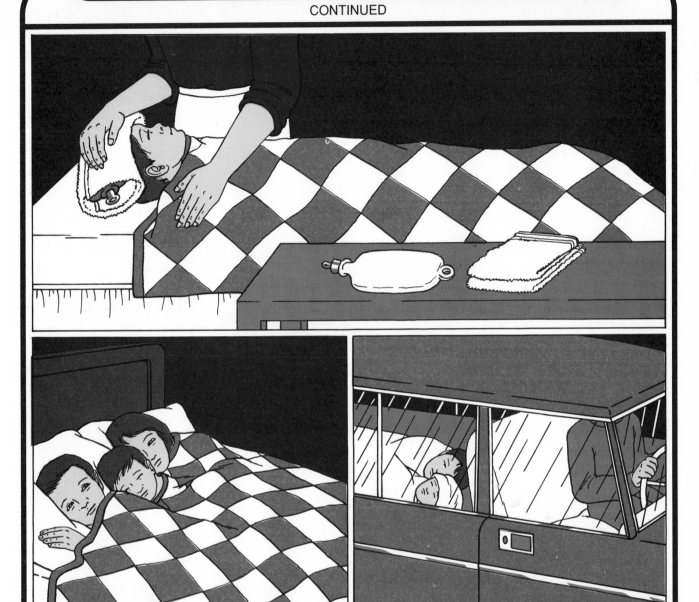

4 **If travel is delayed or impossible and medical aid cannot reach you, rewarm the child:** Expose him to warm air and apply gentle heat to the head, neck, torso and groin with hot-water bottles wrapped in towels. Or warm his body with your own through skin-to-skin contact. If possible, maximize the warming process by placing him between two people. **It is crucial that you prevent further heat loss.** If possible, continue skin-to-skin warming or application of gentle heat during travel to medical aid.

- **Send for help immediately.** Have someone call 911 or Operator; see **EMS,** page 272.

- **Do not** walk near the open ice.

- Tell the child not to try to climb out but to slide his arms onto the ice and hold on until you reach him.

- When safely back on firm footing, check for **HYPOTHERMIA (COLD EXPOSURE);** see pages 332-335. A child who has been in icy water for only a short time can become hypothermic very quickly.

- If necessary, see **DROWNING: FIRST AID,** pages 259-260.

1A Try to reach the child from land with a hand, leg, clothing, rope, ladder, sled, board, etc. Tell him to hold onto the reaching assist and slide on his stomach — not walk upright — back to firm footing.

CONTINUED ON NEXT PAGE

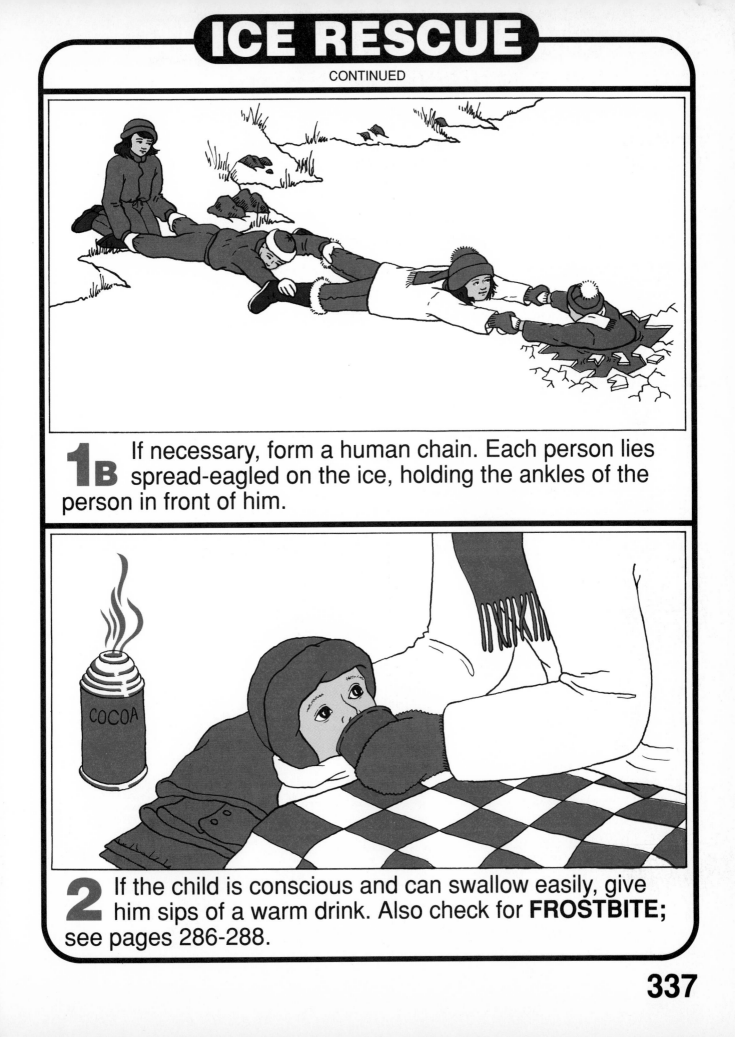

1B If necessary, form a human chain. Each person lies spread-eagled on the ice, holding the ankles of the person in front of him.

2 If the child is conscious and can swallow easily, give him sips of a warm drink. Also check for **FROSTBITE;** see pages 286-288.

337

MOUTH INJURIES

GUMS, PALATE & TEETH

- Wash your hands thoroughly and, if possible, put on sterile latex gloves before starting first aid.

- Check if there are more serious injuries to the head or neck. If necessary, see **HEAD INJURIES: CLOSED HEAD INJURIES,** page 289, and **BACK & NECK INJURIES,** pages 135-136.

- Clear the mouth of broken teeth. Wrap the teeth in a cool, moist cloth, and bring them to the doctor or dentist for possible replanting.

- Lean the child slightly forward so he does not inhale blood.

GUMS & PALATE

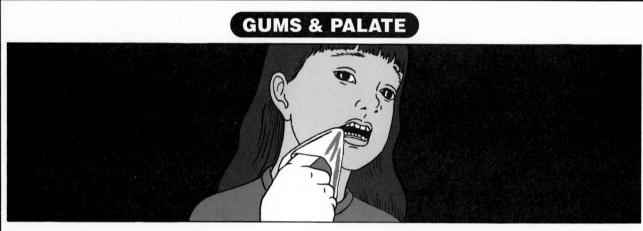

Control bleeding by direct pressure with a sterile dressing or clean cloth.

TEETH

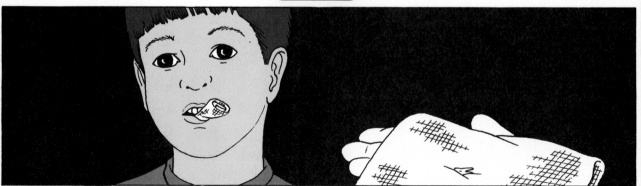

Control bleeding by direct pressure on the tooth socket with a sterile dressing or clean cloth. Have the child bite down firmly to hold the dressing in place.

MOUTH INJURIES

TONGUE & LIPS

IMPORTANT

- Wash your hands thoroughly and, if possible, put on sterile latex gloves before starting first aid.

- Check if there are more serious injuries to the head or neck. If necessary, see **HEAD INJURIES: CLOSED HEAD INJURIES,** page 289, and **BACK & NECK INJURIES,** pages 135-136.

- Clear the mouth of broken teeth. Wrap the teeth in a cool, moist cloth, and bring them to the doctor or dentist for possible replanting.

- Lean the child slightly forward so he does not swallow blood.

TONGUE

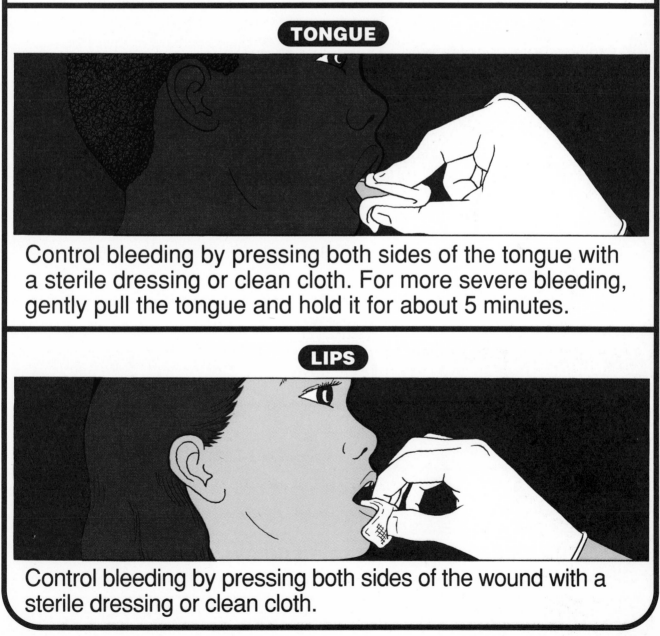

Control bleeding by pressing both sides of the tongue with a sterile dressing or clean cloth. For more severe bleeding, gently pull the tongue and hold it for about 5 minutes.

LIPS

Control bleeding by pressing both sides of the wound with a sterile dressing or clean cloth.

339

MUSCLE CRAMP (CHARLEY HORSE)

IMPORTANT

- Try to relax the affected area. Tension can worsen the muscle spasm.

- **Seek medical aid** if the cramp persists or recurs.

SIGNS & SYMPTOMS

Sudden spasm and pain in a muscle, usually the calf or thigh. May worsen with movement and limit use of the affected area. Often occurs following overexertion, injury or exposure to cold or dampness. In severe cases, discomfort may last several days or longer.

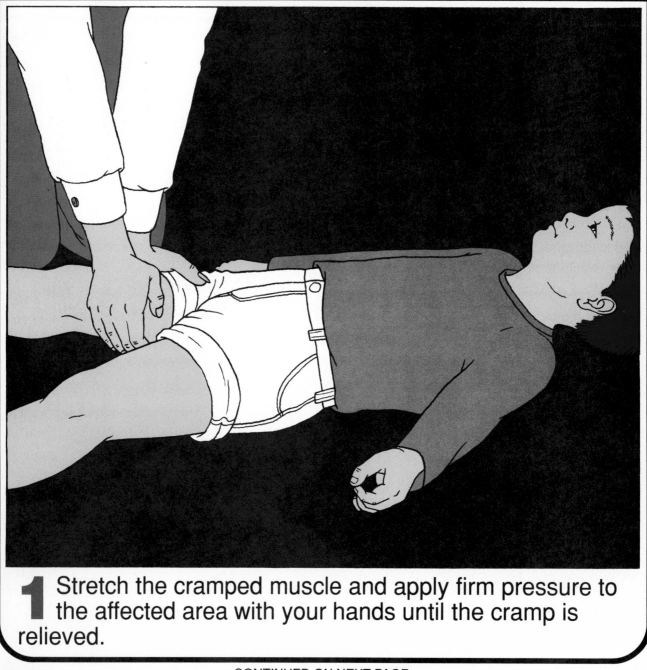

1 Stretch the cramped muscle and apply firm pressure to the affected area with your hands until the cramp is relieved.

CONTINUED ON NEXT PAGE

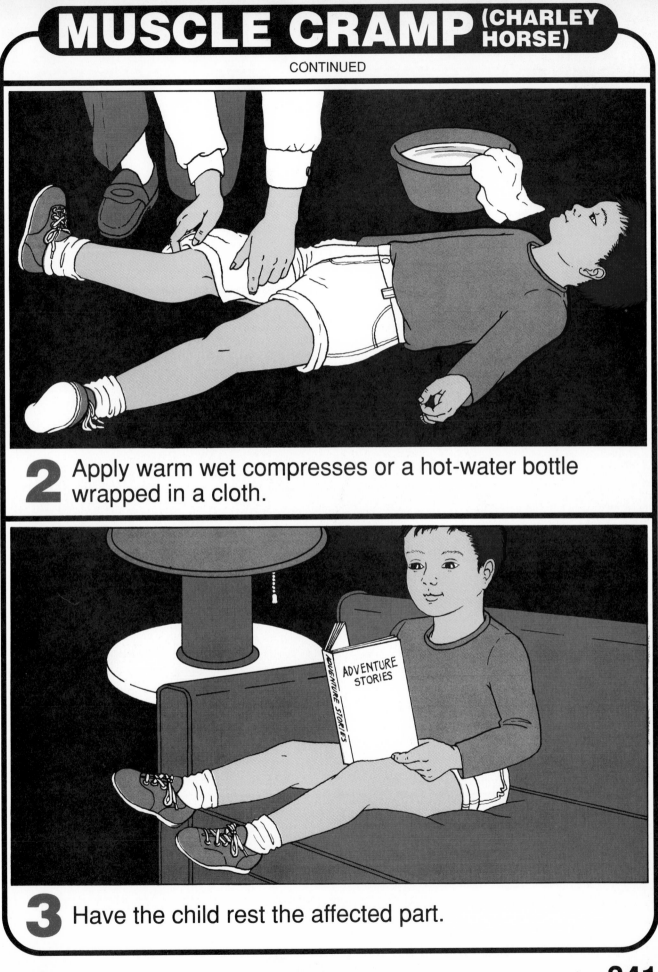

2 Apply warm wet compresses or a hot-water bottle wrapped in a cloth.

3 Have the child rest the affected part.

NOSE INJURIES

BROKEN NOSE, FOREIGN OBJECTS & NOSEBLEED

IMPORTANT

- **Seek medical aid** if you suspect a neck or serious head injury. If necessary, call **EMS;** see page 272.

- If the nose is bleeding, wash your hands thoroughly and, if possible, put on sterile latex gloves before starting first aid.

- Calm and reassure the child.

- Tell the child to inhale through his mouth, **not** his nose.

BROKEN NOSE

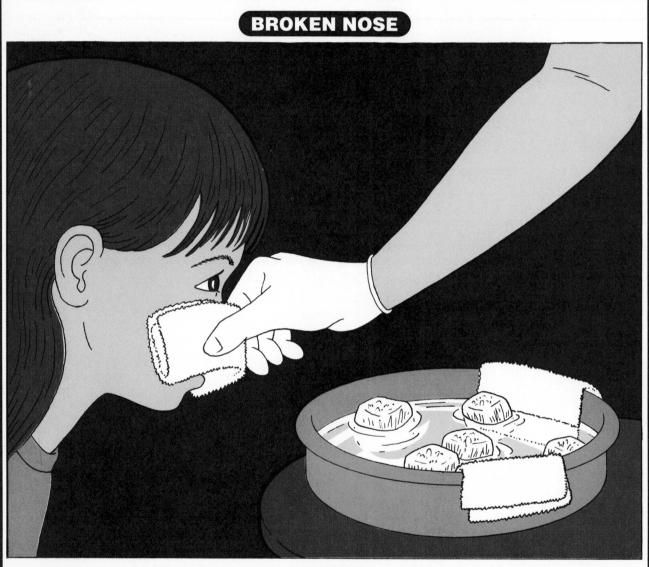

Control the bleeding as for **NOSEBLEED;** see next page. Gently press cold compresses over the nose. **Do not** splint or try to straighten the nose. **Seek medical aid.**

CONTINUED ON NEXT PAGE

FOREIGN OBJECTS

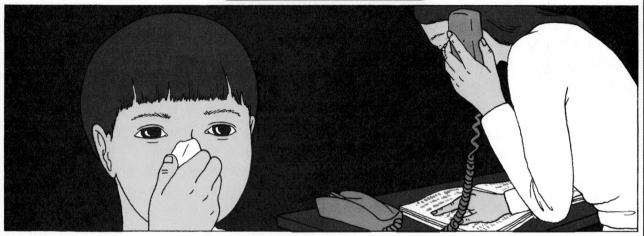

Make sure the child inhales through his mouth, **not** his nose. Have him blow his nose gently, keeping both nostrils open. If the object does not come out easily, **do not** try to remove it. **Seek medical aid immediately.**

NOSEBLEED

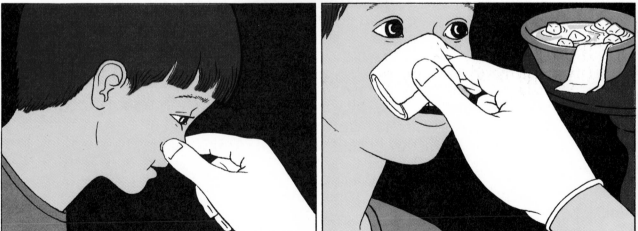

Lean the child forward and gently apply pressure to the lower, soft part of the nose for about 5 minutes, then apply cold compresses against the nose. If bleeding persists, repeat the procedure. **Seek medical aid** if bleeding continues. **Do not** let the child blow his nose for several hours after bleeding stops.

343

POISONING

SWALLOWED POISONS

IMPORTANT

- **Call your local Poison Control Center immediately. If unavailable, seek other medical aid. Call 911 or Operator; see EMS, page 272. Do not** wait for symptoms to develop. **Do not** attempt to use any home remedies.

- Try to identify the poison. Save the poison container or contaminated food and a sample of any vomit.

- **Do not induce vomiting unless instructed to do so by the Poison Control Center.**

- Check the child's ABCs (Airway, Breathing and Circulation); see **CHECKING THE ABCs,** pages 224-232.

- Calm and reassure the child.

- **Do not** give her anything to drink if she is unconscious or having convulsions.

- **Ingredients in products may change over time, and antidotes or counterdoses given on labels may be obsolete or incorrect. Always consult your local Poison Control Center.**

SIGNS & SYMPTOMS OF ALKALI POISONING

Burns around the mouth, lips and tongue. Burning sensations in the mouth, throat and stomach. Cramps. Disorientation. Bloody diarrhea.

SIGNS & SYMPTOMS OF PETROLEUM POISONING

Burning irritation. Coughing. Gagging. Coma. May include petroleum product odor on the breath.

SIGNS & SYMPTOMS OF OTHER KINDS OF POISONING

May be intermittent and develop slowly or quickly. **May include:** Headache. Nausea. Dizziness. Drowsiness. Slurred speech. Lack of coordination. Difficulty swallowing. Difficulty breathing. Cold, clammy skin. Thirst. Convulsions. Coma.

1 **Be prepared with as much of the following information as possible when you call your local Poison Control Center:** the child's age, the name of the poison, the amount swallowed, when the poisoning took place, the child's symptoms, whether or not she has vomited, whether or not she has had anything to eat or drink since the poisoning occurred, and how long it will take you to get to the nearest hospital emergency room.

2 **Follow the Poison Control Center's instructions carefully.** You may be advised to dilute the poison with water, induce vomiting with a prescribed dosage of syrup of ipecac or possibly administer a prescribed dosage of activated charcoal.

POISONING

INHALED POISONS

- **Seek medical aid and oxygen immediately.** Call 911 or Operator; see **EMS,** page 272.

- **Also call your local Poison Control Center.**

- Check the child's ABCs (Airway, Breathing and Circulation); see **CHECKING THE ABCs,** pages 224-232.

- If possible, shut off the source of the fumes and ventilate the area. Open doors and windows, turn on an exhaust fan, etc.

- If the skin or eyes are affected, see **BURNS: CHEMICAL,** pages 218-219, and **EYE INJURIES: CHEMICALS IN THE EYE,** page 277.

SIGNS & SYMPTOMS

Irritated eyes, nose, throat or lungs. Coughing. Headache. Shortness of breath. Nausea. Dizziness. Convulsions. Unconsciousness. Caused by smoke, auto exhaust or chemical fumes from paint, solvents and industrial gases.

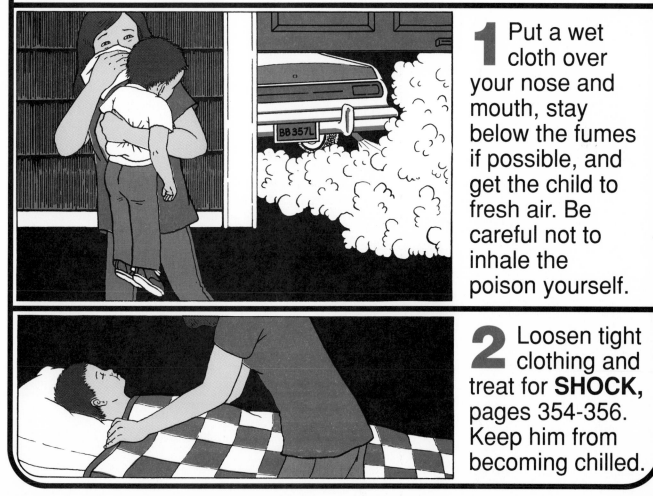

1 Put a wet cloth over your nose and mouth, stay below the fumes if possible, and get the child to fresh air. Be careful not to inhale the poison yourself.

2 Loosen tight clothing and treat for **SHOCK,** pages 354-356. Keep him from becoming chilled.

CONTACT

IMPORTANT

- **Seek medical aid if there is a severe reaction or the child is highly allergic.**
- Check the child's ABCs (Airway, Breathing and Circulation); see **CHECKING THE ABCs,** pages 224-232.
- Observe for **SHOCK,** pages 354-356.

SIGNS & SYMPTOMS

Burning and itching. Rash. Blisters. Swelling. Headache. Fever.

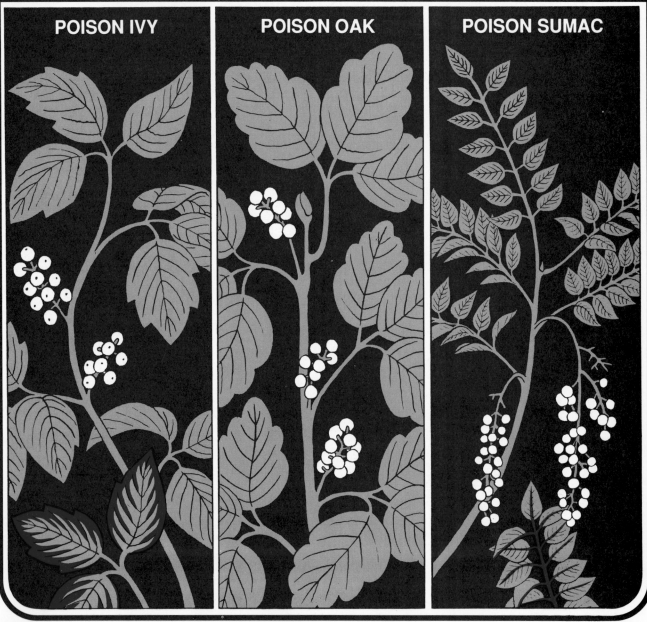

POISON IVY POISON OAK POISON SUMAC

CONTINUED ON NEXT PAGE

346

CONTACT
CONTINUED

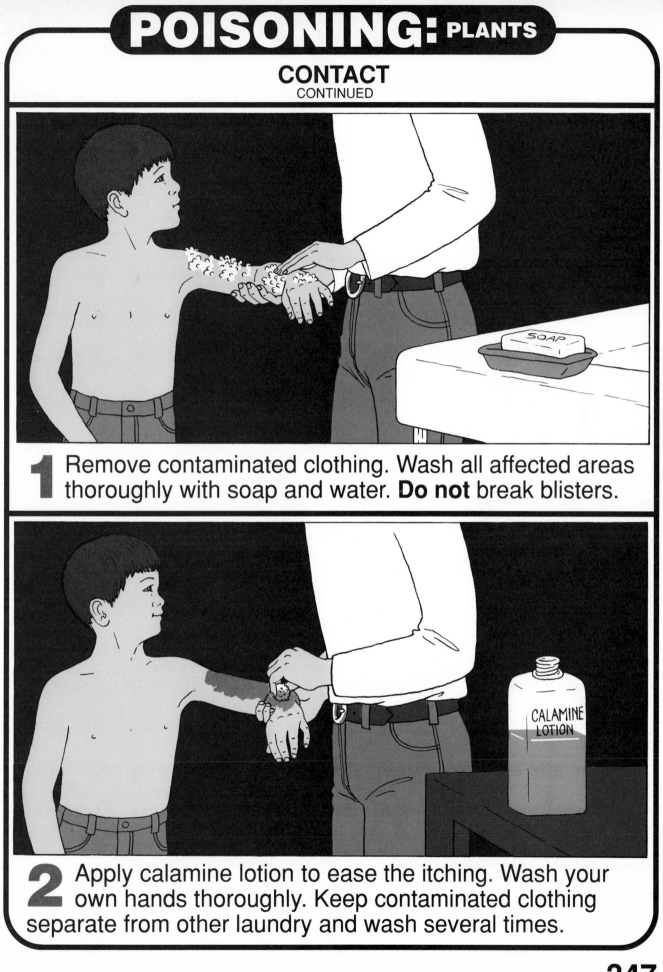

1 Remove contaminated clothing. Wash all affected areas thoroughly with soap and water. **Do not** break blisters.

2 Apply calamine lotion to ease the itching. Wash your own hands thoroughly. Keep contaminated clothing separate from other laundry and wash several times.

347

INGESTED

- **Call your local Poison Control Center immediately. Also seek medical aid.** Call 911 or Operator; see **EMS,** page 272.

- Check the child's ABCs (Airway, Breathing and Circulation); see **CHECKING THE ABCs,** pages 224-232.

- **Do not** give the child anything to drink if he is unconscious.

BANEBERRY

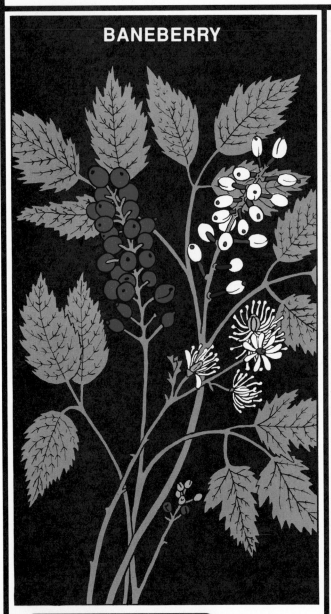

BITTERSWEET

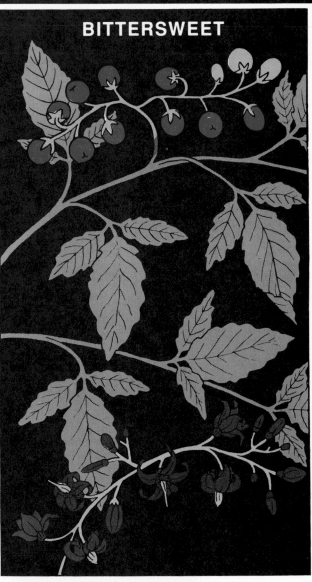

SIGNS & SYMPTOMS

Dizziness. Cramps. Vomiting. Headache. Delirium.

SIGNS & SYMPTOMS

Burning sensation in the throat. Nausea. Dizziness. Dilated pupils. Weakness. Convulsions.

CONTINUED ON NEXT PAGE

INGESTED
CONTINUED

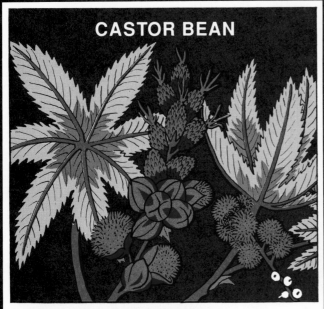

CASTOR BEAN

SIGNS & SYMPTOMS

Burning sensations in the mouth and throat. Nausea. Vomiting. Cramps. Stupor. Convulsions.

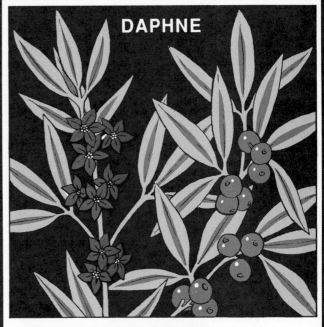

DAPHNE

SIGNS & SYMPTOMS

Burning sensations in the mouth, throat and stomach. Cramps.

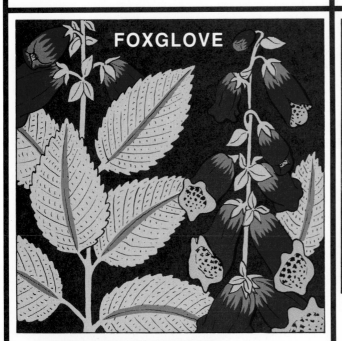

FOXGLOVE

SIGNS & SYMPTOMS

Nausea. Upset stomach. Dizziness. Disorientation.

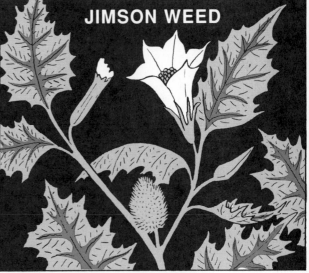

JIMSON WEED

SIGNS & SYMPTOMS

Extreme thirst. Difficulty speaking. Impaired vision. Rapid heartbeat. Dilated pupils. Delirium. Increased body temperature. Coma.

CONTINUED ON NEXT PAGE

349

INGESTED
CONTINUED

LARKSPUR (DELPHINIUM)

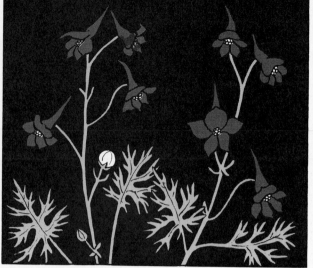

SIGNS & SYMPTOMS

Tingling in the mouth and on the skin. Upset stomach. Anxiety. Severe depression.

LILY-OF-THE-VALLEY

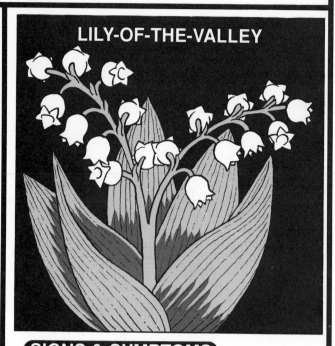

SIGNS & SYMPTOMS

Upset stomach. Dizziness. Vomiting. Disorientation.

MONKSHOOD

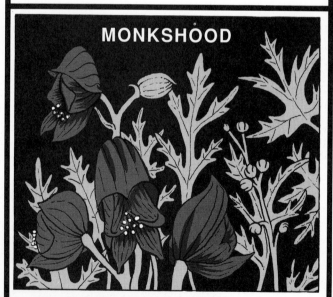

SIGNS & SYMPTOMS

Tingling or numbness of the lips and tongue. Excessive salivating. Dizziness. Nausea. Vomiting. Dimmed vision.

NIGHTSHADE

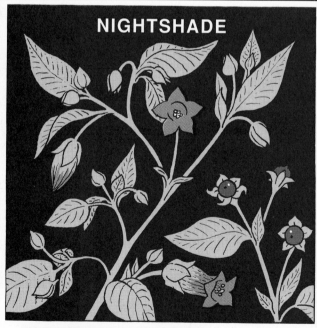

SIGNS & SYMPTOMS

Thirst. Upset stomach. Numbness. Rapid heartbeat.

CONTINUED ON NEXT PAGE

INGESTED
CONTINUED

POISON HEMLOCK

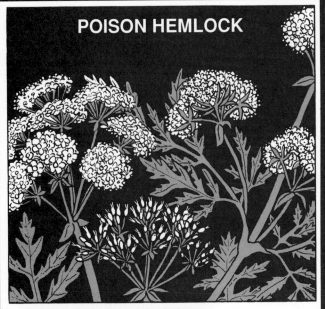

SIGNS & SYMPTOMS

Burning sensations in the mouth and throat. Weakness. Paralysis of the arms and chest. Stupor.

POKEWEED

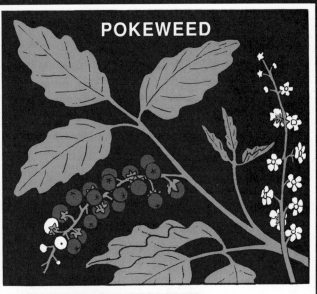

SIGNS & SYMPTOMS

Burning sensations in the mouth and throat. Nausea. Cramps. Upset stomach. Vomiting. Drowsiness. Impaired vision.

WATER HEMLOCK

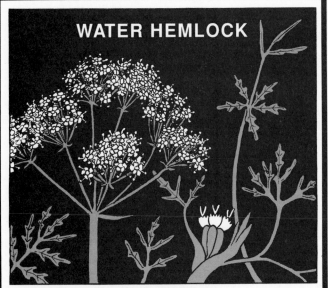

SIGNS & SYMPTOMS

Excessive salivating. Foaming at the mouth. Stomach pain. Frenzy. Shivering. Irregular breathing. Delirium. Convulsions. Coma.

YEW

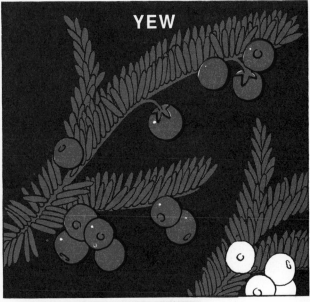

SIGNS & SYMPTOMS

Nausea. Stomach pain. Vomiting. Shivering. Difficulty breathing. Diarrhea.

MUSHROOM POISONING

IMPORTANT

- **Call your local Poison Control Center immediately if you know or suspect that a poisonous mushroom has been ingested. Also seek medical aid.** Call 911 or Operator; see **EMS,** page 272.

- Save a sample of the vomit and, if possible, the mushroom.

- **Do not** give the child anything alcoholic to drink.

- **If he is unconscious, do not** give him **anything** to drink.

- Observe for **SHOCK,** pages 354-356.

SIGNS & SYMPTOMS

Depending on the type and amount of mushroom eaten, symptoms may develop rapidly (from minutes to about 2 hours) or slowly (from 6 to 24 hours). **May include:** Difficulty breathing. Profuse salivation or drooling. Tearing of the eyes. Headache. Nausea. Sweating. Tiny pupils. Vomiting. Stomach cramps. Severe diarrhea. Dizziness and confusion. Coma. **In delayed reactions, symptoms may also include:** Passage of little or no urine. After 2 to 3 days, jaundiced (yellowed) skin and eyes.

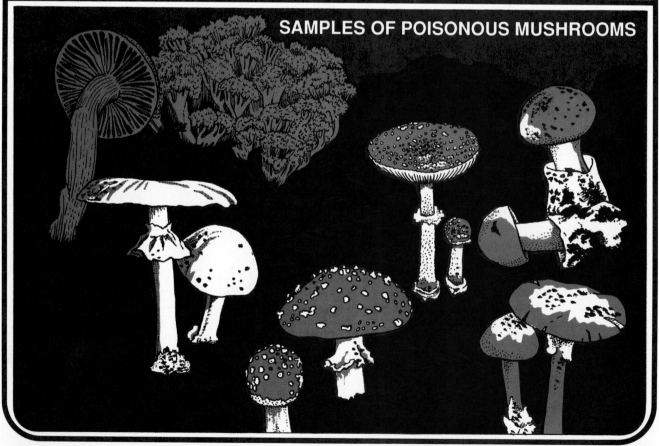

SAMPLES OF POISONOUS MUSHROOMS

RECOVERY POSITION

IMPORTANT

- The recovery position is the safest position for a child who is unconscious but breathing. It promotes good circulation, keeps his airway open so he can breathe easily, and prevents him from inhaling blood or vomit or choking on his tongue.

- **Do not** use if the child isn't breathing.

- **Do not** use if he has been seriously injured or you suspect a neck or back injury.

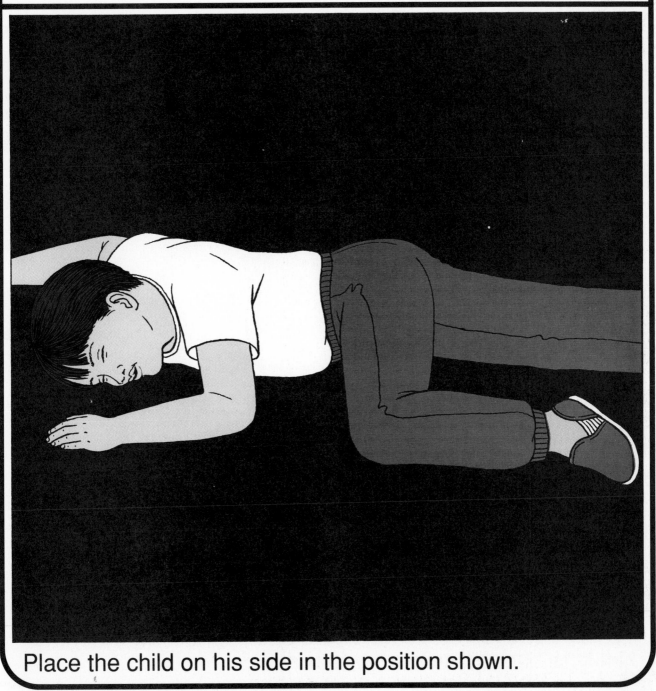

Place the child on his side in the position shown.

353

SHOCK

IMPORTANT

- **Always treat a seriously injured child for shock. Seek medical aid immediately.** Call 911 or Operator; see **EMS,** page 272.

- Conserve body heat, but **do not** overheat.

SIGNS & SYMPTOMS

Pale or bluish lips, gums and fingernails. Clammy skin, mottled in color. Weakness. Breathing is weak and shallow or deep but irregular. **May also include:** Anxiety. Apathy. Nausea. Thirst.

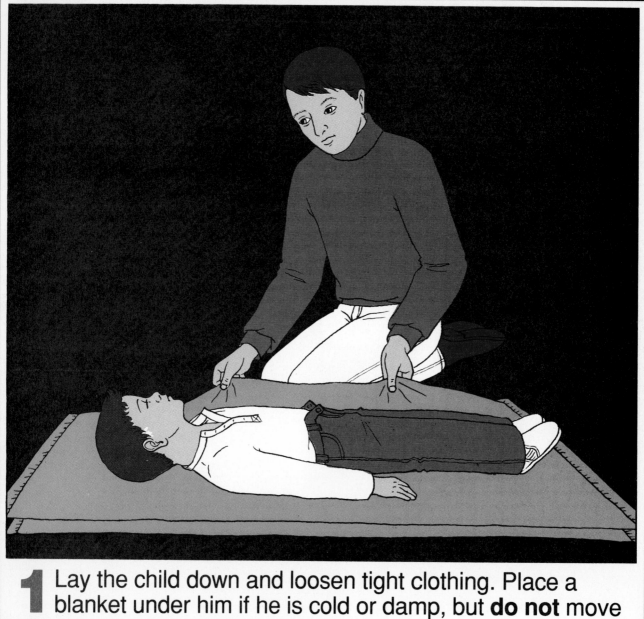

1 Lay the child down and loosen tight clothing. Place a blanket under him if he is cold or damp, but **do not** move him if his back or neck is injured.

354

CONTINUED ON NEXT PAGE

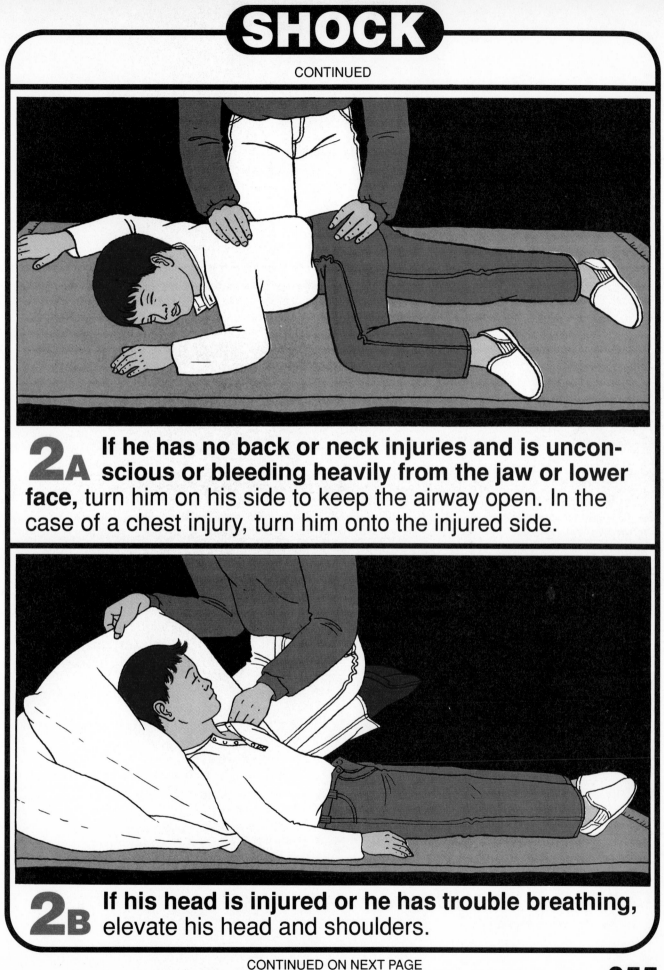

2A **If he has no back or neck injuries and is unconscious or bleeding heavily from the jaw or lower face,** turn him on his side to keep the airway open. In the case of a chest injury, turn him onto the injured side.

2B **If his head is injured or he has trouble breathing,** elevate his head and shoulders.

CONTINUED ON NEXT PAGE

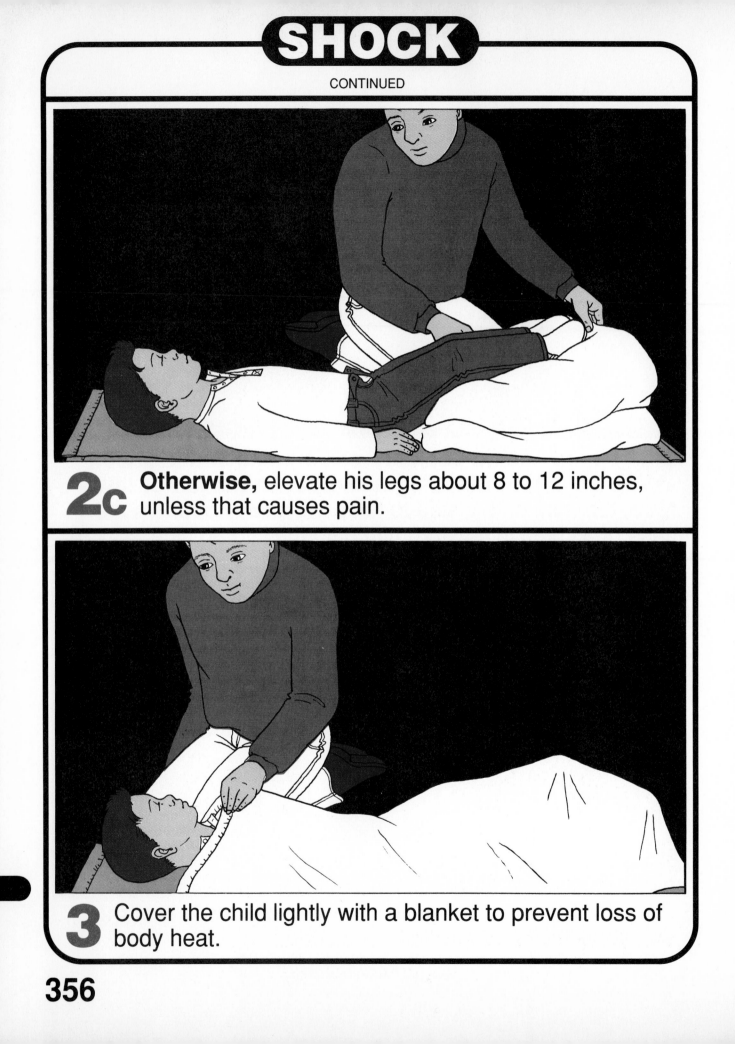

2c **Otherwise,** elevate his legs about 8 to 12 inches, unless that causes pain.

3 Cover the child lightly with a blanket to prevent loss of body heat.

SPLINTERS

- **Seek medical aid if the splinter is deeply embedded, if you are unable to remove all of it, or if signs of infection develop later.**

- Wash your hands thoroughly before you attempt to remove the splinter.

- Check with your doctor to make sure the child's tetanus immunization is still current.

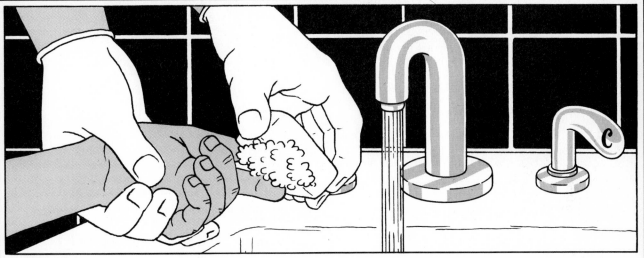

1 Gently wash the area around the splinter with soap and water.

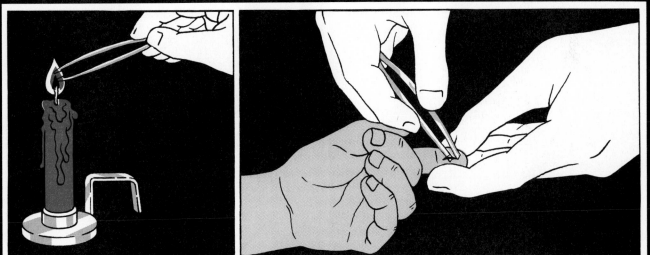

2A **If the splinter is protruding from the skin:** Sterilize a pair of tweezers by holding them over an open flame or soaking them for 10 minutes in rubbing alcohol or boiling water. Then gently remove the splinter at the same angle at which it entered.

CONTINUED ON NEXT PAGE

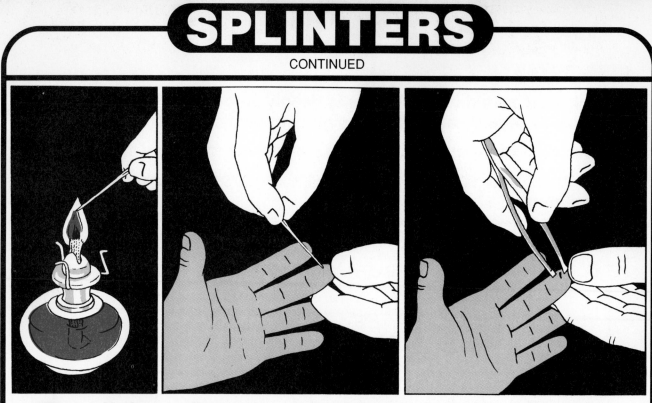

2B **If the splinter is embedded just under the skin:** Sterilize a needle by holding it over an open flame or soaking it for 10 minutes in rubbing alcohol or boiling water. Then gently loosen the skin around the splinter and remove it with a sterilized pair of tweezers at the same angle at which it entered.

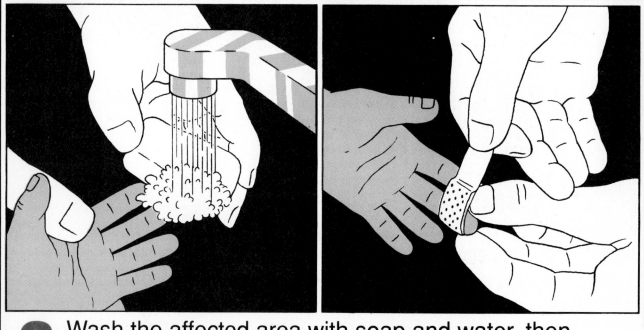

3 Wash the affected area with soap and water, then cover with a bandage.

SPRAINS & STRAINS

IMPORTANT

- A **sprain** is a stretched or torn ligament or muscle tendon in the region of a joint. A **strain** is a pulled or stretched muscle.

- **Seek medical aid** if you suspect a broken bone. See **BREAKS: FRACTURES & DISLOCATIONS,** pages 183-200.

- **Seek medical aid** if the pain is severe, the pain or swelling does not decrease after 24 hours, the injured part does not function, or circulation is affected in other parts of the body.

- **Do not** give the child any medication to relieve the pain, including aspirin, unless a doctor so advises.

- Keep the child off the injured parts. He can slowly begin normal activity when the pain is almost gone. Vigorous activity should be resumed only gradually.

SIGNS & SYMPTOMS

Pain. Rapid swelling. Tenderness when touched. Bruising. Possible loss of efficient movement.

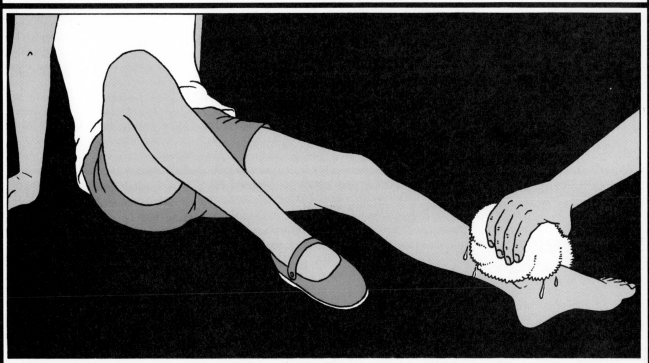

1 To minimize swelling, immediately apply cold, wet compresses or an ice bag wrapped in a towel for 15 to 30 minutes. (**Do not** place ice directly on the skin.) Reapply as needed for the next few hours or until swelling subsides.

CONTINUED ON NEXT PAGE

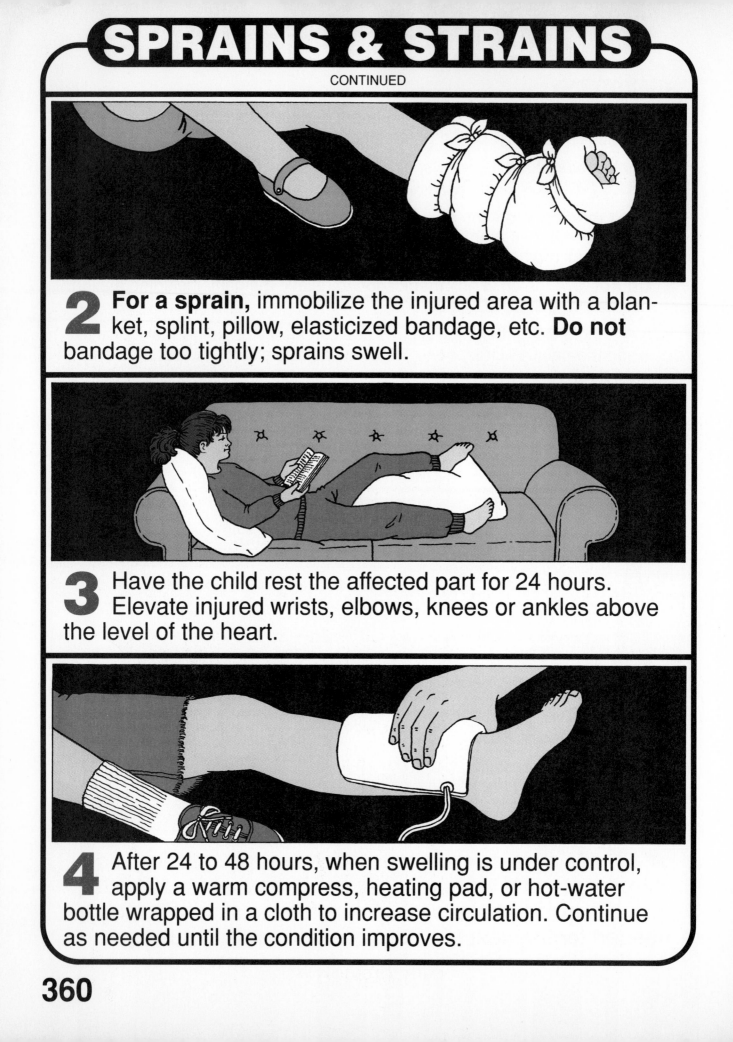

2 **For a sprain,** immobilize the injured area with a blanket, splint, pillow, elasticized bandage, etc. **Do not** bandage too tightly; sprains swell.

3 Have the child rest the affected part for 24 hours. Elevate injured wrists, elbows, knees or ankles above the level of the heart.

4 After 24 to 48 hours, when swelling is under control, apply a warm compress, heating pad, or hot-water bottle wrapped in a cloth to increase circulation. Continue as needed until the condition improves.

STOMACH INJURIES

IMPORTANT

- **Seek medical aid immediately. For a serious injury,** call 911 or Operator; see **EMS,** page 272.

- Check the child's ABCs (Airway, Breathing and Circulation); see **CHECKING THE ABCs,** pages 224-232.

- Wash your hands thoroughly and, if possible, put on sterile latex gloves before starting first aid.

- Check with your doctor to make sure the child's tetanus immunization is still current.

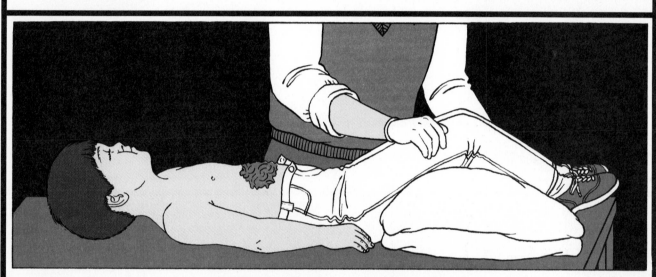

1 Relax the stomach muscles by placing the child on his back with a pillow or blanket under his knees.

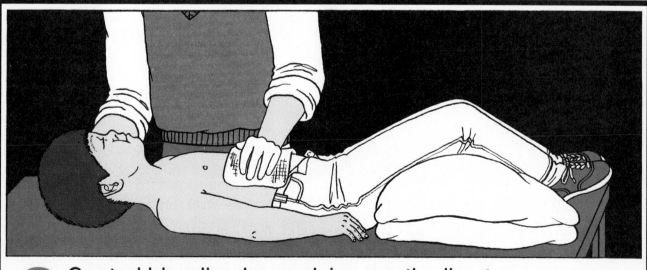

2 Control bleeding by applying gentle direct pressure on the wound with sterile gauze or a clean cloth.

CONTINUED ON NEXT PAGE

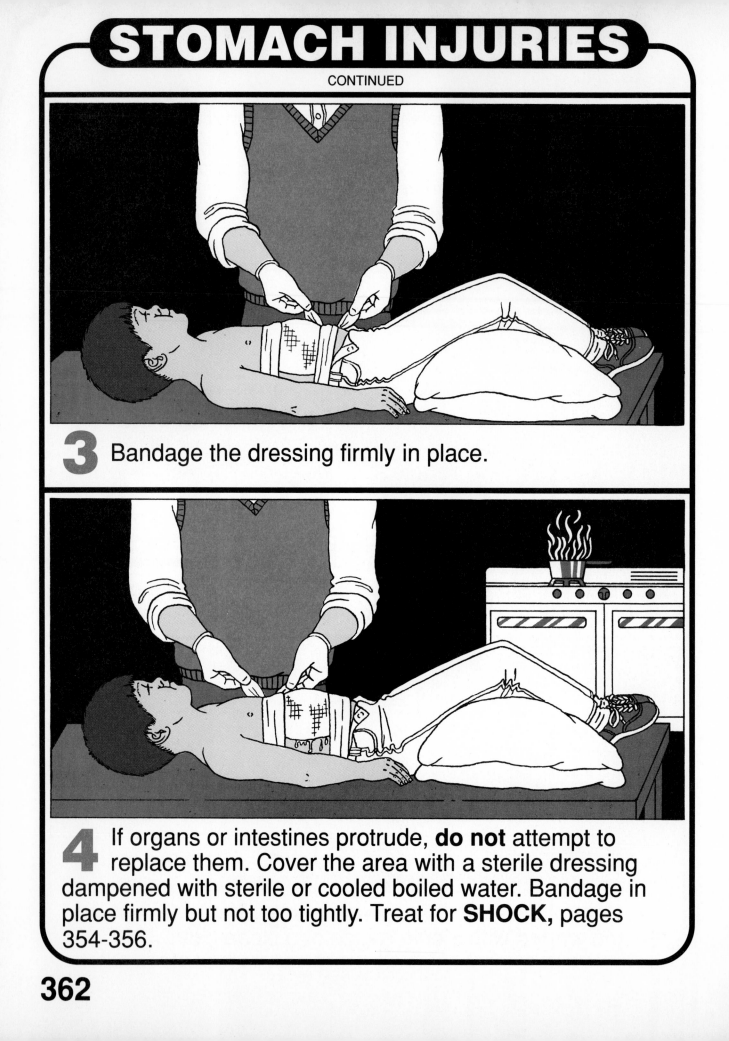

3 Bandage the dressing firmly in place.

4 If organs or intestines protrude, **do not** attempt to replace them. Cover the area with a sterile dressing dampened with sterile or cooled boiled water. Bandage in place firmly but not too tightly. Treat for **SHOCK,** pages 354-356.

SUNBURN

IMPORTANT

- **Seek medical aid immediately** if the child has a rash, chills or fever, is weak, pale, dizzy or nauseous, or shows signs of sunstroke; see **SUNSTROKE,** pages 364-365.

- **Seek medical aid immediately** if the eyes are sunburned.

- Consult your doctor if the sunburn is severe or blisters become infected.

- **Do not** break blisters.

- **Do not** use ointments unless advised to do so by your doctor.

- Observe for **SHOCK;** see pages 354-356.

SIGNS & SYMPTOMS

Reddened, tender skin. Pain. Swelling. Blisters. Burning sensation.

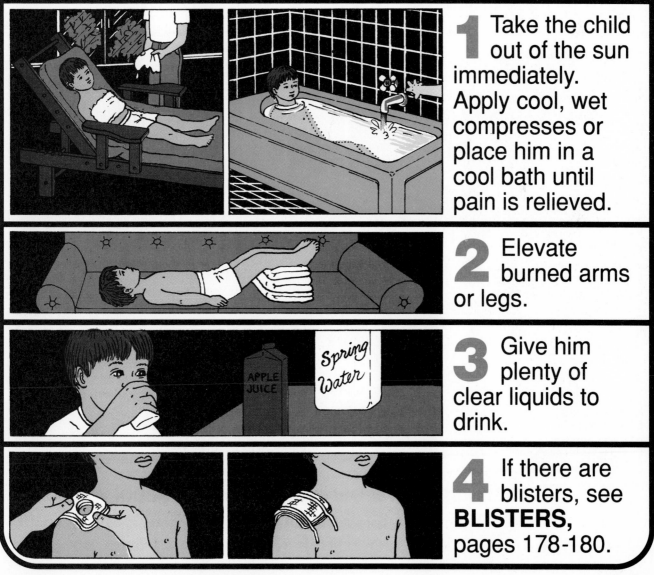

1 Take the child out of the sun immediately. Apply cool, wet compresses or place him in a cool bath until pain is relieved.

2 Elevate burned arms or legs.

3 Give him plenty of clear liquids to drink.

4 If there are blisters, see **BLISTERS,** pages 178-180.

363

SUNSTROKE (HEATSTROKE)

IMPORTANT

- **Seek medical aid immediately.** Call 911 or Operator; see **EMS,** page 272.

- **Act quickly. Body temperature must be lowered at once.** Recheck temperature every 10 minutes. **Do not** reduce temperature below 101° F (38.3° C). **Repeat first aid if temperature rises.**

- **Do not** give the child any medications, including aspirin.

- **Do not** give him an alcohol rub.

- Observe for **SHOCK,** pages 354-356, and **CONVULSIONS & SEIZURES,** page 253.

SIGNS & SYMPTOMS

Red, hot and dry skin. Extremely high temperature. No sweating. Rapid pulse. **May also include:** Disorientation. Convulsions. Unconsciousness.

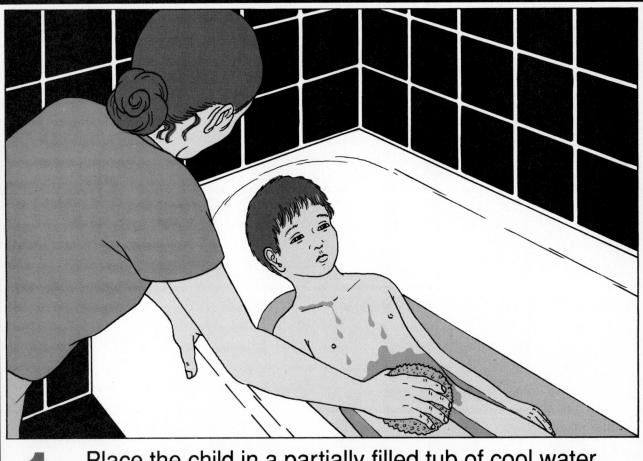

1A Place the child in a partially filled tub of cool water. Using light, brisk strokes, sponge his entire body until temperature is reduced to 101° F (38.3° C).

CONTINUED ON NEXT PAGE

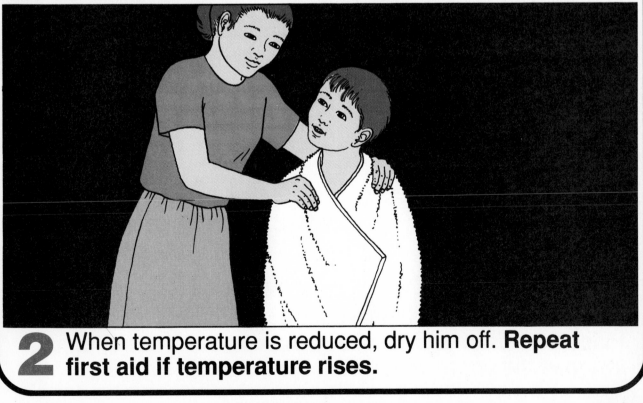

1B Or cool the child by wrapping him in wet, cold towels or sheets, spraying him with a hose, placing him in front of an air conditioner, or applying cold compresses to his neck, armpits and groin until temperature is reduced to 101° F (38.3° C).

2 When temperature is reduced, dry him off. **Repeat first aid if temperature rises.**

TAKING THE PULSE

IMPORTANT

- In an emergency it may be necessary to check the child's pulse to determine whether the heart has stopped beating and emergency first aid for heart failure should therefore begin. In this case, **it is extremely important to find the pulse if one is present since first aid for heart failure is potentially dangerous and should never be performed needlessly. Do not** rush. Check the pulse slowly and carefully, taking between 5 and 10 seconds to find it.

- **Do not** use your thumb to check the pulse since its own pulse may be mistaken for that of the child.

- If possible, check the pulse when the child is at rest. The pulse is normally strong and regular. The rate typically rises to reflect increases in activity, body temperature, anxiety, etc. Illness or injury may produce a pulse that is irregular, slow and/or weak.

NORMAL PULSE RATES (AT REST)

Infant: 100 to 130 beats a minute
Small Child: 80 to 100 beats a minute
Older Child: 60 to 90 beats a minute

INFANTS (UNDER 1 YEAR OLD)

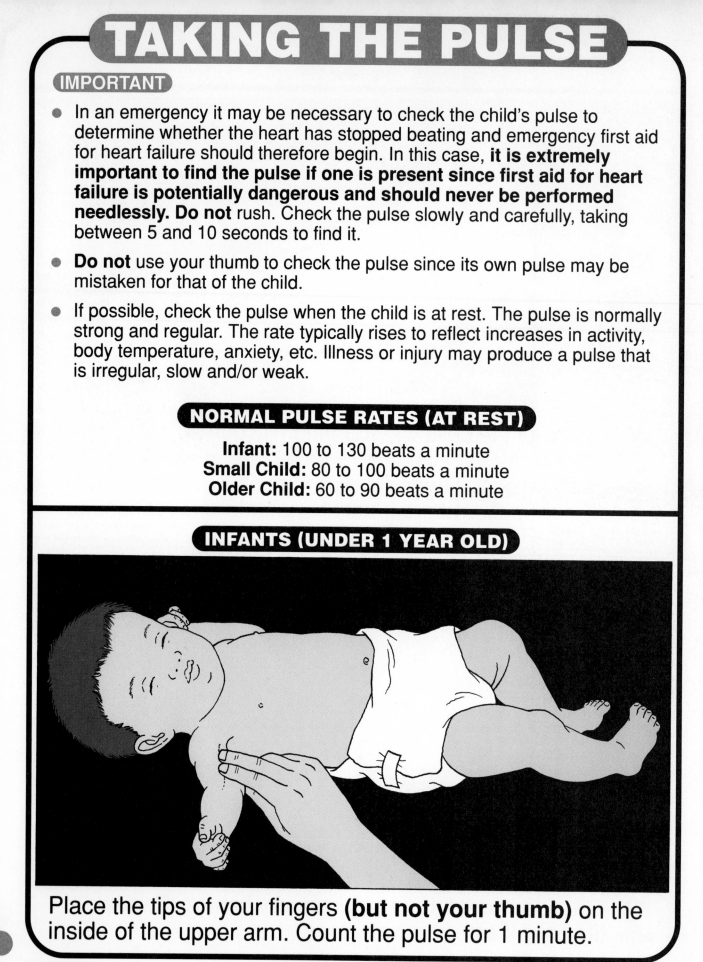

Place the tips of your fingers **(but not your thumb)** on the inside of the upper arm. Count the pulse for 1 minute.

366

CONTINUED ON NEXT PAGE

CONTINUED

CHILDREN (OVER 1 YEAR OLD)

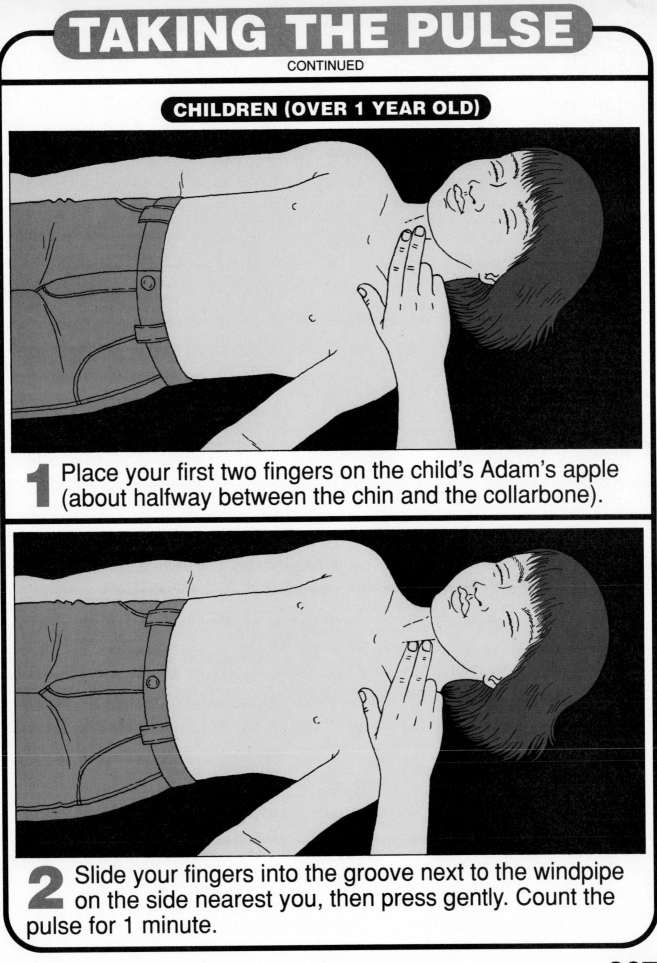

1 Place your first two fingers on the child's Adam's apple (about halfway between the chin and the collarbone).

2 Slide your fingers into the groove next to the windpipe on the side nearest you, then press gently. Count the pulse for 1 minute.

IMPORTANT

- Always hold a thermometer by the top end, not by the bulb.

- Both before and after use, carefully wash the thermometer in soap and cool **(not hot)** water, then wipe it off with rubbing alcohol and a clean cloth.

- When it isn't being used, store the thermometer in its case to keep it from breaking. A cracked or chipped thermometer should be thrown away.

- Before taking the child's temperature, hold the top end of the thermometer, and using quick wrist flips, shake it downward until it reads below 96°F/35.6°C.

- To read the thermometer, hold it under a strong light, then rotate it slowly until you can see the silver or red line of mercury. The point where the mercury stops is the temperature.

- A child's normal temperature is 98.6°F/37°C plus or minus 1 degree. Most thermometers indicate the "normal" temperature with a red line or arrow.

- A **rectal thermometer,** which has a short fat bulb, should be used for infants, and children under about 6 years old. Temperatures taken rectally read about 0.5 to 1°F/0.2 to 0.5°C higher than temperatures taken orally.

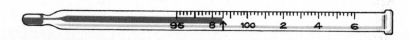

- An **oral thermometer,** which has a long thin bulb, is suitable for an older child who is able to keep it under his tongue without biting down.

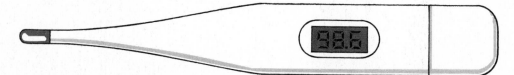

- Never use a rectal thermometer orally or an oral thermometer rectally.

- If you use a **digital thermometer,** follow the accompanying instructions.

- The best times to take a child's temperature are early in the morning and late in the afternoon. However, if the child has a fever, retake his temperature every 4 to 6 hours.

- High temperatures do not necessarily indicate a serious illness, but it is advisable to tell your doctor about any temperature over 101°F/38.3°C (100.2°F/37.9°C in an infant).

CONTINUED ON NEXT PAGE

TAKING THE TEMPERATURE RECTALLY

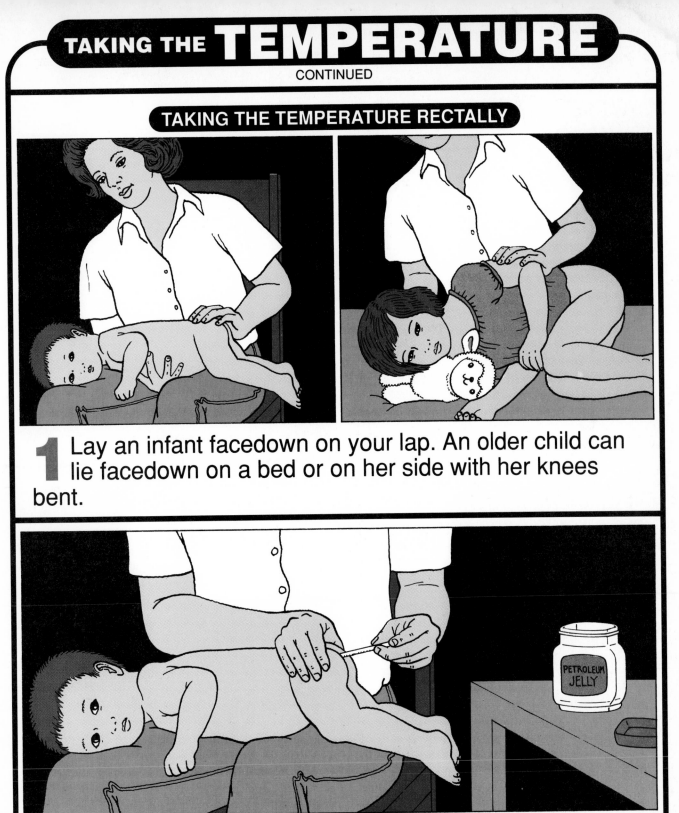

1 Lay an infant facedown on your lap. An older child can lie facedown on a bed or on her side with her knees bent.

2 Dip the bulb of the thermometer in petroleum jelly, gently spread the child's buttocks, then carefully insert the thermometer into her rectum until the bulb is covered (no more than 1 inch). **Do not** use force. If the thermometer resists going in, change the angle slightly.

CONTINUED ON NEXT PAGE

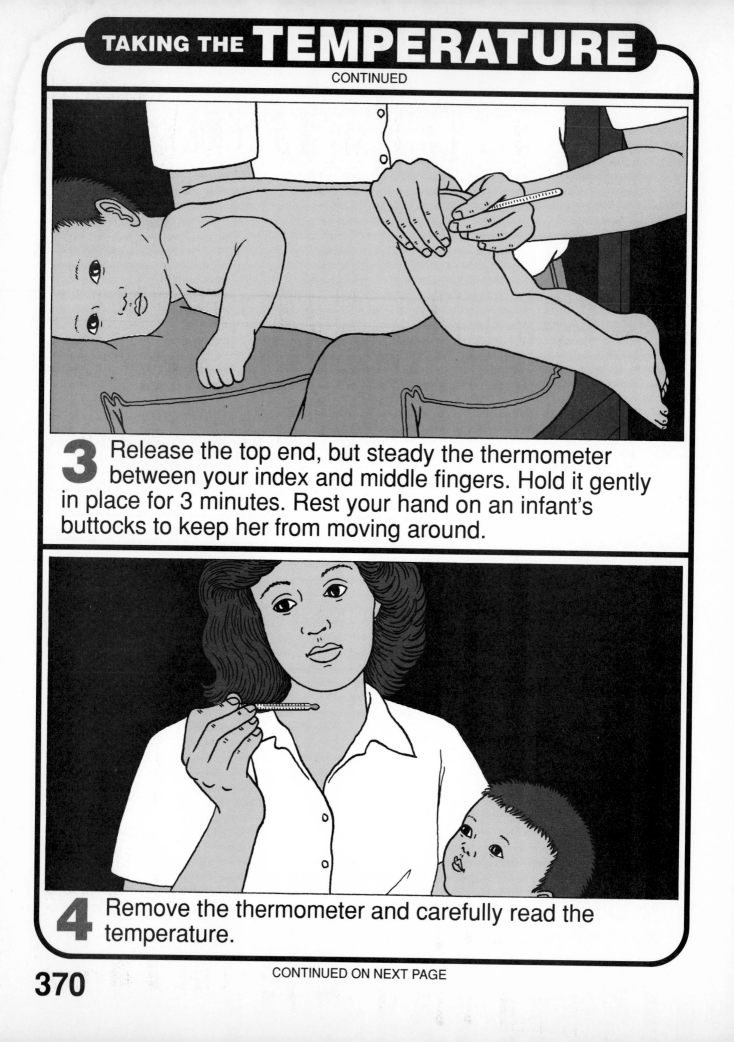

3 Release the top end, but steady the thermometer between your index and middle fingers. Hold it gently in place for 3 minutes. Rest your hand on an infant's buttocks to keep her from moving around.

4 Remove the thermometer and carefully read the temperature.

CONTINUED ON NEXT PAGE

TAKING THE TEMPERATURE ORALLY

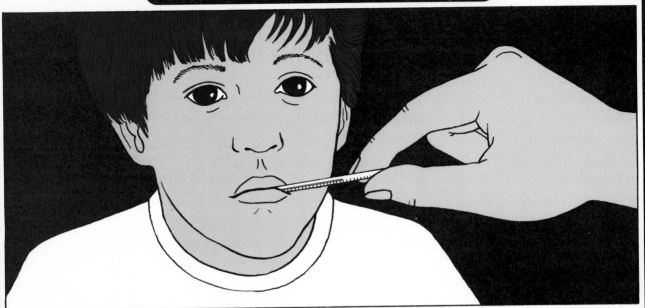

1 Wait at least 30 minutes after the child has bathed or had anything to eat or drink, then gently insert the thermometer under his tongue and a little to one side. Have him close his lips over it but not bite down with his teeth. Make sure he doesn't talk, or breathe through his mouth.

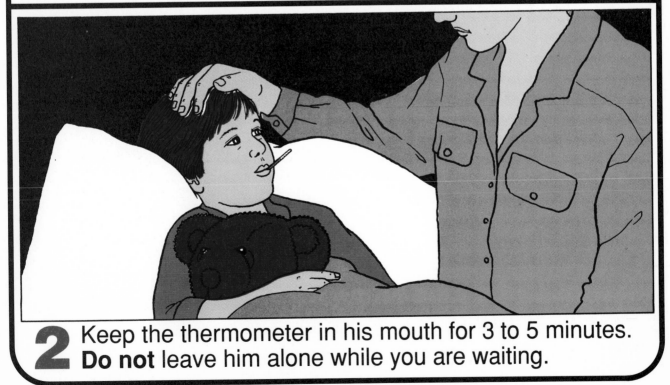

2 Keep the thermometer in his mouth for 3 to 5 minutes. **Do not** leave him alone while you are waiting.

CONTINUED ON NEXT PAGE

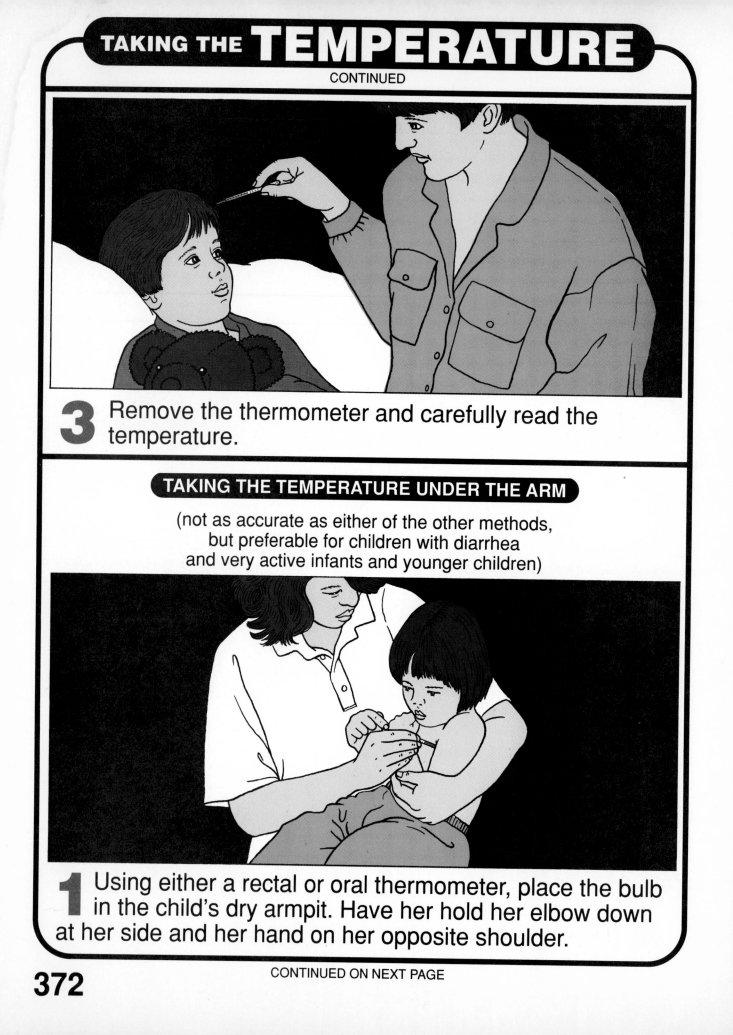

3 Remove the thermometer and carefully read the temperature.

TAKING THE TEMPERATURE UNDER THE ARM

(not as accurate as either of the other methods,
but preferable for children with diarrhea
and very active infants and younger children)

1 Using either a rectal or oral thermometer, place the bulb in the child's dry armpit. Have her hold her elbow down at her side and her hand on her opposite shoulder.

CONTINUED ON NEXT PAGE

372

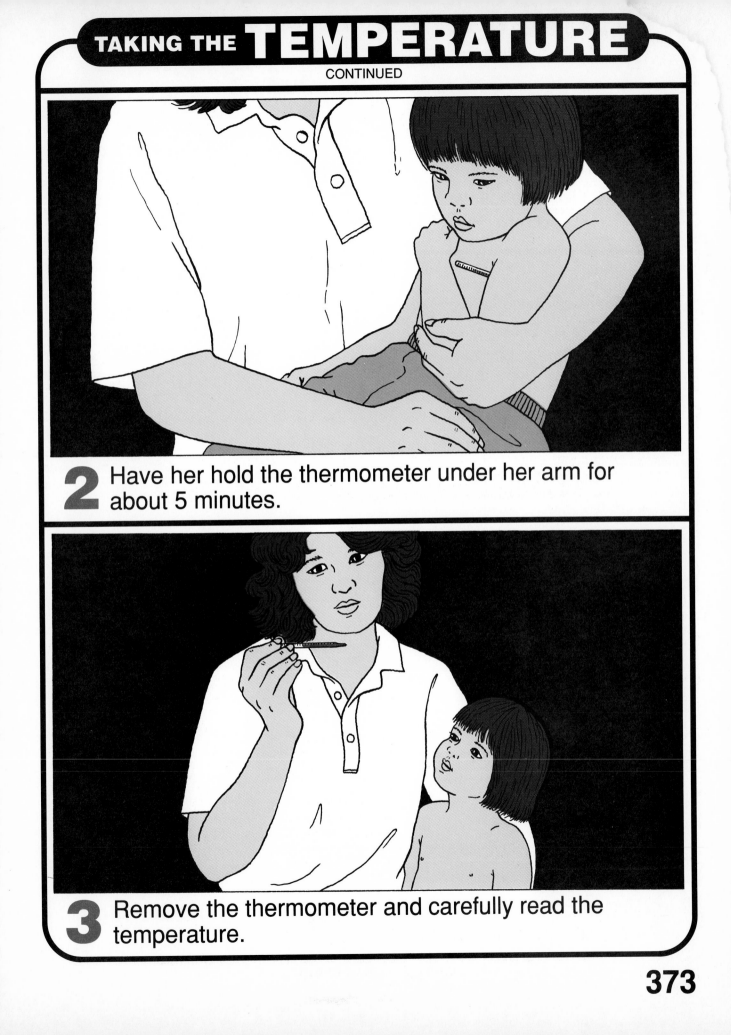

2 Have her hold the thermometer under her arm for about 5 minutes.

3 Remove the thermometer and carefully read the temperature.

373

BACK & NECK INJURIES

IMPORTANT

- **Seek medical aid immediately if you suspect an injury to the neck or back.** Call 911 or Operator; see **EMS,** page 272.

- **Immobilize the child until help arrives;** see **BACK & NECK INJURIES,** pages 135-136. **Do not move him unless it is a matter of life or death and no medical aid is available.** It is almost always better to wait for proper equipment and expert help.

- If you must transport the child, get as much assistance as possible, and follow the method given below.

- If you are alone and he must be quickly moved a short distance to remove him from immediate danger (fire, toxic fumes, etc.), use the **Clothes Drag Technique** or **Blanket Pull;** see page 378. Take extreme care not to bend or twist his body. Try to steady his head with your forearms. If he is lying facedown, **do not** turn him over, but drag him to safety by his shoulders.

- Calm and reassure the child while you move him. Be as gentle as possible.

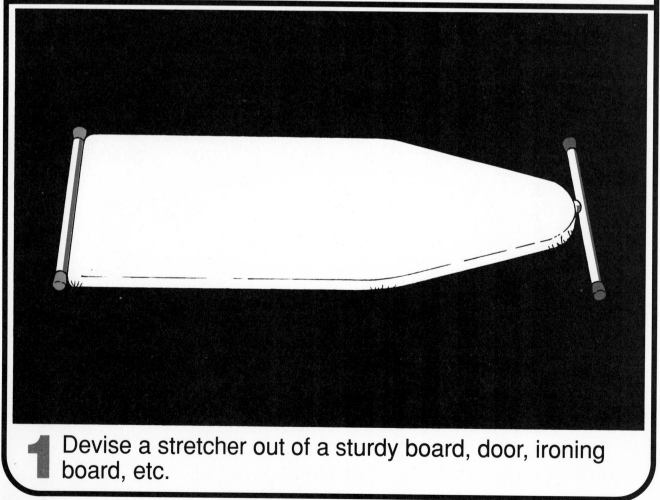

1 Devise a stretcher out of a sturdy board, door, ironing board, etc.

CONTINUED ON NEXT PAGE

BACK & NECK INJURIES
CONTINUED

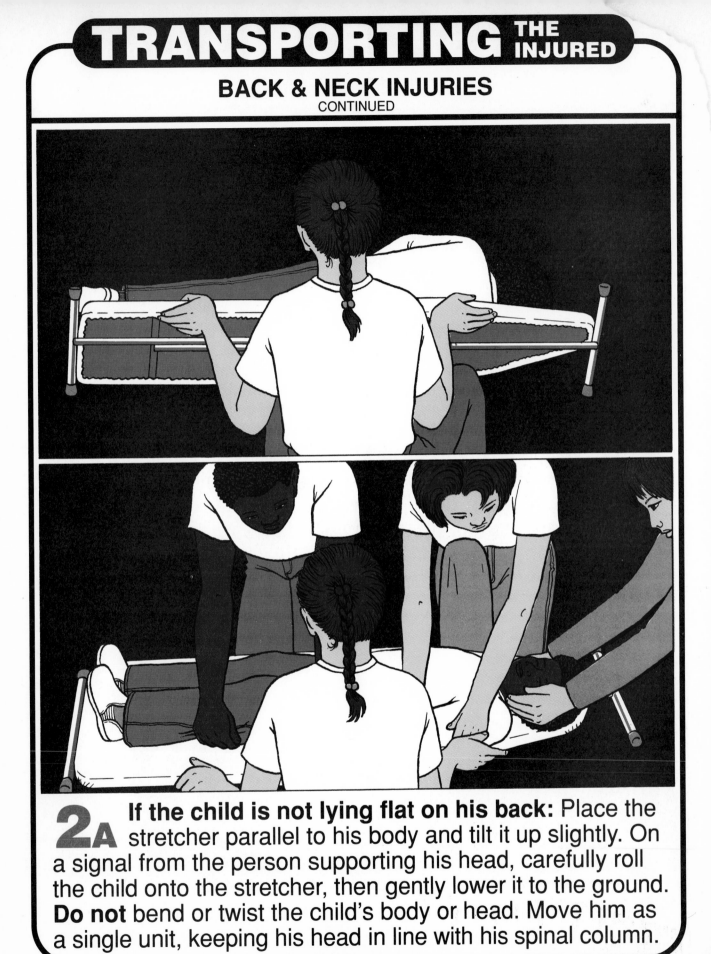

2A **If the child is not lying flat on his back:** Place the stretcher parallel to his body and tilt it up slightly. On a signal from the person supporting his head, carefully roll the child onto the stretcher, then gently lower it to the ground. **Do not** bend or twist the child's body or head. Move him as a single unit, keeping his head in line with his spinal column.

CONTINUED ON NEXT PAGE

BACK & NECK INJURIES
CONTINUED

2B **If the child is lying flat on his back:** Place the stretcher on the ground next to him. On a signal from the person supporting his head, lift him onto it as carefully as possible. **Do not** bend or twist the child's body or head. Move him as a single unit, keeping his head in line with his spinal column.

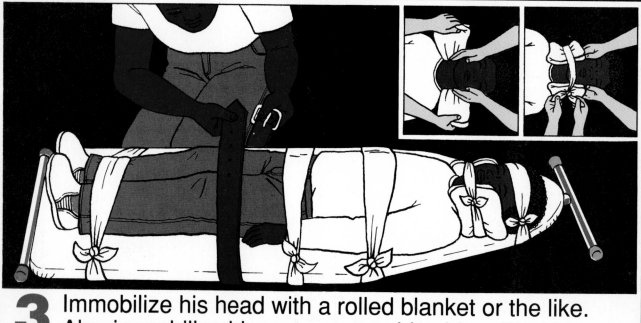

3 Immobilize his head with a rolled blanket or the like. Also immobilize his arms next to his sides. Bind him to the stretcher with bandages, belts, etc.

PULLS, CARRIES & STRETCHERS

IMPORTANT

- **If the child is seriously injured, call an ambulance immediately;** see **EMS,** page 272. **Do not move him unless it is a matter of life or death and no ambulance is available.** It is almost always better to wait for proper equipment and expert help.

- If you must move the child, get as much assistance as possible.

- Extreme care must be taken in moving a child with an injured neck or spine. For the proper procedures, see **TRANSPORTING THE INJURED: BACK & NECK INJURIES,** pages 374-376.

- Before moving an injured child, consider how the various methods given below may affect his injuries, and choose the one least likely to cause further harm.

- Calm and reassure the child while you move him. Be as gentle as possible.

IF YOU ARE ALONE

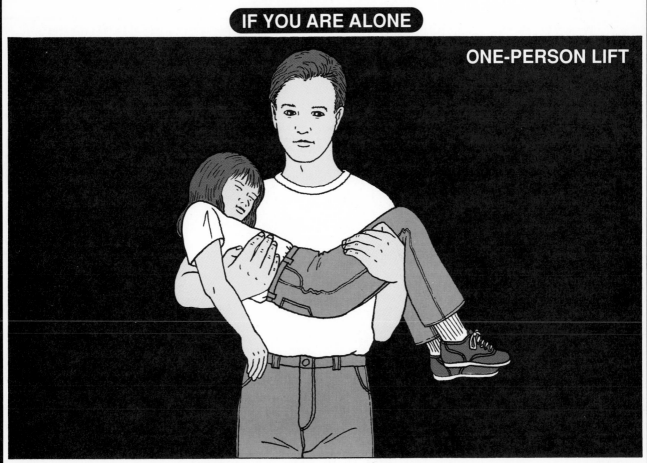

ONE-PERSON LIFT

Place one arm under the child's knees and the other securely around her back. If possible, have her hold onto your neck.

CONTINUED ON NEXT PAGE

TRANSPORTING THE INJURED

PULLS, CARRIES & STRETCHERS
CONTINUED

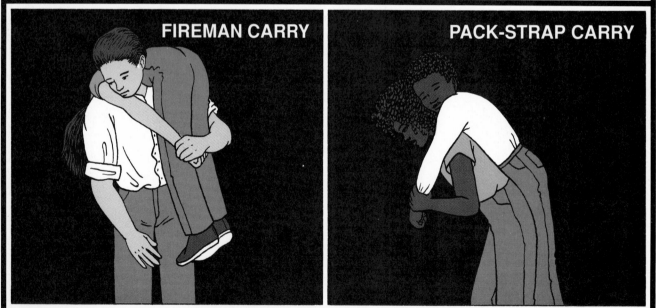

CLOTHES DRAG

BLANKET PULL

FOOT DRAG

To be used when the child is too heavy to carry and must be quickly moved a short distance to remove him from immediate danger (fire, toxic fumes, etc.). The **Foot Drag** works well on a smooth surface, but if the surface is rough, the **Clothes Drag** is preferable.

FIREMAN CARRY

PACK-STRAP CARRY

To be used for longer distances. Employ the **Pack-Strap Carry** if the **Fireman Carry** is likely to aggravate the child's injuries.

CONTINUED ON NEXT PAGE

PULLS, CARRIES & STRETCHERS
CONTINUED

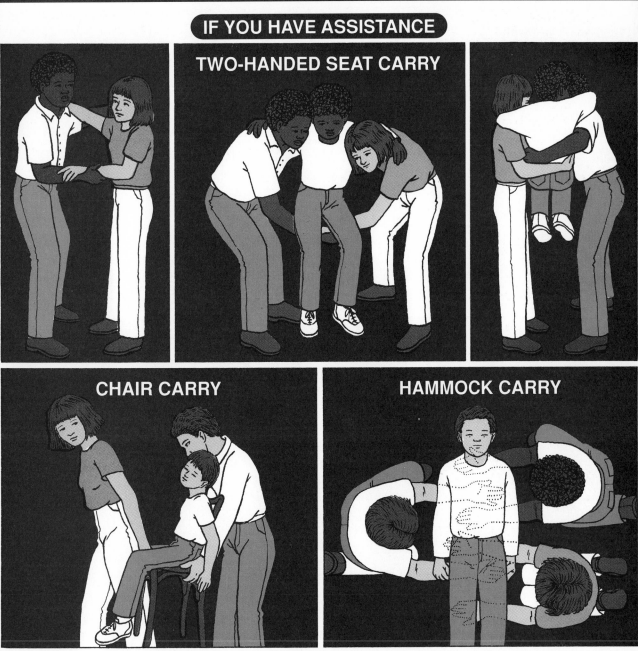

IF YOU HAVE ASSISTANCE

TWO-HANDED SEAT CARRY

CHAIR CARRY

HAMMOCK CARRY

Only use the **Two-Handed Seat Carry** if the child is conscious and able to hold on tightly with both hands. The **Chair Carry** is especially good for climbing stairs and moving through narrow, winding hallways. If you use the **Hammock Carry,** make sure all parts of the child's body are firmly supported and kept in a straight line. Take care not to bend, twist or shake the injured parts.

CONTINUED ON NEXT PAGE

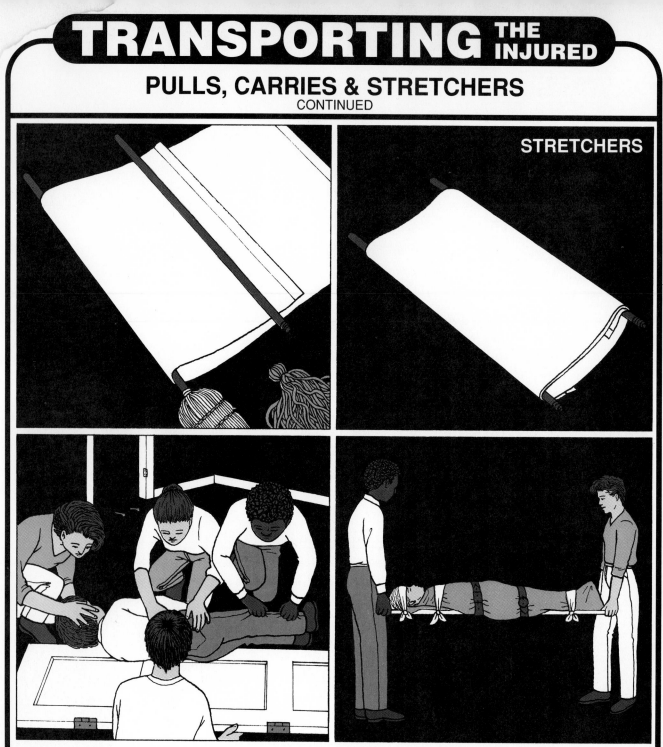

STRETCHERS

A stretcher can be improvised from a blanket and broomsticks, oars, poles, etc. Fold the blanket as shown, and the child's weight will keep it from unwrapping. A sturdy board, door, ironing board, etc. can also be made to serve as a stretcher. If you use this method, be sure to tie the child down securely so he won't roll off. When transporting a child on an improvised stretcher, try to get 1 or 2 people to walk alongside it to share the weight and hold the child in place.

UNCONSCIOUSNESS

IMPORTANT

- **Seek medical aid immediately if the child does not respond when you call him loudly, tap him on the shoulder or shake him gently.** Call 911 or Operator; see **EMS,** page 272. Note how long he remains unconscious and any changes in his state.

- Check the child's ABCs (Airway, Breathing and Circulation); see **CHECKING THE ABCs,** pages 224-232.

- **Do not** move the child unless absolutely necessary. You may cause further harm. If necessary, see **TRANSPORTING THE INJURED,** pages 374-380.

- **Do not** give him anything to drink.

- If the cause of unconsciousness is not known, check for signs of injury, hidden bleeding, bites or stings, poisons, drugs, etc. Look for emergency medical information tags around the neck or wrist, or a card in the wallet identifying the possible cause. On hot days or following vigorous exercise, the child may be suffering from heatstroke or heat exhaustion; see **SUNSTROKE (HEATSTROKE),** pages 364-365, and **HEAT EXHAUSTION,** page 326.

SIGNS & SYMPTOMS

Can vary from a brief loss of consciousness, from which the child can be easily roused, to a deep coma. Depending on the cause, the face, gums or inner linings of the eyelids may appear either flushed, white or blue.

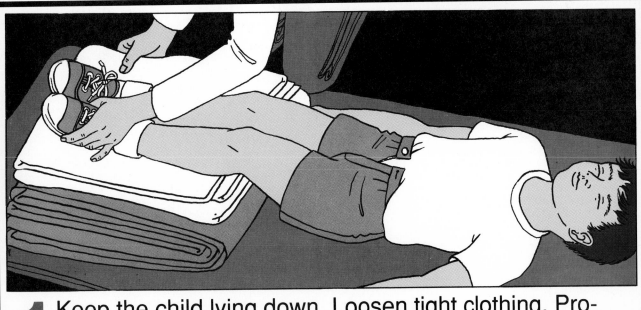

1 Keep the child lying down. Loosen tight clothing. Provide good ventilation. Elevate his legs 8 to 12 inches.

CONTINUED ON NEXT PAGE

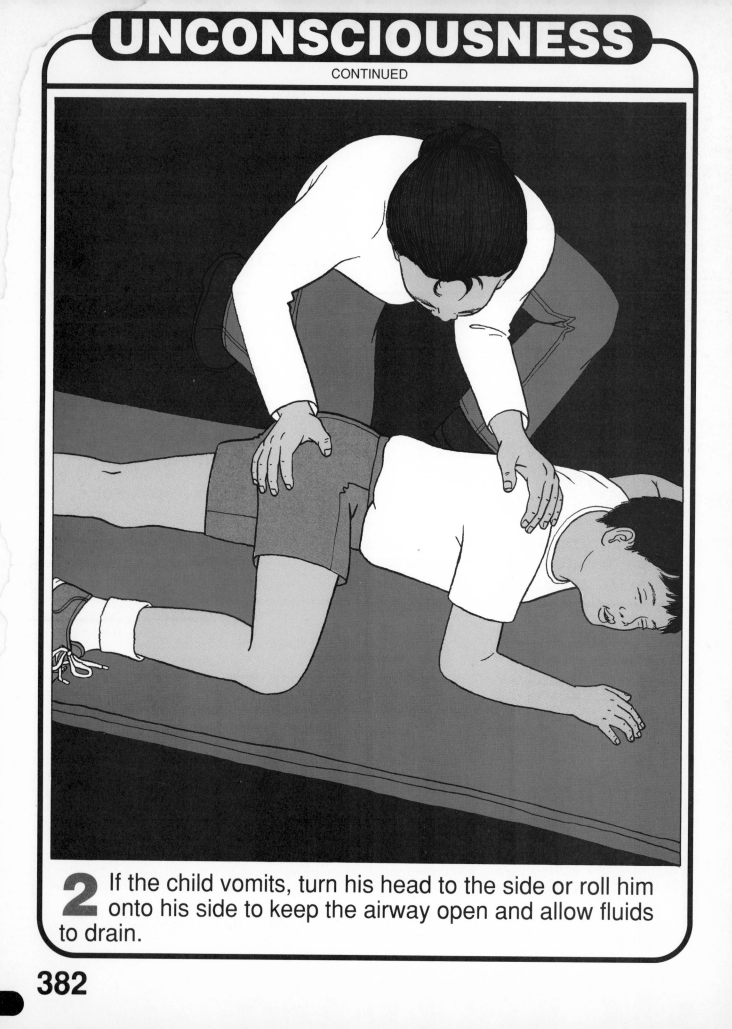

2 If the child vomits, turn his head to the side or roll him onto his side to keep the airway open and allow fluids to drain.

WHEEZING

IMPORTANT

- **Seek medical aid immediately** if there is pink or frothy phlegm. If necessary, call 911 or Operator; see **EMS,** page 272.

- If the child turns blue or has difficulty breathing, see **BREATHING: ARTIFICIAL RESPIRATION,** pages 201-215.

- If wheezing is the result of an inhaled foreign object, see **CHOKING,** pages 239-252.

- Wheezing could be a symptom of **ANAPHYLACTIC SHOCK;** see pages 131-132, or an **ASTHMA ATTACK;** see pages 133-134.

- Consult your doctor if wheezing persists or worsens.

SIGNS & SYMPTOMS

Difficult, noisy breathing. May be accompanied by whistling sounds.

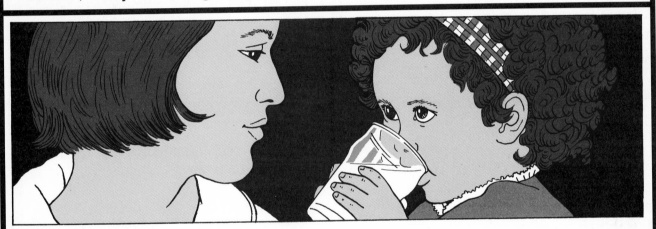

1 Offer the child clear, room-temperature liquids.

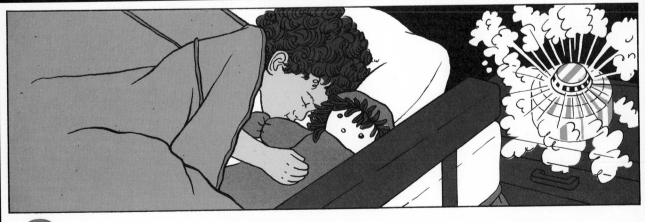

2 Use a cool-mist vaporizer when she is sleeping.

EMERGENCY TELEPHONE NUMBERS

This list of emergency numbers should be filled in immediately, then photocopied so you can also post it next to each of your telephones. **Keep the numbers up-to-date.** Be sure to show this page to your baby-sitter whenever you go out.

EMERGENCY MEDICAL SERVICES (EMS): _____

RESCUE SQUAD OR EMERGENCY AMBULANCE: _____

POISON CONTROL CENTER: _____ **POLICE:** _____

FIRE DEPARTMENT: _____ **TAXI:** _____

EMERGENCY SHELTER: _____

HOSPITAL EMERGENCY ROOM: Name: _____

    Address: _____ Phone: _____

PEDIATRICIAN: Name: _____ Office: _____ Home: _____

FAMILY DOCTOR: Name: _____ Office: _____ Home: _____

ALTERNATE DOCTOR: Name: _____ Office: _____ Home: _____

SPECIALIST: TYPE: _____ Name: _____ Office: _____

SPECIALIST: TYPE: _____ Name: _____ Office: _____

DENTIST: Name: _____ Office: _____ Home: _____

NEAREST DRUGSTORE: Name: _____ Hours: _____ Phone: _____

ALL-NIGHT DRUGSTORE: Name: _____ Phone: _____

FATHER'S PHONE AT WORK: _____ **MOTHER'S PHONE AT WORK:** _____

OTHER FAMILY MEMBERS' PHONES:

Name: _____ Home: _____ Work: _____

Name: _____ Home: _____ Work: _____

NEIGHBORS & FRIENDS:

Name: _____ Address: _____ Phone: _____

Name: _____ Address: _____ Phone: _____

Name: _____ Address: _____ Phone: _____

MISCELLANEOUS NUMBERS:

Name: _____ Address: _____ Phone: _____

Name: _____ Address: _____ Phone: _____

Name: _____ Address: _____ Phone: _____

Name: _____ Address: _____ Phone: _____

COAL SUPPLIER: _____ **GAS COMPANY:** _____

ELECTRIC COMPANY: _____ **OIL COMPANY:** _____

FIREWOOD SUPPLIER: _____ **WATER DEPARTMENT:** _____

OTHER NUMBERS: _____